CHRONIC CONDITIONS AND CAREGIVING IN CANADA: SOCIAL SUPPORT STRATEGIES

Edited by Miriam J. Stewart

While the number of Canadians suffering from chronic illness continues to increase, recent health care cutbacks are resulting in more responsibility for the care of these patients being taken on by families. This book shows how various forms of social support can benefit those experiencing chronic illness and those involved in caregiving.

Chronic Conditions and Caregiving in Canada is based on the results of a nationally funded research program conducted by teams of multidisciplinary researchers. This collection includes innovative assessment and intervention studies involving patients with diabetes, cystic fibrosis, spina bifida, HIV-AIDS, cardiac conditions, and stroke. The studies evaluate various forms of social support on the basis of a model that is outlined in the first chapter. Several chapters explore barriers to accessing support and key strategies for seeking support. The final chapters summarize the findings and outline the challenges that still face researchers in the field.

Some of the forms of support explored by contributors include peer support for family caregivers of seniors suffering from stroke and heart failure; telephone support for hemophiliacs with AIDS and their caregivers, and for parents of children with chronic conditions; and support for spouses of patients with cardiac conditions. This volume is an invaluable resource for students, teachers, and practitioners in health-related disciplines.

Miriam J. Stewart is Professor of Nursing in Public Health Sciences and Director of the Centre for Health Promotion Studies at the University of Alberta.

Chronic Conditions and Caregiving in Canada: Social Support Strategies

Edited by
Miriam J. Stewart

UNIVERSITY OF TORONTO PRESS
Toronto Buffalo London

Toronto Buffalo London

Printed in Canada

ISBN 0-8020-4129-9 (cloth)
ISBN 0-8020-7974-1 (paper)

Printed on acid-free paper

Canadian Cataloguing in Publication Data

Main entry under title:

Chronic conditions and caregiving in Canada : social support strategies

ISBN 0-8020-4129-9 (bound) ISBN 0-8020-7974-1 (pbk.)

1. Chronically ill – Social networks – Canada. 2. Caregivers – Social networks – Canada. I. Stewart, Miriam.

RC108.C476 1999 362.1'96044 C99-932731-3

University of Toronto Press acknowledges the financial assistance to its publishing program of the Canada Council for the Arts and the Ontario Arts Council.

University of Toronto Press acknowledges the financial support for its publishing activities of the Government of Canada through the Book Publishing Industry Development Program (BPIDP).

Contents

Preface

Chronic illness has escalated at an alarming rate in Canada. Current initiatives in health and other sectors have shifted the major responsibility for caring for persons with chronic conditions to their families. An interdisciplinary team of investigators conducted a nationally funded program of research to determine if social support plays a role in chronic illness and caregiving and to test the impact of different support strategies on health and functioning.

Assessment studies guided the design of follow-up interventions by identifying predominant stressful situations, coping strategies, appraisal of support from social networks, support needs, and desired interventions. The conceptual underpinnings of the social support research program and issues in assessment and intervention research are outlined in the initial chapter. Key findings from assessment and intervention studies, designed to identify and meet the support needs of people with chronic conditions and caregivers, are delineated in the next six chapters. The authors of these chapters capture a range of concerns associated with chronic illness and caregiver demands. Across the lifespan, diverse populations face issues concerning diabetes, cystic fibrosis, spina bifida, HIV/AIDS, cardiac conditions, and stroke. Suitable intervention strategies for these populations involved dyads and groups and employed different modalities – face-to-face, telephone and computer mutual aid, and home visits. Participants confirmed that these programs were innovative and important. Moreover, the interventions encompassed lay and professional collaboration, consistent with recent calls for partnership in reform initiatives. In chapter 8 the authors document barriers and incentives for professional partnership with support groups and self-help groups. Issues pertaining to accessibility and mobilization of support for caregivers and persons with chronic conditions are explored in chapters 9 and 10. Finally, conceptual, methodological, and practical insights and implications for intervention research are highlighted in the two concluding chapters.

Lessons learned from these assessment and intervention studies can inform programs and policies. It is hoped that this book will be of interest to academics, practitioners, and policy decision makers in health and health-related sectors.

MIRIAM STEWART

Acknowledgments

It is gratifying to acknowledge the University of Toronto Press for publishing *Chronic Conditions and Caregiving in Canada: Social Support Strategies*. This book would not have been possible without the superb contributions of Judith Ritchie, Mary-Lou Ellerton, Renee Lyons, Benjamin Gottlieb, Gail Tomblin Murphy, Geraldine Hart, Anne Neufeld, and seventeen co-authors. They are acknowledged as experts in the themes identified in their chapters.

Mary Anne Martell's skill and perseverance in typing contributions to this publishing venture and in helping to coordinate communications among authors are greatly appreciated.

The program of research reported in this text was funded through my Scholar Award from the Medical Research Council of Canada and the National Health Research and Development Program. The individual projects were supported by a variety of funding sources acknowledged at the end of each chapter.

The book is dedicated to my daughters, Evelyn and Shauna, and to my parents, Dorothy and Ross Mortimer, important sources of social support.

CHRONIC CONDITIONS AND CAREGIVING IN CANADA: SOCIAL SUPPORT STRATEGIES

1

A Framework for Social Support Assessment and Intervention in the Context of Chronic Conditions and Caregiving

Miriam J. Stewart and Lynn Langille

Abstract. The increasing number of Canadians living with chronic conditions and caregiving require social support. The sources, functions, and appraisal of social support help to determine support needs of persons with chronic conditions and their caregivers. Social support is conceptualized as a coping resource. There is a reciprocal relationship between social support and coping strategies and between social support and the stress of illness and caregiving. Support moderates the impact of stress on health outcomes and influences health status, health behaviour, and use of health services. Assessment of support needs and desires should guide the design of diverse dimensions of support interventions – level, mode, content, timing, and duration. Intervention processes and procedures should be documented. Outcome measures should reflect participants' life situations and expectations of support interventions. We conducted assessment and intervention studies to determine the role of support in chronic illness and caregiving and the impact of support strategies. The conceptual underpinnings of this research program and key issues in assessment and intervention research are elucidated in this chapter.

Introduction

The incidence of chronic illness has grown at an alarming rate in Canada. Current reform and renewal initiatives in health and other sectors have shifted the major responsibility of caring for persons with chronic conditions to families. These trends have important implications for the health of Canadians and for the determinants – social, economic, educational, cultural, and geographic – of their health. Social support is a significant social determinant of the health and functioning of the growing number of Canadians with chronic conditions and their family caregivers. Furthermore, it is a primary protective factor influencing their resilience in the face of chronic stressors.

Chronic conditions are a leading public health concern in North America. The number of people with chronic health conditions in the United States was almost 100 million in 1995; 44 per cent had more than one condition (Hoffman, Rice, & Sung, 1996). Almost 5 million Canadians report having a disability, a handicap, or continuing limitation in certain activities because of a health problem (Health Canada, 1997). Moreover, over half of all Canadian adults have at least one chronic condition (Statistics Canada, 1996). According to the National Population Health Survey, chronic conditions are those that have been diagnosed by a health professional and last six months or more (Statistics Canada, 1996). Chronic pain is directly associated with chronic conditions; almost 17 per cent of Canadian adults experience chronic pain or discomfort (Millar, 1996).

Sex and age exert important influences on vulnerability to chronic conditions. The higher prevalence of chronic conditions among women is congruent with their greater use of the health care system (Millar, 1996). Indeed, women often report multiple chronic conditions (Statistics Canada, 1996). Older Canadians are also more likely to suffer from chronic conditions (Health Canada, 1997). The National Population Health Survey revealed that one-third of Canadians aged sixty-five to seventy-four had health problems that restricted their activities (Statistics Canada, 1996). Furthermore, the number of elderly persons reporting two or more diagnosed chronic conditions increases with age (Millar, 1996). In 2011 about 1 million elderly people in Canada will have some level of disability (Rosenberg & Moore, 1997). Similarly, rates of chronic conditions in the United States are highest among the elderly (88 per cent), but chronic conditions are also prevalent among middle-aged adults (68 per cent), younger adults (35 per cent), and children (25 per cent) (Hoffman, Rice, & Sung, 1996).

Persons with chronic conditions must cope with 'recurrent exacerbations, higher health care costs, and more days lost from work than others, and the risk of long-term limitations and disabilities' (Hoffman et al., 1996, 1477). The total cost of illness, disability, and premature death in Canada for 1993 was an estimated $156.9 billion. Direct costs accounted for $71.7 billion. Most direct health care services (e.g., visits to physicians, prescriptions, hospitalizations) and costs per capita involve chronic conditions. Indirect costs totalled $85.1 billion; almost half of this amount was attributable to the loss of productivity resulting from long-term disability (Moore, Mao, Zhang, & Clarke, 1997). Cardiovascular disease and injuries have the greatest economic impact, generating $8.3 and $7.6 billion dollars, respectively, in direct costs (Health Canada, 1997). The leading causes of short-term disability in

Canada are respiratory diseases ($4.4 billion, 24.8 per cent), injuries ($3.2 billion, 18.5 per cent), and musculoskeletal diseases ($1.8 billion, 10 per cent) (Moore et al., 1997). The number of people affected by chronic conditions may be as high as 148 million in the United States by 2030, with resultant direct costs approaching $800 billion (Hoffman et al., 1996).

Most Canadians living with chronic conditions are cared for and supported by family members. There are 2.8 million family caregivers in Canada (Statistics Canada, 1997): 'The danger is not that families will abandon their ill relatives but that the health care system will abandon its caregivers' (Boise, Heagerty, & Eskenazi, 1996). Family caregivers who stop work to provide care are significantly older and have lower incomes and fewer social supports. Moreover, relinquishment of work roles may be a precursor to social isolation and social vulnerability (Pohl, Given, Collins, & Given, 1994).

Clearly, Canadians with chronic conditions and their caregivers require support. Our interdisciplinary team of investigators conducted a nationally funded program of research to determine the role of support in chronic illness and caregiving, and the impact of different support strategies. Specifically, the aims of the Social Support Research Program were to assess support experienced by persons with chronic conditions and their caregivers; to examine the conceptual links among social support, coping, and stress; and to test the impact of support interventions on health outcomes. Accordingly, assessment studies and intervention studies were designed to identify and meet the support needs of populations affected by chronic conditions, across the lifespan, and of their caregivers.

Theoretical Foundations of Social Support Research Program

Social support has been studied from diverse disciplinary and theoretical perspectives (Stewart, 1993), such as epidemiology, sociology, and social psychology. The complex dimensions of the construct of social support, its conceptual links with stress and coping, and its impact on health outcomes were articulated in the theoretical framework guiding our program of research.

Social Support

Social support was defined as *interactions with family members, friends, peers, and health professionals that communicate information, esteem, practical aid, or emotional help. When these communications are perceived as supportive, they may enhance coping, moderate the impact of stressors, and*

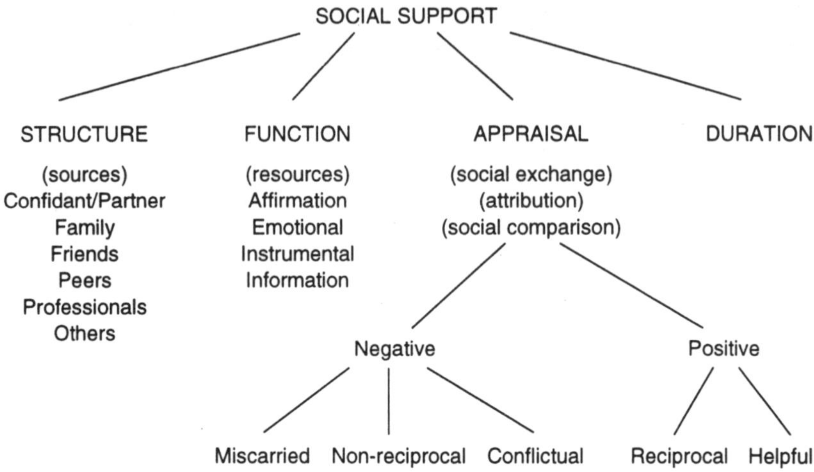

Figure 1.1 Conceptualization of Social Support Construct in Framework

promote health (Stewart, 1993). The multifaceted dimensions of the social support construct – structure, function, and appraisal – were investigated in the research program described in this book.

Sources of Support

The *structure* of social support comprises lay sources such as partners/spouses, family members, friends, neighbours, co-workers, volunteers, and self-help mutual aid groups, as well as professional sources such as health professionals (see figure 1.1). Professionals can provide intermittent, specialized support (Norbeck, 1988) or can mobilize lay support (Stewart, 1993).

Structure, encompassing social integration and social networks, has effects through social regulation or control, relational demands and conflicts, and social support. Social support, according to House, Umberson, and Landis (1988), pertains only to the emotional or practical sustenance gained from relationships. One powerful indicator of social support is an intimate, confiding relationship (Thoits, 1995). Thus, social support and social networks are distinct. Social structure variables that influence support include community size, socio-economic status, ethnicity, age, marital status, sex (House, Umberson, & Landis, 1988), and the size and density of the social network.

In one recent study, persons with cancer were supported by small, dense networks, primarily consisting of family members (Courtens, Stevens,

Crebolder, & Philipsen, 1996). In another investigation, family caregivers (of cognitively impaired older persons) with kin-focused social networks reported little satisfaction with support and a high degree of conflict, whereas caregivers who belonged to diverse social networks reported high satisfaction with support and little or no conflict (Fudge, Neufeld, & Harrison, 1997). In the sociological perspective particular attention is paid to the size, composition, and density of social networks.

Functions of Support

The functional content of relationships involves the flow of resources from social networks. The specific functions of support resources are emotional, instrumental (practical), informational, and affirmational (House et al., 1988) (see figure 1.1). These types of support functions, provided by social networks or support interventions, should be specific to stressors encountered (Cutrona, 1990). Furthermore, specific types of support are most helpful when they are provided by particular sources (Dakof & Taylor, 1990).

Assessment of types of support functions provided by social networks can inform interventions (House & Kahn, 1985). The specific resource received may affect health beneficially, depending on its appropriateness for the person and situation. In the functional approach it is suggested that support needs vary with stressors and situational factors, but the sources of social support and the interpersonal context of social provisions are not considered (Pierce, Sarason, & Sarason, 1990). Early debate, relevant to the functional approach, focused on whether social support is a unidimensional (e.g., Brown, 1986) or multidimensional construct (e.g., Barrera, 1986).

Appraisal of Support

Social support may be perceived as potentially available from the social network or actually may be delivered and received (Sarason, Sarason, & Pierce, 1990). It is important to distinguish the psychological sense of support (i.e., perceived support) from the actual expression and exchange of support (i.e., received support) (Dunkel-Schetter & Bennett, 1990). Received support is appraised or evaluated with respect to direction and to drawbacks or benefits (figure 1.1).

Support can be unidirectional/non-reciprocal or bidirectional/reciprocal. Norms of equity and reciprocity (Tilden & Gaylen, 1987) suggest that support should be bidirectional. As social-psychological theories of equity and social exchange indicate, support may involve benefits and costs for both recipients and providers. Yet reciprocity has been neglected in many social-support studies (Winemiller, Mitchell, Sutcliffe, & Cline, 1993), despite the fact that ill people experience non-reciprocal relationships with their social networks, which diminishes their self-esteem and increases their sense of indebtedness (Simmons, 1994). Many family caregivers of the chronically ill also experience lack of reciprocity (Gottlieb, 1989) and a sense of obligation. Obligatory social ties can produce harmful effects, whereas voluntary ties may have more manageable or escapable demands, allowing benefits to exceed costs (Thoits, 1995). When Canadian General Social Survey data were used to examine instrumental support exchanged with individuals outside the household, the complexity of simultaneously examining the provision and receipt of support was revealed (Hirdes & Strain, 1995).

Support from the network may have negative as well as positive effects (Brenner, Norwell, & Limacher, 1989). Indeed, most social relationships have supportive and stressful elements (Rook, 1990). Furthermore, some ties with friends and families are sources of stress and conflict rather than support. Drawbacks of support affect both support providers and support recipients. Support providers might experience overload, overexposure to chronic and acute stressors, overprotection, overinvolvement, and overcommitment. For example, in one study, focused on spouses of disabled stroke survivors, wives' responsibilities increased, their satisfaction with household responsibilities decreased, and their marital unhappiness increased significantly following the husband's stroke (Enterlante & Kern, 1995). Difficulties for the support recipient include feared loss of support, advice that constrains options, learned helplessness, relational costs, and diminished trust (La Gaipa, 1990). Support provided may be perceived as unhelpful, particularly when it undermines the recipient's self-esteem. Nevertheless, there has been insufficient research about the negative effects of social networks, and measures of social support typically disregard the inadequate and inappropriate aspects of relationships.

Perceptions of low support may reflect the *absence* of a supportive relationship or the presence of a negative, *conflictual* relationship (Coyne & Bulger, 1990). Even successful relationships involve lapses in support, miscarried efforts (Sarason et al., 1990), and failed support modes or functions (Eckenrode & Gore, 1990). Attribution, social exchange, and social comparison theories have been invoked to interpret *miscarried* or inadequate helping (Buunk & Hoorens, 1992).

Conflict and negative interactions correlate more strongly with low perceived support than with positive interactions (Schuster, Kessler, & Aseltine, 1990). As drawbacks of support may also have more powerful influences on health than the more general benefits of support (Burg & Seeman, 1994;

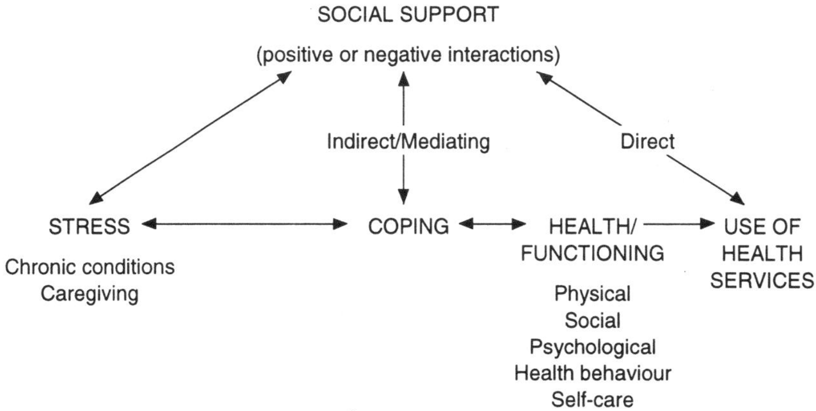

Figure 1.2 Social Support Research Program Framework

House et al., 1988; Rook, 1990), both the supportive and the non-supportive features of clients' interactions and relationships should be assessed.

Duration of Support

Support can either endure or dissipate over time (see figure 1.1). The changes in an individual's network (Bernard, Johnson, Killworth, McCarthy, Shelley, & Robinson, 1990) and patterns of support in chronically stressful situations, such as illness or caregiving, can be significant. For example, the size of cancer patients' networks as well as the amount of their emotional support decreased over time (Courtens et al., 1996).

The conceptual framework for the research program depicts the relationships between social support and stress (i.e., stressful demands or situations), social support and coping, and social support and health (see figure 1.2).

Relationship between Stress and Social Support

As indicated by the two-way arrow, stress and social support have a reciprocal relationship (figure 1.2). In the previous section, it was noted that conflictual interactions, miscarried helping, and inadequate support can be stressful. Social relationships are not necessarily supportive and, indeed, can sometimes become stressors (De Ridder & Schreurs, 1996), as reflected in the arrow from support to stress. For instance, in a study of social-psychological correlates of women's health, the least healthy women had more arguments with their children and more conflicts with spouses, and stress was the strongest predictor of their health (Thomas, 1995). In another investigation, elderly married women were in the poorest health and most vulnerable to stress, suggesting the potential role of relationship conflict (Preston, 1995). Similarly, family caregivers who had poorer relationships with heart transplant recipients experienced more distress (Canning, Dew, & Davidson, 1996). A family stress perspective (e.g., Boss, 1988; Funk, 1993) can help to interpret the pervasive influences of illness stressors on persons with chronic conditions and their family caregivers.

Conversely, support can mediate or moderate the impact of stressful situations on health and functioning outcomes (see figure 1.2). Stress-moderating processes determine an individual's reaction to or appraisal of stress (Eckenrode & Gore, 1990). A study of persons with rheumatoid arthritis suggested that social support had a significant effect on stress and adaptation through the mediating effect of control (Spitzer, Bar Tal, & Golander, 1995). In another investigation, people who received positive support from their spouses and did not appraise the stress associated with diagnosis of rheumatoid arthritis as a challenge had the lowest levels of depression (Schiaffino & Revenson, 1995). Appraisal of stressors, personality, and social support were associated with health outcomes of spouse caregivers of dementia patients (Monahan & Hooker, 1995).

Implicit in this framework is the acknowledgment that stressful situations can be chronic as well as acute. Furthermore, support has a moderating effect on the appraisal of the stressfulness of chronic illness and caregiving. Social-psychological theories are instructive in understanding the links between stress and social support.

Social Support and Coping

This research program recognizes the limitations of an individualistic perspective that ignores the social context of coping (Folkman, Chesney, McKusick, Ironson, Johnson, & Coates, 1991; De Ridder & Schreurs, 1996). Other people affect the way chronically ill persons and caregivers cope, irrespective of whether they seek support. The two-way arrow between social support and coping in the framework (figure 1.2) depicts the reciprocal relationship of support and coping. The social-psychological literature yields insights into this relationship.

Social support is conceptualized as a coping resource or coping assistance (Thoits, 1986, 1995). Social support is considered a social 'fund' from which people may draw when handling stressors (Thoits, 1995). As illustrated by the arrow from social support to coping, supportive persons can alter appraisal of stressors, sustain coping efforts, and influence choice of coping strategies. Social support also may augment coping resources available to deal with stressful encounters (Stewart, 1993). Furthermore, the receipt of support can change the trajectory of coping. Finally, perceived availability of social support is related to coping effectiveness (Bennett, 1993).

Conversely, the arrow from coping to support indicates that the ways an individual copes provide important clues to potential supporters about whether support is needed and, if it is, about the types of support needed (Silver, Wortman, & Crofton, 1990). People who use avoidance and distancing tend to have fewer support resources, whereas support seeking has been linked to greater provision of support (Dunkel-Schetter & Skokan, 1990). Indeed, coping portrayals can influence the course of interpersonal interactions and the nature and quality of support received (Silver et al., 1990). Chronically ill persons' ability to mobilize support depends on their coping skills and on the quality of their relationships (De Ridder & Schreurs, 1996). Thus, social support influences coping abilities and coping strategies influence support sought and received.

Coping helps people to manage stressful situations associated with chronic conditions and caregiving. Coping refers to 'efforts to master conditions of harm, threat, or challenge when routine or automatic response is not readily available' (Monat & Lazarus, 1985, 5). It has also been defined as 'constantly changing cognitive and behavioural efforts to manage specific external and/or internal demands that are appraised as taxing or exceeding the resources of the person' (Lazarus & Folkman, 1984, 141). Coping strategies, in addition to being emotion or problem focused, may be relationship focused (Coyne & Downey, 1991). Thus, coping with a chronic condition or caregiving can be conceptualized as managing distress (emotion focused), completing instrumental tasks (problem focused), and attending to each others' needs (relationship focused) (Coyne & Smith, 1991; Lazarus & Folkman, 1984). In close support relationships, one partner's coping influences the coping behaviours of the other (Gottlieb & Wagner, 1991). Recent studies of coping and support in marital relationships suggest that there should be a match between support needed/wanted and support given and that there are gender differences in coping and support-giving strategies and in desired types of support (Thoits, 1995).

According to the framework (figure 1.2), both coping and social support influence health. In one study, daily stressors, coping by seeking social support, and indirect coping strategies (i.e., avoidance, wishful thinking, self-blame) were significantly associated with physical symptomatology. Indirect coping, seeking social support, and extroversion were correlated with psychological symptomatology. Social support given and received and indirect coping were significantly related to EBV antibody titres (Kelly, Carter, Guarnaccia, & Ennis, 1996).

Impact of Social Support on Health

Social support influences health status (House et al., 1988; Kaplan & Toshima, 1990), health behaviour (Bloom, 1990), and use of health services (Birkel & Repucci, 1983). In the framework, the two-way arrow between social support and health depicts a bidirectional relationship (figure 1.2).

Health Status

The bidirectional relationship between health status and social support reflects the reciprocal nature of person and environment (Lough & Schank, 1996). The arrow from support to health indicates that integration in a social network and the ability to draw support resources from the network can maintain health and facilitate physical recovery (Bloom, 1990). For example, socially integrated persons are less likely to have high rates of schizophrenia, depression, tuberculosis, hypertension, accidents, and pregnancy complications (Ford & Procidano, 1990; House et al., 1988).

Although social integration is generally associated with better health outcomes, such as recovery following a myocardial infarction, the quality of existing ties and relationships influences health benefits (Seeman, 1996). Kaplan and Toshima (1990) reviewed evidence that social support enhances health outcomes and reduces mortality, whereas stressful social relationships can prolong physical dysfunction. Indeed, the negative qualities of relationships may have a stronger impact than the positive qualities on health and well-being. To illustrate, negative aspects of close relationships may increase sickness absence (Rael, Stansfeld, Shipley, Head, Feeney, & Marmot, 1995), and negative interactions are more predictive of depressed mood and poor emotional health than supportive interactions are (Coyne & Downey, 1991; Rook, 1990). In this context, poor marital satisfaction was strongly associated with depression (Burg & Seeman, 1994). Women's satisfaction with the functioning of their families contributed to lower levels of global stress and constituted a barrier against mental health disturbances, such as depression, sleeplessness, and anxiety (Sprusinska, 1994). Similarly, emotional adjustment to breast cancer was predicted by women's satisfaction with spouses' responses to their interactional and emotional needs and with support from other adults; their satisfaction with formal support (i.e., health care) predicted perceived health status (Hoskins, Baker, Sherman, Bohlander, Bookbinder, Budin, Ekstrom, Knauer, & Maislin, 1996). In a study of nurses' health, a poor relationship with a supervisor was associated with health problems, whereas a confiding relationship with a friend reduced the likelihood of health problems (Walters, Lenton, French, Eyles, Mayr, & Newbold, 1996). Recent research demonstrates that social isolation and non-supportive social interactions can result in higher cardiovascular and neuroendocrine activity and lower immune function, while socially supportive interactions have the opposite effect (Seeman, 1996).

Absent and insufficient support also has a detrimental impact on health outcomes. To illustrate, inadequate social support resulted in insufficient improvement in walking ability following hip-fracture surgery (Mutran, Reitzes, Mossey, & Fernandez, 1995). Sleep problems were significantly greater among African-American elderly women with more chronic illnesses and lower levels of emotional support (Bazargan, 1996). In another study, absence of instrumental support and lower levels of social network contact predicted decline in seniors' health (McAvay, Seeman, & Rodin, 1996).

Consistent with the buffering model (Quittner, Glueckouf, & Jackson, 1990), our intervention trials in the research program hypothesize that support has a moderating impact on health outcomes in the context of chronic stressors, such as illness and caregiving (see figure 1.2). Other research focused on chronic conditions supports this hypothesis. A study of women with multiple sclerosis revealed that social support reduced their uncertainty and enhanced their self-esteem and mastery (Crigger, 1992). Improvements in self-efficacy among older adults were influenced primarily by the availability of financial and emotional support resources (McAvay et al., 1996). As perceived available support increases, social-psychological adjustment to chronic illness improves (White, Richter, & Fry, 1992).

Social support also influences family caregivers' health outcomes. Social support predicted the health of caregivers of seniors (Pohl et al., 1994). A study of caregivers of seniors with Alzheimer's disease revealed that satisfaction with social support was related to improved ratings of subjective health (McNaughton, Patterson, Smith, & Grant, 1995). In another investigation, deteriorated physical health of family caregivers of Alzheimer's patients was explained by caregiver overload, while relinquishment of the caregiver role was influenced by use of formal support (Bourgeois, Schulz, & Burgio, 1996).

Social support influences the health of seniors: people in this age group experience more chronic conditions than others do. Social support for elderly people decelerated deterioration of their health (Choi & Wodarski, 1996). In a study of health and social networks as predictors of survival in old age, physical health status and activity patterns had the most significant effects on subsequent longevity, while the impact of social networks was greatest for women in the oldest age group (Ljungquist & Sundstrom, 1996). A study of community-dwelling elderly women revealed that perceptions of positive health status and adequate social support did not decline with age (Lough & Schank, 1996).

The arrow from health to social support (figure 1.2) illustrates how health and illness affect availability and quality of social support. Illness can be a major stressor, involving loss of social mobility, capacity to work, status, independence, and relationships. The continued need for social support in chronic stressful situations, such as those caused by illness, can deplete support, drain the social network resources that contribute to support, and result in alienation and estrangement from the network (Stewart, 1993). Thus, support can diminish over time in chronic stressful situations involving ill health. To illustrate, in one study prior depression among older adults was associated with a decline in relationships with family and friends (McAvay et al., 1996). In another study, the health status of diabetic women significantly influenced perceived social support (White et al., 1992). Indeed, poor health may limit opportunities for the chronically ill to develop and maintain social networks.

Health Behaviours

The arrow from social support to health outcomes (figure 1.2) also reveals the projected impact of support on health behaviour. Social network members may influence health behaviour directly through provision of information and indirectly through encouragement to comply with regimens or to maintain healthy behaviours. Network members may provide advice, act as role models, and constrain people from inappropriate health behaviours (Bloom, 1990). Zimmerman and Connor (1989) found that the greatest influences on health behaviour were supportiveness, encouragement, and modelling by family members, friends, and coworkers. A review of intervention studies revealed positive effects of support from family and others on smoking cessation, weight loss, blood pressure control, and dietary intake (Stewart, 1993). In another investigation, support from spouses and visiting homemakers had substantial effects on elderly persons' compliance with regimens for hypertension (Foshu, 1995).

Use of Health Services

As the arrow from support through health to use of health services depicts, the impact of social support on health services use is distal, whereas its effect on health status and on health behaviour is proximal. Social-network members can influence use of health services by providing desired support, by acting as screening and referral agents, and by transmitting values about help seeking (Birkel & Repucci, 1983). Positive beliefs about help seeking are associated with support mobilization (Dunkel-Schetter & Bennett, 1990) from laypersons and professionals.

The complex connections of social support and social networks with use of health services are illustrated in the following studies. The extent of elderly persons' informal support was influenced more by their social network size than by their demand for health care arising from declining health (Choi & Wodarski, 1996). In another investigation, the use of health care services by disabled older persons was related to caregiver depression and social isolation (Bass, Noelker, & Rechlin, 1996).

Summary

The *epidemiological perspective* on social support is evident in the preceding analysis of the influence of social networks on health outcomes and in the description of prevalence and incidence data on chronic conditions in the following chapters. Clearly, the discovery of relationships between health outcomes and social support may help practitioners to target and improve interventions (Monahan & Hooker, 1995).

Social Support Interventions

Social support is a salient concept for intervention because of its impact on health and health behaviour, its response to consumer demands, and its suitability to evolving health system emphases. Recognition of the importance of social support is reflected in recent health system reform trends, such as health promotion. For example, a key health promotion strategy entails strengthening social networks and social support (World Health Organization, 1997). Interventions that augment the supportive resources available to community members are congruent with health-promotion premises involving mutual aid, healthy environments, and public participation (Stewart & Tilden, 1995).

Trends related to the financing of health care have also made social networks central to health-care delivery. Families shoulder much of the responsibility for the care of ill persons, who now have briefer hospital stays, live longer, and have more chronic conditions. Clearly, the evolving health needs of contemporary society and health-care financial constraints cannot be addressed by professional sources alone. Although support interventions that involve lay networks and peers, as well as professionals, are needed in the context of system restraint and renewal, there has been a paucity of intervention research focused on social support (Gottlieb, 1992; Stewart, 1993). Therefore, assessment and intervention studies focused on persons with chronic conditions and their family caregivers were launched within the Social Support Research Program.

Assessment Guides Intervention

Judicious decisions about appropriate support strategies can be informed by careful assessment of the social environment in which the target population is embedded, personal characteristics of members of that population, and the population's unmet needs for certain types of support that promote health or health behaviours (Gottlieb, in press). Supplementary support through the introduction of new ties is advisable when the existing social network is impoverished, drained, or in conflict; reinforces undesirable behaviour; or lacks experiential knowledge; and when specialized knowledge and expert opinion are required. Intervention within the natural network is warranted when assessment reveals that the behaviour of network members influences attainment of health goals, the presenting problem is stigmatized, and the existing network needs strengthening to meet long-term continuing support needs (Gottlieb, in press). For example, family caregivers have varied support needs and expectations that typically have not been assessed (Lavoie, 1995). Assessment intended to inform support interventions for caregivers and persons with chronic conditions should consider the following questions:

- *Who is providing support?* Different people serve different supportive functions within the social network.
- *Who should be the targets of supportive interventions?* Most interventions are directed towards individual-level change. Existing social contexts or relationships should also be the foci of intervention (Lanza & Revenson, 1993).
- *Who are the members of the target population deficient in the types of support needed?* The target group for a support intervention should be individuals at risk due to inadequate social support. For example, an intervention with African-American women was preceded by assessment of their risk of inadequate support (Norbeck, Dejoseph, & Smith, 1996).

- *Who are the parties to deliver the required support?* (Gottlieb, 1988).
- *What are the supportive requirements aroused by the stressor or deficiencies in supportive provisions?* (Gottlieb, 1988)

Intervention Issues

Specificity of Interventions

Few support groups reviewed by Toseland (1989) were targeted to specific populations, although specificity of support to stressors has been advocated (e.g., Cutrona, 1990). In this context, Norbeck et al. (1996) contend that medical risk factors will not inform selection of participants for psychosocial interventions, including support groups. Specific issues such as time of diagnosis, gender, course of illness, changing needs, adaptive tasks confronting the chronically ill, caregiver roles, and caregiver characteristics (Bourgeois et al., 1996; De Ridder & Schreurs, 1996) should guide the composition of support groups and dyads.

Intervention Agents

Intervention agents (e.g., group leader, facilitator, home visitor) have received little attention from researchers. Their personalities, skills, and orientations influence the development of dyadic and group relationships (Bourgeois et al., 1996). Peers and professionals can act as intervention agents who provide supplementary support or mobilize support from the social network. Debates surrounding peer versus professional leadership prevail in the self-help group literature (Stewart, Banks, Crossman, & Poel, 1994). Alternative health care providers also can offer supplementary, intermittent support.

Level, Mode, and Content

Interventions can occur at different *levels* (e.g., individual, dyad, group). Although many of the support interventions described in this book focus on the group level, the peer visitor support intervention for family caregivers of seniors with stroke (chapter 6) is at the dyadic level.

The varied *modes* of intervention include face-to-face, telephone, and computer. Face-to-face interventions are delineated in chapters 4, 6, and 8; telephone modes are exemplified in chapters 2, 5, 7, and 8; and the computer modality is depicted in chapter 3.

Telephone support has begun to be used with adults dealing with stressful situations such as caregiving and illness; it is particularly advantageous for those whose participation in face-to-face groups would be hampered by distance, disability, stigma, or multiple demands. The advantages of telephone support are its anonymity, accessibility, and appeal to those who have no access to or do not wish to participate in a face-to-face group. Telephone support interventions have resulted in information gain and increased support satisfaction for caregivers of persons with Alzheimer's disease (Goodman & Pynoos, 1990); improved self-care by persons with osteoarthritis (Rene, Weinberger, Mazzuca, Brandt, & Katz, 1992), and increased self efficacy, diminished social isolation, and enhanced feelings of normality among people with HIV (Rounds, Galinsky, & Despard, 1995; Weiner, DuPont Spencer, Davidson, & Fair, 1993).

On-line computer networks can provide relief from isolation, practical information for coping, and positive role models, and can enhance empowerment and access to professional support when needed (Hillis & Lefebvre, 1994). Other benefits include increased emotional support and improved communication (Hassett, Lawden, & Rutan, 1992). Social isolation from peers was the strongest predictor of participation in a computer-mediated support network for adolescent mothers (Dunham, 1997). Over 70 per cent of self-help groups in the United States have developed their on-line availability over the past few years. Many of these self-help/support groups focus on adults with chronic conditions and their caregivers (Madara & White, 1997). Clearly, technology can enhance access to support interventions.

The *content* of the intervention should also address the specific support needs and wishes of participants. For example, focus groups and individual interviews conducted with pregnant women with support deficits revealed that emotional support was more crucial than informational support. Consequently, a randomized clinical trial was designed to test the impact of an emotionally supportive relationship with a nurse. The intervention encompassed four standardized face-to-face sessions every two weeks in the women's homes and telephone contact in the interval between home visits (Norbeck et al., 1996). In another intervention study, the presence of a caring, concerned person who provided emotional support for persons waiting for a cardiac catheterization was as effective as procedural information (Peterson, 1991). Friedland's (1992) support intervention following stroke consisted of six to twelve sessions involving survivors and their social-network members. 'Social support intervention therapists' helped network members to enhance support or create new support. The content of the program seemed as important as its intensity or duration (Friedland, 1992). Moreover, methodological challenges pertaining to heterogeneity of intervention groups, variability of intervention across individuals, and timing of intervention can be compounded in evaluations of multi-component interventions.

Evaluations may yield inadequate insight into the relative effectiveness of specific features of the intervention (Bourgeois et al., 1996). For example, a review of group interventions for family caregivers revealed that although almost all included education and support, little information was available on the efficacy of different approaches (Toseland, 1989).

Timing and Duration

When should support interventions take place? The times when caregivers seek and/or receive support intervention in the caregiving trajectory can have an impact on outcomes (Bourgeois et al., 1996). Similarly, the timing of intervention within the illness trajectory can affect caregiver, family, and client outcomes. People with chronic conditions often have to cope with increasing disability, intermittent recurrence, and periodic pain. Consequently, varied types and amounts of support may be helpful at different times, and altering adaptive tasks faced at specific stages should be considered (Lanza & Revenson, 1993). In one study, stroke survivors were on average eleven months post-stroke and nine months post-discharge from hospital. The investigator concluded that support interventions should begin earlier, before previously existing supports begin to deplete, preferably during hospitalization (Friedland, 1992). If social support is to influence recovery, it must be present early in the recovery process (Mutran et al., 1995).

Duration of interventions is also significant. Most support groups in one review were time limited, yet caregiving is often a long-term occupation (Toseland, 1989). Short-lived support groups are unsuited for people in chronically stressful circumstances that isolate them from natural sources of support. For this reason, participants frequently want to continue meeting beyond the planned duration (Gottlieb, 1992).

Documentation of Intervention Processes

There are few concrete guidelines for structural aspects of interventions such as timing, duration, number and frequency of sessions, and group composition (Bourgeois et al., 1996; Sidani and Biaden 1998). Processes and procedures in support interventions should be documented carefully (Toseland, 1989), yet evaluations of interventions rarely focus on implementation (Lavoie, 1995). Support intervention processes should be described, measured, and monitored to ensure delivery of the prescribed intervention and permit replication.

Outcomes and Outcome Measures

Outcomes should be selected judiciously in the context of specific stressful situations and participants' expectations. For instance, in the study of pregnant women, low birth weight in the intervention condition was 9.1 per cent, compared with 22.4 per cent in the control condition (Norbeck et al., 1996). Another intervention study, focused on cardiac catheterization, revealed that educational and social groups significantly reduced anxiety levels, in contrast to no change in the control condition (Peterson, 1991). In most studies of group interventions, positive outcomes, such as reduction of isolation and loneliness, are reported (Toseland, 1989).

Nevertheless, the selection of outcomes to be measured is complex and challenging. Lavoie (1995) observed 'a certain opposition between the research results based on standardized measures determined a priori and evaluations made by clinicians or based on self-assessment indicators.' Studies reviewed by Toseland (1989) failed to establish a clear link between satisfaction measures and other important indices (e.g., alleviation of stress or psychological disturbances, increased access to and use of informal support systems and community resources, improved self-care ability). Global measures of generic social-psychological factors (e.g., stress, burden, depression, life satisfaction, coping) became popular mechanisms to capture intervention effects (Bourgeois et al., 1996). Measuring specific behavioural changes may be more fruitful, however, than measuring global psychological changes (Toseland, 1989). Most important, outcome measures should accurately reflect the specific focus of the intervention (Gottlieb, 1996).

In conclusion, the conceptual links between social support and health outcomes, the paucity of support intervention research despite the desperate need for support experienced by chronically ill persons and their caregivers, the importance of prior assessment of support needs and desires, and emerging insights regarding support intervention research informed the design of projects described in the next seven chapters of this book.

Acknowledgments

The Social Support Research Program was made possible by a Scholar Award to the first author from the Medical Research Council of Canada and the National Health

Research Development Program (NHRDP). The projects encompassed within the program were supported by grants primarily from national research funding agencies. The germane funding sources for these assessment and intervention projects are reported in the Acknowledgments at the end of each chapter.

Note

The conceptual framework delineated in this chapter is described in Stewart et al. (1997).

References

Barrera, M. (1986). Distinctions between social support concepts, measures and models. *American Journal of Community Psychology, 14*(4), 435–447.

Bass, D.M., Noelker, L.S., & Rechlin, L.R. (1996). The moderating influence of service use on negative caregiving consequences. *Journal of Geronotology, Series B. Psychological Sciences and Social Sciences, 51*(3), S121–131.

Bazargan, M. (1996). Self-reported sleep disturbance among African-American elderly. The effects of depression, health status, exercise, and social support. *International Journal of Aging and Human Development, 42*(2), 143–60.

Bennett, S.J. (1993). Relationships among selected antecedent variables and coping effectiveness in postmyocardial infarction patients. *Research in Nursing and Health, 16*, 131–139.

Bernard, H., Johnson, E., Killworth, P., McCarthy, C., Shelley, G., & Robinson, S. (1990). Comparing four different methods for measuring personal social networks. *Social Networks, 12*, 179–215.

Birkel, R.C., & Repucci, N. (1983). Social networks, information seeking, and the utilization of services. *American Journal of Community Psychology, 11*(2), 185–205.

Bloom, J.R. (1990). The relationship of social support and health. *Social Science and Medicine, 39*, 635–637.

Boise, L., Heagerty, B., & Eskenazi, L. (1996). Facing chronic illness: The family support model and its benefits. *Patient Education and Counseling, 27*, 75–84.

Boss, P. (1988). *Family stress management.* Newbury Park, CA: Sage.

Bourgeois, M.S., Schulz, R., & Burgio, L. (1996). Interventions for caregivers of patients with Alzheimer's Disease: A review and analysis of content, process and outcomes. *International Journal of Aging and Human Development, 43*(1), 35–92.

Boyle, J.S. (1989). Constructs of health promotion and wellness in a Salvadoran population. *Public Health Nursing, 6*(3), 129–134.

Brenner, G.F., Norwell, W.R., & Limacher, M. (1989). Supportive and problematic social interactions: A social network analysis. *American Journal of Community Psychology, 12*, 831–836.

Brown, M.A. (1986). Social support, stress and health: A comparison of expectant mothers and fathers. *Nursing Research, 35*, 72–76.

Burg, M.M., & Seeman, T.E. (1994). Families and health: The negative side of social ties. *Annals of Behavioural Medicine, 16*(2): 109–115.

Buunk, B.P., & Hoorens, V. (1992). Social support and stress: The role of social comparison and social exchange processes. *British Journal of Clinical Psychology, 31*, 445–57.

Canning, R.D., Dew, M.A., & Davidson, S. (1996). Psychological distress among caregivers of heart transplant recipients. *Social Science and Medicine, 42*(4), 599–608.

Choi, N.G., & Wodarski, J.S. (1996). The relationship between social support and health status of elderly people: Does social support slow down physical and functional deterioration? *Social Work Research, 20*(1), 52–63.

Courtens, A.M., Stevens, F.C., Crebolder, H.F., & Philipsen H. (1996). Longitudinal study on quality of life and social support in cancer patients. *Cancer Nursing, 19*(3), 162–169.

Coyne, J.C., & Bulger, N. (1990). Doing without support as an explanatory concept. *Journal of Social and Clinical Psychology, 9*(1), 148–158.

Coyne, J.C., & Downey, G. (1991). Social factors and psychopathology: Stress, social support and coping processes. *Annual Review of Psychology, 42*, 401–425.

Coyne, J.C., & Smith, D. (1991). Couples coping with a myocardial infarction: A contextual perspective on wives' distress. *Journal of Perspectives on Social Psychology, 61(3)*, 404–412.

Crigger, N.J. (1992). An adaptation model for women with multiple sclerosis. PhD dissertation, University of Florida.

Cutrona, C. (1990). Stress and social support: In search of optimal matching. *Journal of Social and Clinical Psychology, 9*(1), 3–14.

Dakof, G.A., & Taylor, S.E. (1990). Victims' perceptions of social support: What is helpful from whom? *Journal of Personality and Social Psychology, 58*, 80–89.

De Ridder, D., & Schreurs, K. (1996). Coping, social support and chronic disease: A research agenda. *Psychology, Health and Medicine, 1*(1), 71–82.

Dunham, P.J. (1997). Staying connected: A computer-mediated parenting support network for young single mothers. Unpublished report.

Dunkel-Schetter, C. & Bennett, T. (1990). Differentiating the cognitive and behavioral aspects of social support. In B.R. Sarason, I.B. Sarason & G.R. Pierce (Eds.), *Social support: An interactional view* (208, 267–296). New York: Wiley.

Dunkel-Schetter, C., & Skokan, L. (1990). Determinants of social support provision in personal relationships. *Journal of Social and Personal Relationships, 7*(4), 437–450.

Eckenrode, J., & Gore, S. (1990). *Stress between work and family*. New York: Plenum Press.

Enterlante, T.M., & Kern, J.M. (1995). Wives' reported role changes following a husband's stroke: A pilot study. *Rehabilitation Nursing, 20*(3), 155–60.

Folkman, S., Chesney, M., McKusick, L., Ironson, G., Johnson, D.S., & Coates, T.J. (1991). Translating coping theory into an intervention. In J. Eckenrode (Ed.), *The social context of coping* (240–260). New York: Plenum Press.

Ford, G., & Procidano, M. (1990). The relationship of self actualization to social support, life stress and adjustment. *Social Behaviour and Personality, 18*(1), 41–51.

Foshu, G.B. (1995). Social support and compliance with hypertensive regimens among the elderly. *Journal of Mental Health and Aging, 1*(1), 7–20.

Friedland, J.F. (1992). Social support intervention after stroke: Results of a randomized trial. *Archives of Physical Medicine and Rehabilitation, 73*, 573–81.

Fudge, H., Neufeld, A., & Harrison, M.J. (1997). Social networks of women caregivers. *Public Health Nursing, 14*(1), 20–7.

Funk, S. (1993). *Key aspects of caring for the chronically ill*. New York: Springer.

Goodman, C.G., & Pynoos, J. (1990). A model telephone information and support program for caregivers of Alzheimer's patients. *Gerontologist, 30*, 399–404.

Gottlieb, B.H. (1988). Marshalling social support: The state of the art in research and practice. In B.H. Gottlieb (Ed.), *Marshalling social support: Formats, processes and effects*. London: Sage.

Gottlieb, B.H. (1989). A contextual perspective on stress in family care of the elderly. *Canadian Psychology, 30*(3), 596–607.

Gottlieb, B.H. (1992). Quandaries in translating support concepts to intervention. In H.O.F. Veiel & U. Baumann (Eds), *The meaning and measurement of social support* (293–309). New York: Hemisphere.

Gottlieb, B.H. (1996). Social support intervention research: Review and prospectus. Presentation at Social Support Research Program Symposium, Halifax, NS, 25 October.

Gottlieb, B.H. (in press). Selecting and planning support interventions. In S. Cohen, B. Gottlieb, & L. Gordon (Eds), *Social support measurement and intervention: A guide for health and social scientists*. New York: Oxford University Press.

Gottlieb, B.H., & Wagner, F. (1991). Stress and support processes in close relationships. In J. Eckenrode (Ed.), *The social context of coping* (165–187). New York: Plenum Press.

Hassett, M., Lawden, C., & Rutan, D. (1992). Use of computer network bulletin board system by disabled persons. *Proceedings – Annual Symposium on Computer Applications in Medical Care* (151–155 University of Maryland School of Nursing, Baltimore).

Health Canada. (1997). *Report on the health of Canadians.* Prepared by the Federal, Provincial and Territorial Advisory Committee on Population Health. Ottawa: Advisory Committee.

Hillis, B., & Lefebvre, A. (1994). Putting children and adolescents with disabilities in touch with the world. *Communication Outlook,* Fall.

Hirdes, J.P., & Strain, L.A. (1995). The balance of exchange in instrumental support with network members outside the household. *Journal of Geronotology, Series B. Psychological Sciences and Social Sciences, 50*(3), S134–142.

Hoffman, C., Rice, D., & Sung (1996). Persons with chronic conditions. *Journal of the American Medical Association, 276*(18), 1473–9.

Hoskins C.N., Baker, S., Sherman, D., Bohlander, J., Bookbinder, M., Budin, W., Ekstrom, D., Knauer, C., & Maislin, G. (1996). Social support and patterns of (adjustment to breast cancer including commentary by L.L. Northouse and J. Swirsky). *Scholarly Inquiry for Nursing Practice, 10*(2), 99–123.

House, J.S., & Kahn, R.L. (1985). Measures and concepts of social support. In S. Cohen & S.L. Syme (Eds), *Social support and health* (83–108). Orlando, FL: Academic Press.

House, J.S., Umberson, D., & Landis, K. (1988). Structures and processes of social support. *Annual Review of Sociology, 14,* 293–318.

Kaplan, R.M., & Toshima, T. (1990). The functional effects of social relationships on chronic illnesses and disability. In B.R. Sarason, I.B. Sarason, & G.R. Pierce (Eds), *Social support: An interactional view* (427–453). New York: Wiley.

Kelly, K.S., Carter, A.P., Guarnaccia, C.A., & Ennis, M. (1996). Stress, social support, psychological resources, health and antibody titres to Epstein-Barr virus in active older women. *Journal of Mental Health and Aging, 2*(1), 29–37.

La Gaipa, J.J. (1990). The negative effects of informal support systems. In S. Duck (Ed.), *Personal relationships and social support* (122–139). London: Sage.

Lanza, A.F., & Revenson, T.A. (1993). Social support interventions for rheumatoid arthritis patients: The cart before the horse? *Health Education Quarterly, 29*(1), 97–117.

Lavoie, J.-P. (1995) Support groups for informal caregivers don't work! Refocus the groups or the evaluations? *Canadian Journal on Aging, 14*(3), 580–603.

Lazarus, R., & Folkman, S. (1984). *Stress appraisal and coping.* New York: Springer.

Ljungquist, B., & Sundstrom, G. (1996). Health and social networks as predictors of survival in old age. *Scandinavian Journal of Social Medicine, 24*(2), 90–101.

Lough, M.A., & Schank, M.J. (1996). Health and social support among older women in congregate housing. *Public Health Nursing, 13*(6), 434–441.

Madara, E., & White, B. (1997). On-line mutual support: The experience of a self-help clearinghouse. *Information Referral: The Journal of the Alliance of Information and Referral Systems, 19*, 91–102.

McAvay, G.J., Seeman, T.E., & Rodin, J. (1996). A longitudinal study of change in domain-specific self-efficacy among older adults. *Journal of Geronotology, Series B. Psychological Sciences and Social Sciences, 51*(5), 243–253.

McNaughton, M.E., Patterson, T.L., Smith, T.L., & Grant I. (1995). The relationship among stress, depression, locus of control, irrational beliefs, social support and health in Alzheimer's disease caregivers. *Journal of Nervous and Mental Diseases, 183*(2), 78–85.

Millar, J. (1996). Chronic pain. *Health Reports, 7*(4), Cat. #82-003. Ottawa: Statistics Canada.

Monahan, D.J., & Hooker, K. (1995). Health of spouse caregivers of dementia patients: The role of personality and social support. *Social Work, 40*(3), 305–314.

Monat, A., & Lazarus, R. (1985). *Stress and coping* (2nd ed.). New York: Columbia University Press.

Moore, R., Mao, Y., Zhang, J., & Clarke, K. (1997). Economic burden of illness in Canada, 1993: Executive summary and recommendations. *Chronic Diseases in Canada, 18*(2), 95–96.

Mutran, E.J., Reitzes, D.C., Mossey, J., & Fernandez, M.E. (1995). Social support, depression, and recovery of walking ability following hip fracture surgery. *Journal of Gerontology, Series B. Psychological Sciences and Social Sciences, 50*(6): S354–361.

Norbeck, J.S. (1988). Social support. *Annual Review of Nursing Research, 6*, 85–109.

Norbeck, J.S., Dejoseph, J.F., & Smith, R.T. (1996). A randomized trial of an empirically-derived social support intervention to prevent low birth weight among African American women. *Social Science and Medicine, 43*(6), 947–954.

Peterson, M. (1991). Patient anxiety before cardiac catheterization: An intervention study. *Heart & Lung, 20*(6), 643–647.

Pierce, G.R., Sarason, B.R., & Sarason, I.G. (1990). Integrating social perspectives: Working models, personal relationships and situational factors. In S. Duck (Ed.), *Personal relationships and social support* (173–189). London: Sage.

Pohl, J.M., Given, C.W., Collins, C.E., & Given, B.A. (1994). Social vulnerability and reactions to caregiving in daughters and daughters-in-law caring for disabled aging parents. *Health Care for Women International, 15*(5), 385–395.

Preston, D.B. (1995). Marital status, gender roles, stress, and health in the elderly. *Health Care for Women International, 16*(2), 149–165.

Quittner, A.L., Glueckouf, R.L., & Jackson, D.N. (1990). Chronic parenting stress: Moderating versus mediating effects of social support. *Journal of Personality and Social Psychology, 56*(6), 1266–1278.

Rael, E.G., Stansfeld, S.A., Shipley, M., Head, J., Feeney, A., & Marmot, M. (1995). Sickness absence in the Whitehall II study, London: The role of social support and material problems. *Journal of Epidemiology and Community Health, 49*(5), 474–481.

Rene, J., Weinberger, M., Mazzuca, S.A., Brandt, K.D., & Katz, B.P. (1992). Reduction of joint pain in patients with knee osteoarthritis who have received monthly telephone calls from lay personnel and whose medical treatment regimens have remained stable. *Arthritis and Rheumatism, 35*, 511–515.

Rook, K. (1990). Parallels in the study of social support and social strain. *Journal of Social and Clinical Psychology, 9*(1), 118–132.

Rosenberg, M., & Moore, E. (1997). The health of Canada's elderly population: Current status and future implications. *Canadian Medical Association Journal, 157*(8), 1025–1032.

Rounds, K.A., Galinsky, M.J., & Despard, M.R. (1995). Evaluation of telephone support groups for persons with HIV disease. *Research on Social Work Practice, 5*, 442–459.

Sarason, R.B., Sarason, I.G., & Pierce, G.R. (1990). *Social support: An interactional view*. New York: Wiley.

Schiaffino, K.M., & Revenson, T.A. (1995). Relative contributions of spousal support and illness appraisals to depressed mood in arthritis patients. *Arthritis Care Research, 8*(2), 80–87.

Schuster, T., Kessler, R., & Aseltine, R. (1990). Supportive interactions, negative interactions and depressed mood. *American Journal of Community Psychology, 18*, 423–438.

Seeman, T.E. (1996). Social ties and health: The benefits of social integration. *Annals of Epidemiology, 6*(5), 442–51.

Sidani, S., & Biaden, C. (1998). *Evaluating nursing interventions: A theory-driven approach.* Thousand Oaks, CA: Sage.

Silver, R., Wortman, C., & Crofton, C. (1990). The role of coping in support provision: The self presentational dilemma of victims of life crises. In R.B. Sarason, I.G. Sarason, & G.R. Pierce (Eds), *Social support: An interactional view* (397–426). New York: Wiley.

Simmons, S. (1994). Social networks: Their relevance to mental health nursing. *Journal of Advanced Nursing, 19*(5), 281–289.

Spitzer, A., Bar Tal, Y., & Golander, H. (1995). Social support: How does it really work? *Journal of Advanced Nursing, 22*(5), 850–854.

Sprusinska, E. (1994). The Family APGAR Index: Study on the relationship between family function, social support, global stress and mental health perception in women. *International Journal of Occupational Medicine and Environmental Health, 7*(10), 23–32.

Statistics Canada. (1996). Health Facts from the 1994 National Population Survey. *Canadian Social Trends, 40*, Spring.

Statistics Canada. (1997). Who cares? Caregiving in the 1990's. *The Daily*, 19 August, 5–6.

Stewart, M. (1993). *Integrating social support in nursing*. Newbury Park, CA: Sage.

Stewart, M., & Tilden, V. (1995). Nursing science and social support: Contributions and challenges. *International Journal of Nursing Research, 32*(6), 535–544.

Stewart, M., Banks, S., Crossman, D., & Poel, D. (1994). Partnerships between health professionals and self help groups: Meanings and mechanisms. *Prevention in Human Services, 11*(2), 199–240.

Stewart, M., Ellerton, M.L., Hart, G., Hirth, A., Mann, K., Meagher-Stewart, D., & Tomblin-Murphy, G. (1997). Insights from a nursing research program on social support. *Canadian Journal of Nursing Research, 29*(3), 93–110.

Thoits, P.A. (1986). Social support as coping assistance. *Journal of Consulting and Clinical Psychology, 54*, 416–423.

Thoits, P.A. (1995). Stress, coping and social support processes: Where are we? What next? *Journal of Health and Social Behavior, Spec No*, 53–79.

Thomas, S.P. (1995). Psychosocial correlates of women's health in middle adulthood. *Issues in Mental Health Nursing, 16*(4), 285–314.

Tilden, V., & Gaylen, R. (1987). Cost and conflict: The darker side of social support. *Western Journal of Nursing Research, 9*(1), 9–18.

Toseland, R.W. (1989). Group interventions to support family caregivers: A review and analysis, *Gerontologist, 29*(4), 438–448.

Walters, V., Lenton, R., French, S., Eyles, J., Mayr, J., & Newbold, B. (1996). Paid work, unpaid work and social support. A study of the health of male and female nurses. *Social Science and Medicine, 43*(11), 1627–1636.

Weiner, L.S., DuPont Spencer, E.D., Davidson, R., & Fair, C. (1993). National telephone support groups: A new avenue toward psychosocial support for HIV-infected children and their families. *Social Work with Groups, 16*(3), 55–71.

White, N.E., Richter, J.M., & Fry, C. (1992). Coping, social support, and adaptation to chronic illness. *Western Journal of Nursing Research, 14*(2), 211–224.

Winemiller, D.R., Mitchell, M.E., Sutcliffe, J., & Cline, D.J. (1993). Measurement strategies in social support: A descriptive review of the literature. *Journal of Clinical Psychology, 49*(5), 638–648.

World Health Organization. (1997). *Milestones on the road to a global alliance.* Geneva: WHO.

Zimmerman, R.S., & Connor, C. (1989). Health promotion in context: The effects of significant others on health behavior change. *Health Education Quarterly, 16*(1), 57–75.

2

Social Support for Children with a Chronic Condition

Mary-Lou Ellerton, Miriam J. Stewart, and Judith A. Ritchie

Abstract. Children with a chronic condition are at risk for problems pertaining to emotional health, and behavioural and social adjustment. In this exploratory study social support experienced by children with a chronic illness was described and their use of social support in coping with developmental and illness-related stress was examined. Sixty-two school-age children participated (sixteen with diabetes, fifteen with cystic fibrosis, sixteen with spina bifida, and fifteen with no chronic condition). Children were interviewed about their social networks, support functions provided by the networks, and their appraisal of support. The children described support and support-seeking in specific stressful situations. Academic and peer issues were everyday stressors for all children; restrictions imposed by their condition accounted for the most illness-related stress. Healthy children reported the largest networks, the most peer supporters, and the greatest amount of support. Family members provided the majority of the support given to children with a chronic condition. Children with spina bifida identified the fewest supporters for every type of support function and less support from non-family members, including peers. The results have helped to shape plans for a computer-based support intervention for children, such as those with spina bifida, whose capacity for social interaction is impaired by a chronic condition and whose physical limitations prohibit accessibility to telephone and face-to-face support.

Introduction

The increasing incidence of chronic illness in childhood is attributed largely to improved survival rates for perinatal conditions and better treatment for conditions that were once life threatening (Drotar, 1981). In Canada, an estimated 500,000 children under the age of twenty years have a chronic condition, representing 7 per cent of all children (Canadian Institute of Child

Health, 1994). The Health Activity Limitation Survey (HALS) (Statistics Canada, 1991), which examined the rates and demographic characteristics of disabled children in Canada, revealed that the rates of disability vary from as low as 4.8 per cent for children in Newfoundland to as high as 9.3 per cent for children in Alberta.

Advances in the management of chronic childhood illness have improved life for many children with chronic conditions over the last decade. Even some medically fragile children are now able to live at home with their families and are being accommodated within the public school systems. Nevertheless, research on chronic childhood illness and disability reveals that these children are at risk for a lower quality of life due to emotional health, behavioural, and social adjustment problems (Cadman, Boyle, Szatmari, & Offord, 1987; Pless & Pinkerton, 1975; Pless, 1984; Satterwhite, 1978). For almost half of these children, their condition prevents or limits their participation in school and recreational activities (Statistics Canada, 1991). Thirty-five per cent have conditions that interfere with sensory function, and another 11 per cent have psychological, emotional, or mental health conditions that limit their activities. Similar findings emerged from an epidemiological study of Ontario children aged four to sixteen years (Cadman et al., 1987). In that study, children with chronic illness and disability were at substantially higher risk for psychiatric and social-adjustment problems than healthy children. Isolation was also more prevalent in the children with chronic illness and disability.

The HALS study uncovered the limitations that a chronic condition places on children's access to educational and recreational activities and on their opportunities for social interaction. It also pointed to the heavy demands for support that chronic childhood illness places on family and community resources. Although there has been some study of the factors associated with psychological and social outcomes in children with chronic conditions (e.g., Perrin, Stein, Walker, & Weitzman, 1993), the impact of social support on the lives of these children is only beginning to be understood. Little is known about the significance of children's inability to experience meaningful interactions with peers and significant adults for their physical and mental health.

In this chapter we examine the impact of physical illness on children's health and functioning, as well as the linkages between social support and children's health. The assessment study described in this chapter explores how children with a chronic condition use social support in managing the difficult aspects of life associated with normal developmental challenges and with their illness. A suitable support intervention for those most at risk for social isolation is proposed.

Psychological Adjustment in Children with a Chronic Condition

Epidemiological studies conducted in Canada and the United States suggest that children with disabilities have twice the incidence of psychosocial adjustment problems as healthy children (Cadman et al., 1987; Drotar & Bush, 1985; Gortmaker, Walker, Weitzman, & Sobol, 1990). To assess adjustment in children with chronic illness a variety of psychological measures have been used, dealing with self-esteem (Appleton, Minchom, Ellis, Elliott, Ball, & Jones, 1994), loneliness (Hurtig & White, 1986), social competence (Breitmayer, Gallo, Knafl, & Zoeller, 1992; Wallander, Varni, Babani, Banis, & Wilcox, 1988), and behaviour problems (Hurtig & White, 1986). It is shown in these studies that children with chronic illness are at increased risk for anxiety, depression, peer conflict, hyperactivity, and aggression (Cadman et al., 1987; Gortmaker et al.,1990). However, evidence of a direct relationship between chronic childhood illness and psychological adjustment is scarce (Wallander & Thompson, 1995).

Studies of chronic childhood illness and adjustment are fraught with controversy. Some studies have demonstrated that children with chronic illness are no different than their healthy peers in rates of mental health and adjustment problems (King, Schultz, Steel, Gilpin, & Cathers, 1993; La Greca, 1990; Nassau & Drotar, 1995). Others have found that these children resist stress generated by their illness (MacLean, Perrin, Gortmaker, & Pierre, 1992; Wallander et al., 1988). More often, the research has found higher rates of adjustment difficulties in the areas of social interaction, social isolation, and social competence, (Breitmayer et al., 1992; Wallander et al., 1988).

Some illness conditions have been shown to have stronger correlations with adjustment than others. For instance, children with neurological conditions score lower on measures of social competence and feel more isolated than healthy children and children with non-central nervous system conditions (Breslau, 1985; Wallander et al., 1988). Children with visible conditions, such as cancer and limb anomalies, have reported loneliness, social isolation, and even ridicule from peers (Baum & Forehand, 1984; Ross & Ross, 1984). Children with restricted physical activity, including those with spina bifida and cerebral palsy, may be withdrawn and less socially skilled than their healthy peers (Hurtig & White, 1986). Even invisible illnesses, such as asthma and diabetes, involve treatments and restrictions that interfere with children's social activities and friendship development (Graetz & Shute, 1995; MacLean et al., 1992; Simmons, Corey, Cowan, Keenan, Robertson, & Levinson, 1985). In summary, although most children with disabilities are not substantially different from healthy children in the acquisition of severe emotional illness, the presence of chronic illness places them at risk for psychological maladjustment. Furthermore, problems with social interactions are more profound. This signifies the need for social support.

Social Support and Psychological Adjustment in Children

Although there has been little research into the effects of social support on helping children to manage stress associated with chronic illness, there is an emerging body of literature that suggests that social support is a significant factor in children's capacity to overcome stressful life situations such as divorce, family poverty, parental mental illness, and adolescent pregnancy (Patterson & Geber, 1991; Wolchik, Sandler, & Braver, 1987a; Zelkowitz, 1981). Compas, Slavin, Wagner and Vannatta (1986) reported relationships between low levels of social support and depression, somatization, and anxiety in adolescents coping with major life events. Social support in early school age has a direct effect on adolescent adjustment (Kaplan, Robbins, & Martin, 1983) and social-psychological functioning (Bryant, 1985). Belle, Dill, and Burr (1991) reported higher self-esteem in children with a positive network orientation (i.e., expectation of support).

Belle and Longfellow (1983) distinguished between psychological outcomes for children associated with confiding in parents (e.g., higher self-esteem, lower levels of loneliness), confiding in peers (e.g., less loneliness), and confiding in no one (e.g., lower self-esteem). Other researchers have also found separate effects for family and peer support on the child's management of difficult life events (Kaplan et al., 1983) and the additive effect of family and peer support (Wallander & Varni, 1989). The literature is consistent about the significance of a healthy balance of family and peer support (Bryant, 1994; Wolchik, Beals, & Sandler, 1989) for children's adjustment.

Fewer studies have been conducted about the effects of social support on the adjustment of children with chronic illness. The results of these few studies suggest an important role for family and friends in positive psychological outcomes (e.g., Perrin, Ayoub, & Willett, 1993; Wallander & Varni, 1989).

Children's Social Networks

As the natural caretakers of their children, parents are their primary supporters throughout childhood and well into adolescence (Belle & Longfellow, 1983; Bryant, 1994). Parents who share activities with their children and applaud their decision making have children who are better adjusted, have fewer conflicts with their parents, and choose well-adjusted friends (Hetherington, Clingempeel, Anderson, Deal, Hagan, Hollier, & Lindner, 1992). The support derived from a satisfactory mother-child relationship is the strongest correlate of a child's network orientation in solving a problem and is the key to children's responsiveness to potential supporters (Belle et al., 1991; Reid, Landesman, Treder, & Jaccard, 1989).

Although families are generally considered to be the most crucial influence on children's adjustment and the main source of their emotional, instrumental, and guidance support, the role of peers cannot be underestimated. Peer conflicts and negative evaluations from peers are troubling aspects of day-to-day life for children (Asher, Hymel, & Renshaw, 1984; Compas, Malcarne, & Fondacara, 1988; Cowen, Pederson, Babigian, Izzo, & Trost, 1973). Children's peer networks increase in late school-age years and maintain their significance for companionship and recreation throughout adolescence (Bryant, 1985; Fuhrman & Buhrmester, 1985). In peer friendships, the norms of cooperation and reciprocity provide children with opportunities to develop socially in ways that are not possible in adult-child interaction alone (Cauce, 1986; Krappmann, 1992).

Children's use of people in their support networks changes according to their development. Support-seeking directed towards parents declines with age in favour of peer help (Nelson-Le Gall & Gumerman, 1984; Pflederer, 1990). Girls and boys use their social networks differently (Walker & Greene, 1987; Wolchik et al., 1989).

Impact of Social Support on Children with Chronic Illness

In general, social support for children with chronic illness has not been well studied. The existing research suggests an important role for family and friends in positive psychological outcomes (Wallander et al., 1988) and better adjustment in children with a chronic condition (Wallander & Varni, 1989). In a study of adjustment in children with limb deficiencies, peer support was more significantly related to children's adjustment than parent or teacher support (Varni, Setoguchi, Rappaport, & Talbot, 1992). Studies of children with end-stage renal disease (Melzer, Leadbeater, Reisman, Jaffe, & Lieberman, 1989) and children with cancer (Noll, Bukowski, Rogosch, LeRoy, & Kulkarni, 1990) revealed that children with chronic illness had smaller peer networks and more social isolation than their healthy peers.

Satisfying peer relationships is an important factor in compliance with disease protocols (La Greca & Hanna, 1983). Newly diagnosed diabetic adolescents' acceptance of their condition was related to social functioning

(Jacobson, Hauser, Wertlieb, Wolfsdorf, Orleans, & Vierya, 1986). Low levels of social support from classmates predicted low self-esteem and depression in children with limb deficiencies (Varni et al., 1992). Similarly, for children with spina bifida, self-esteem was related to peer and teacher support as well as parent support (Appleton, Minchom, Ellis, Elliott, Ball, & Jones, 1994). The relative roles of parent and peer support in children's adjustment is important for children who, by virtue of their condition are dependent on their families and restricted in their capacity for social interaction with their peers. In this context, other studies reveal that differences in children's adjustment emerge more from the sources of support than from functions (Cauce, Reid, Landesman, & Gonzales, 1990; Fuhrman & Buhrmester,1985). For instance, there was less depression and fewer behavioural problems in children with strong family support and less anxiety in those with strong non-family support (Wolchik et al., 1989).

Support Seeking in Children

For some children, the demands of physical illness may act as a stimulus for the acquisition of social support resources, leading to increased capabilities for managing stress (Patterson & Geber, 1991). The ability to solicit social support is an important skill, even for children. Children's social-cognitive problem-solving strategies (i.e., those manifest in support seeking) are important components of satisfying relationships with others, especially peers, and are associated with fewer emotional problems (Compas et al., 1988; Varni et al., 1992). Even very young children can be selective and demonstrate initiative in help seeking (Barnett, Darcie, Holland, & Kobasigawasa, 1982). Others (Pearlin, 1989; Thoits, 1985) contend that support is not purposefully sought, but rather is a natural and spontaneous outcome of relationships.

In summary, there is convincing evidence that social support is a significant factor in healthy psychological development in children and a deciding factor in the adjustment of children coping with major stressful life events. Support from family and peers is a necessary foundation upon which children learn to develop a positive network orientation for life. Children with a chronic condition are vulnerable to loneliness and low levels of support, particularly from peers, while having fewer resources with which to seek support. Nevertheless, very little is known about whether networks differ in size, composition, or support functions for children with chronic illness; how the children seek support; and how their receipt of support changes with stressful situations. Moreover, few studies exist in which the effects of support interventions on their support needs and social and emotional adjustment are examined.

Support Interventions

Social support interventions for children living in conditions of significant stress or adversity have demonstrated improved self-esteem and self-efficacy (Garmezy, 1991). For instance, a supportive transition program for children advancing from elementary to secondary school reduced antisocial behaviour and improved life skill development in participating students (Felner & Adams, 1988). A school-based program designed to improve social competence in adolescents improved their interpersonal as well as their problem-solving skills (Caplan, Weissberg, Grober, Sivo, Grady, & Jacoby, 1992). However, interventions for chronically ill children are rare. The only 'interventions' targeting children with chronic health conditions include an asthma day camp (Meng, 1997) and a school-based self-management program (Magyary & Brandt, 1996). Although these interventions have the potential to enhance interaction with peers, this was not their intent. Individualistic self-care was emphasized, rather than social support. Although many researchers have studied adjustment in children with chronic illness and the relationships between psychological outcomes and support, there are no published reports of social-support interventions that promote their adjustment through interactions with peers. Clearly, children with chronic conditions could benefit from *accessible* support interventions delivered by vehicles such as the telephone or computer.

Advances in computer technology have made significant contributions to the accessibility of computers by persons with a variety of disabilities. For instance, programs that convert ASCII files to Braille format and those that enlarge characters offer accessibility to visually impaired persons. Similarly, there are programs that convert computer 'beeps' to light flashes on the monitor for the hearing impaired and voice recognition programs and word predictor programs to facilitate input of messages for those with musculoskeletal disabilities (Chiang, 1994). The early evidence regarding the effects of computer-based social support for persons with disabilities who cannot participate in face-to-face support groups is encouraging. Fullmer and Walls (1994) reported almost 3,000 message postings on five computer discussion groups for persons with disabilities on topics as diverse as pain management, accessibility, and funding. Electronic support groups for persons with disabilities resulted in enhanced emotional support and improved communication (Hassett, Lowder, & Rutan, 1992). Most reports of computer use, however, are focused on disabled adults. Moreover, in the few that pertain to adolescents with chronic conditions the use of computers for learning and assistive technology and augmentative communication (Hassett et al., 1992; Holder-Brown & Parette, 1992) are emphasized, not social support and support seeking. The potential of computers to foster social skills and diminish loneliness and social isolation in adolescents with a disability is exemplified in an initiative called 'Ability-Online,' a computer-based public forum for children and adolescents for the electronic exchange of ideas, knowledge, and experiences (Lefebvre, 1992). Children equipped with a computer, a modem, and a telephone line have ready access to disabled and non-disabled children in this service, which has links to over a thousand subscribers every day (Lefebvre & McClure, 1996). The anecdotal evidence about the effectiveness of the program in bridging barriers for children and fostering independence by providing easy access to resources is impressive. To date there has been no evaluation of the effects of the program on the support needs, coping, and loneliness/isolation of the children who use it.

Fit with Framework

In our assessment study of social support in children with chronic illness, we adapted the model that guides the Social Support Research Program (see chapter 1). Children's support was conceptualized as interactions with family, friends, peers, and health professionals that communicate esteem, aid, or emotional help (Stewart, 1993). Support was viewed as a coping resource for managing the particular stressors that children with chronic conditions encounter, which is most helpful when the supporter and the support function respond to the particular requirement of the child for support (Cutrona, 1990; Dakof & Taylor, 1990). For that reason, we assessed the amount and types of support that the children received from particular people in the context of specific situations. We included the child's view of support in managing everyday stress (i.e., stress associated with school, friends, home life), as well as a stressful aspect of living with a chronic illness. Because support may have negative as well as positive features, we assessed both the supportive and non-supportive aspects of children's relationships with family and friends and the type of support they received through those relationships. Based on the findings from our assessment study, we designated loneliness as the most appropriate health outcome for the intervention pilot.

Assessment Study: Support Needs of Children

In the assessment study we used an exploratory design to describe and compare the sources, functions, and appraisal of support in children with a chronic condition and healthy children. We also identified the factors that influence children's experiences with social support. Finally, we examined the children's use of support in managing stress in illness-related situations, as well as in situations that present the child with predictable developmental challenges.

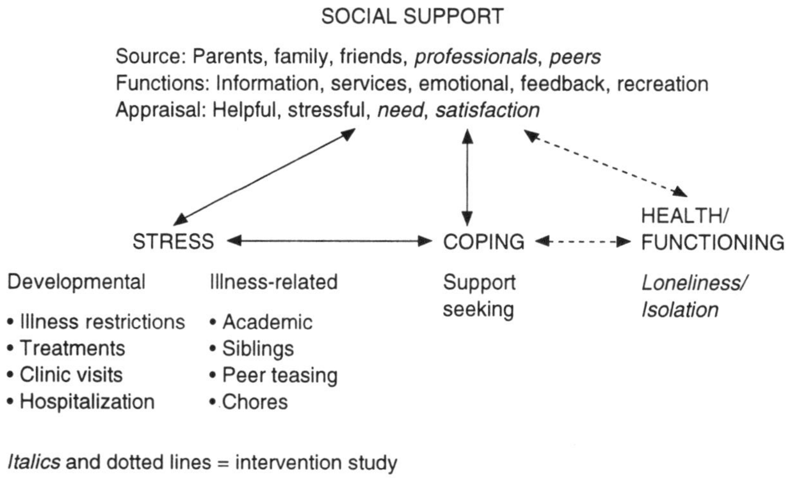

Figure 2.1 Framework for Assessment and Intervention Studies Involving Children with Chronic Conditions

Sample

We interviewed sixty-two children (twenty-eight boys and thirty-two girls) between the ages of eight and sixteen years. Fifteen were healthy children and the remainder had been diagnosed with a chronic condition: diabetes (n = 16), cystic fibrosis (n = 16), and spina bifida (n = 15). The children in the three illness groups were recruited either through letters to their mothers, who had participated in an earlier study (see chapter 3, below), or through hospital specialty clinics for the conditions. The conditions selected represented a range of differences in treatments, lifestyle and mobility restrictions, and visibility. The healthy children were nominated by the mothers of children in the three illness groups from among family friends. All of the children lived at home with their parent(s) and attended school.

Methodology

Most interviews took place in the child's home. When that was not possible, the child was interviewed in a quiet place in the hospital clinic. In the first part of the interview, the child responded to the *Children's Inventory of Social Support* (CISS) (Wolchik, Sandler, & Braver, 1987b), which solicits the child's perceptions of the sources and types of their social support and their satisfaction with the support they receive from family and friends. Several instruments have been used to assess social support in children (see appendix A). Most focus on sources and types of support. However, most do not assess appraisal of negative interactions and are limited to satisfaction with support. We selected the CISS for use in the study for its consistency with the research program framework, its capacity to capture children's assessments of negative support, and its suitability for a wide age range. These features were demonstrated in our pilot with four children that preceded the assessment study. Furthermore, the CISS is adapted from the *Arizona Social Support Inventory Schedule* (ASSIS), a measure used in many studies involving adult samples in our research program (appendix B).

Because many studies of social support have relied strictly on the structure of support and on global assessments that neglect the child's reflections on their experiences, we also asked questions about supportive and non-supportive interactions that the child had experienced during stressful situations. We developed a narrative interview guide that focused on stressful situations and the use of support in those situations. Initially, the child was asked to describe an everyday event that had been difficult or stressful during the past two months and to rate the stressfulness of that situation on a 10cm *Visual Analogue Scale* (VAS). Then the interviewer used probe questions to elicit the coping behaviours used by the child to manage the situation, who had helped them, and what these people said or did that was helpful. Finally, the child responded to the seven 'seeking support' items from the *Self-Report Coping Scale* (SRCS) (Causey & Dubow, 1992) in relation to the stressful event described. The children with chronic conditions repeated the narrative part of the interview process and the 'seeking support' items from the SRCS in responding to a specific stressful event related to their illness.

We calculated descriptive statistics for the demographic variables, and for the size and functions of the children's support networks, their appraisal of support, and their use of social support as a coping strategy. We conducted one-way *Analyses of Variance* (ANOVAs) to explore the relationships between the study variables and the factors of age group, gender, and condition group. *T*-tests were used to examine differences in number of support functions, and appraisal of support by age group and gender. Chi square was used to determine differences in type of helper identified in different types of stressful situations.

We did a content analysis of the children's responses to the narrative interview questions about the type of stressful situations they described and about the type of helper, type of support, and appraisal of support in those situations. The child's complete response to each interview question consti-

TABLE 2.1
Research Design

	Assessment Study	Intervention
Sample	Convenience Children with chronic conditions ($n = 45$) Healthy children ($n = 15$)	Random Older children with chronic conditions ($n = 100$)
Design	Descriptive Correlational	Randomized control trial
Instruments		
Stress	Interview Guide	–
Coping	Self-Report Coping Scale	*Self-Report Coping Scale*
Support	Interview Guide Children's Inventory of Social Support	*Children's Inventory of Social Support*
Health	–	*Loneliness and Social Dissatisfaction*
Data collection	T_1– Interviews	T_1 – pre-test T_2 – post-test after intervention T_3 – delayed post-test 3 months later
Data analysis		
Qualitative	Content analysis of themes	Thematic content analysis of computer transcripts and post-intervention interviews
Quantitative	Descriptive statistics, ANOVAs, t–tests	Summary statistics, *t*-tests, MANOVA

tuted a unit of analysis and was coded according to a category system developed by the researchers. The research design is summarized in table 2.1.

Results

Support Sources, Functions, and Appraisal (CISS)

The children reported an overall average of twenty-one supporters ($sd = 10.1$) in their social networks. The networks ranged from an average of twenty-six persons for the healthy children to only sixteen for the children with spina bifida. The majority of supporters for all children were peers. Typically, negative members of the support network were siblings and classmates; over half of the children reported negative interactions with other children. The average number of support functions (i.e., the sum of the number of people providing each type of support: play, advice, goods/service, emotional support, positive feedback) ranged from a high of sixty-one for the children without a chronic condition to only thirty-three for the children with spina bifida. The children in all groups indicated that they were highly satisfied with their support (M = 8.5 out of a possible score of 10).

Factors Influencing Support

Sources of Social Support: Children without a chronic condition had the largest support networks; post hoc analysis showed the significant difference was between the children without a chronic condition (M = 26) and the children with spina bifida (M = 16). The children with spina bifida had the smallest peer networks, significantly smaller than the peer network size of the children without a chronic condition. These findings are consistent with other researchers' reports that children with disabilities can have weak social networks (Belle, 1989; Lyons, 1989; Taylor, 1988). In a study of the support needs of mothers of children with chronic conditions that preceded this research (see chap. 3, below), mothers described extraordinary efforts to provide supportive environments for their children. In spite of these efforts, the mothers worried that their children lacked the support needed for healthy development. The much smaller networks of the children with spina bifida, particularly their peer network, may exemplify the social consequences of childhood conditions that limit physical activity and/or are visible.

Support Functions: There were differences between the groups of children in the number of support functions reported. Children without a chronic condition reported significantly more support overall than the children in the spina bifida group. The children with no chronic condition and the children with cystic fibrosis reported more non-family support than the children with diabetes and spina bifida did. In this context, the children without a chronic condition reported more support from peers than the children in any of the illness groups did. Moreover, the children without a chronic condition reported more providers of all types of support, namely, play, information, goods, emotional support, and positive feedback. The children with spina bifida had significantly smaller networks (i.e., fewer sources of support) for every type of support than the other children had. Older children (over twelve years) reported more support functions and more informational support than the younger children did. The social competence skills acquired in late childhood and adolescence (Ford & Procidano, 1983), necessary for forming and maintaining relationships, may account for the higher numbers of supporters among the older children.

Appraisal of Support: The children's scores for support satisfaction averaged 8.5 (*sd* = 1.1) on a ten point scale. There were no differences in satisfaction with support from family or non-family (i.e., friends) between the healthy children and those in the illness groups. Although the older children reported more support, they were less satisfied with that support than the younger children were. These lower levels of satisfaction are consistent with the challenges of early adolescence, which include a transition to junior high school, the need to acquire new friends, the decreasing impact of parental attitudes, and the increasing importance of peer influence. The findings related to age shed some light on the appropriate timing of support interventions for chronically ill children and the importance of fostering peer support relationships in adolescence.

Stressful Situations and Related Use of Support

With the exception of the older girls, who gave full descriptions of the stressful situations in their lives and the pertinent support rendered by their networks, most children gave only terse responses to the interview questions. Across all groups, children described major everyday stressful events, which included academic issues (30 per cent), such as problems with homework and struggles with parents over completing assignments, and peer relationships (29 per cent), such as arguments with friends. Other stressful events included conflict with siblings (14 per cent), teasing (13 per cent), and chores (5 per cent). There was more consistency in the chronically ill children's descriptions of stressful events related to their chronic condition than to everyday situations. Nearly half (47 per cent) described stressful events related to restrictions attributable to their condition, followed by situations related to treatments (25 per cent), clinic visits (18 per cent), and hospitalization (9 per cent).

The children with chronic conditions found situations related to everyday life more stressful than those directly associated with their condition. These children shared with their healthy peers normal developmental concerns about schoolwork and social relationships with teachers, peers, and siblings. The everyday stressful situations they identified were the same as those reported by Causey and Dubow (1992) in their study of healthy schoolchildren, and by Bull and Drotar (1991) in their study of school-age children and adolescents in remission from cancer. The findings may demonstrate the essential normality of life for these children despite chronic conditions. On the other hand, a chronic condition undoubtedly exerts an indirect impact on children's lives, so that, for these children, everyday activities are not really 'non-illness' situations. Although the stressful situations in everyday life are the same as those for healthy children, the child with a chronic condition must manage the additional stress associated with the condition. Twelve of the fifteen children with spina bifida had mobility problems and all but two used a wheelchair. An adolescent girl shared the frustration of her immobility through a fantasy about dance: '*I would like to be able to dance – and I can, sort of. But I wouldn't – not in front of anybody. So I just do my dance in my head.*'

In their narratives, these children described lives of loneliness and of physical and social isolation. Several expressed their boredom at sitting on the sidelines during gym class, keeping score or holding ropes in place. Others had difficulty in naming a single friend. Almost all the children with spina bifida reported struggles to join peer activities. One child's voice rose with anger as he described the effort involved in trying to manoeuvre a wheelchair through snow to be with his friends; another boy talked about a leg fracture sustained when he discarded his crutches to participate in a football game. Many of the children voiced their frustration at physical barriers, such as steps and inclines and small doorways, that barred them from social activities with other children.

The children with spina bifida found themselves socially isolated from peers at school, in part because of their limited mobility and in part because most lived in rural communities where they had few opportunities to interact with other children. The loneliness of emotional isolation (absence of a close emotional-attachment figure) has been distinguished from social isolation (absence of an assessable social network) (Weiss, 1974). These children described close bonds and abundant support from family members. Although they were not critical of the lack of supportive relationships with persons outside the family, they revealed their profound loneliness stemming from social isolation. Social support can redress different forms of loneliness and isolation (Rook, 1990).

Support Received in Stressful Situations

The children with a chronic condition identified family members as major supporters in both condition-related and everyday situations. Children without a chronic condition reported that they relied equally on family and friends for support. Consistent with other research on support providers (e.g., Dakof & Taylor, 1990), this study revealed that most support was provided to the children with chronic conditions by family members and within close relationships. Children with a chronic condition reported that they received help from non-family members, including peers, more often with respect to everyday than to condition-related stressful situations. They described receipt of advice (affirmational support), material support, and emotional support with equal frequency (31 per cent) in non-illness situations. In condition-related situations, they reported that more than a third of their support was emotional (36.2 per cent), followed by material goods (practical support) (31.8 per cent), and advice (informational support) (16.4 per cent).

Children in all study groups indicated that they were very satisfied with the help they received. The mean rating for satisfaction with help for children without a chronic condition was 8.04, whereas the average satisfaction rating for children with a chronic condition was greater than 8.5 for both types of stressful situations. When the children were asked to report 'helpful' types of support in particular stressful situations, most described efforts of family or friends to advise them on managing disputes with other children, assist them with school or homework, and enhance their self-esteem.

Support Seeking as a Coping Strategy

Total support-seeking scores (out of a possible score of 35) were modest for both illness-related situations ($M = 20.3$) and everyday situations ($M = 18.2$). The children with a chronic condition used more support seeking in everyday situations than in illness situations. There were no differences in support seeking in everyday stressful situations between the children with a chronic condition and the healthy children. The fact that children with a chronic condition used more support seeking in coping with developmental demands suggests that these children do not define themselves by their condition and seek support that enhances their chances of inclusion in the mainstream of everyday life and friendships. Support seeking, as a coping strategy, has been linked to greater receipt of social support (Dunkel-Schetter & Skokan, 1990).

Key Findings from the Assessment Study

- Family members were the major source of support for all children.
- Healthy children had the largest networks, the most peer supporters, and the greatest amount of support.
- Children with a chronic condition received less support from non-family network members and less peer support.
- Children with spina bifida had the smallest networks for every type of support and the least non-family support, including peer support.
- Healthy children were more satisfied with non-family support than chronically ill children were.
- Academic and peer issues were major sources of everyday stress for all children.

- Restrictions related to illness were major sources of stress due to chronic conditions.
- Children with chronic conditions reported more stress and more coping strategies in everyday than in illness situations.
- Younger children received less support than older children, but they were more satisfied with their support.

Implications for Intervention

Many stressors described by the children developed in the context of coping with peer relationships and the social consequences of their chronic condition. The expressed need for peer friendships suggests the value of assisting children to develop relationships with peers. In peer relationships, children learn to cooperate, appreciate the ideas of others, and develop skills around consensus building and reciprocity. These experiences, unique to friendships with other children, were missing in the lives of the children with chronic conditions, in particular, those with spina bifida. In previous research it has been demonstrated that when children with disabilities have friends and are integrated in schools, they are more self-confident and have improved communication skills, academic performance, participation in social life and extra-curricular activities, social skills, and sense of belonging (Bradley, 1994; Giangreco, Dennis, Cloninger, Edelman, & Schattman, 1993).

Parents were strong and consistent supporters to all the children in this study. The lack of peer support for the chronically ill children has raised questions about the interchangeability of support. Siblings were typically the only accessible child supporters for these children, although these relationships were often conflictual. Other research (Bryant, 1994) concludes that, although high levels of sibling support can improve adjustment somewhat in peer-deprived children, these children have higher rates of maladjustment.

The measurement of support satisfaction may not be as useful as we had thought when we planned the assessment study. Overall satisfaction with support was high for all children in the study. Although participants in support programs are generally appreciative of the support they receive, the extent to which there have been changes to their lives in areas that matter to them may be more important (Benjamin Gottlieb, personal communication, 1996).

Many children with spina bifida expressed their profound isolation and loneliness. Those who did attempt to participate in activities that were inaccessible to them used impressive ingenuity without a corresponding expectation of reciprocal support from others. These support-seeking children described many supporters external to their families, including health professionals. The fact that children accepted the onus for their own involvement in meaningful activities suggests the need to ensure accessibility of services that respond to the support needs of children with a chronic condition.

In summary, this assessment study revealed that, although children look primarily to parents and peers for social support, support from peers is often inaccessible. Moreover, children with a chronic condition used support seeking more as a coping strategy in stressful situations than healthy children did. A further contribution of this study was the assessment of support from the perspective of children themselves, rather than sole reliance on the views of parents or teachers.

Lessons Learned

- Parental support is a primary source of social support for all children, regardless of age or condition.
- Support from peers is often inaccessible to children with a chronic condition.
- Children with limited mobility are the most vulnerable to lack of peer support.
- Children with a chronic condition share the same developmental concerns as healthy children and seek social support to manage those situations.
- Support interventions are most appropriately targeted at children who are isolated by their limited mobility or vulnerable to social and geographical isolation.

Proposed Intervention Study: Computer Mutual Aid for Children with Limited Mobility

Rationale

The findings from our assessment study helped to shape our research team's plans for the intervention phase of our investigation of children's social support. The smaller networks and lower levels of support reported by children with spina bifida suggest that the intervention should respond to the needs of children with chronic illness who are isolated – physically, emotionally, and socially – from participating in interpersonal relationships and developing friendships with peers. Supportive friends help children with chronic illness to manage the continuous demands that can cause feelings of loss of control and helplessness (Pflederer, 1990). Yet, with the exception of summer camps, there are no reported interventions involving peer support that promote psychological adjustment in children with chronic illness. Perhaps the isolation that prevents these children from participation in friendships also represents a barrier to the development of accessible support interventions. Technology, such as the telephone and the computer, can offer accessible avenues of peer support.

A pilot study of a computer-mediated parenting support network with adolescent mothers revealed that close personal relationships and a strong sense of community developed (Dunham, Hurshman, Litwin, Gusella, Ellsworth, & Dodd, 1998). The most important predictor of participation in the network was isolation from peers. Early evidence of the effects of computer-based social support for persons with disabilities is encouraging. As noted earlier, however, most studies of computer interventions are focused on adults, and in the few that pertain to children with disabilities the use of computers for learning is emphasized and the effects on social isolation or support needs are not evaluated.

Objectives

The purpose of the intervention study is to test a computer mutual aid intervention for adolescents with physical disabilities that provides for their support needs and reduces the risk of psychological and behavioural adjustment problems. More specifically, the objectives of the project are to determine (1) the extent to which young adolescents use the computer as a resource for social support; (2) the effect of the intervention on (a) support network size and on amount, type, and appraisal of social support, (b) loneliness and social isolation, and (c) coping with developmental and illness-related stress; (3) the influence of age, sex, and type of illness on adolescents' use of computer-based social support.

Sample

The intervention group will include adolescents aged twelve to eighteen years with spina bifida (n = 25) and cerebral palsy (n = 25); a non-intervention group will include equal numbers of adolescents with these same disabilities (n = 50). Like the young people with spina bifida in our assessment study, many adolescents with cerebral palsy use a wheelchair and are isolated from their peers geographically and socially. Moreover, difficulties with expressive functions limit the capacity of some children with cerebral palsy for social interaction. The eligibility criteria for the study include (1) a diagnosis of spina bifida or cerebral palsy, (2) the capacity to use a computer keyboard with modifications such as a keyguard, and (3) IQ within a normal range and ability to read at a grade six level. The adolescents will be recruited through the clinic staff at the two health centres where the study will take place (one in eastern Canada and one in the Atlantic region) and randomly assigned to the intervention or control condition.

Intervention

The project is a randomized control trial of a computer support intervention. The adolescents will be equipped with a Pentium computer in their homes. Links to the Internet will be confirmed, and training will be provided according to the needs of the individual participant. Adaptive communication systems will be secured for those who cannot use a standard keyboard. The intervention communication tools will be accessed through a single Internet software package and will include electronic mail, news groups, net folders, and chat rooms – all integrated under a simple worldwide interface. Once they are connected to the network, the adolescents will be able to post or answer notices to a bulletin board accessible only to participants in the study, send e-mail messages to the other network members, and participate in an open computer 'chatline' for adolescents on the network. The children will be assisted to progress from simple: 'non-real' time (e-mail) to real time (chatline) over the course of the intervention.

At the outset of the study, adolescents in the intervention group will be introduced to each other and helped to test their equipment during a telephone conference. A health professional, available for support throughout the intervention, and a mentor, a mature adolescent with either spina bifida or cerebral palsy, will be introduced at this initial meeting. During the first session, adolescents may share as much about themselves as they wish. During the six months of the intervention study, the adolescents will be free to use the computer as frequently as they want.

The professional and peer supporters will be trained jointly in communication and facilitation skills by an expert in communications and by one of the investigators using simulated situations and role play. Strategies will be developed for identifying and assisting adolescents who may need more support than the computer network can provide. Monthly check-in sessions involving the communications expert, peer and professional supporters, and one of the investigators will be conducted by teleconference to provide feedback, and monitor the progress of the intervention.

Key Features of the Intervention Study

- Examine the effects of a computer mutual-aid intervention on support needs and coping of children with chronic illness.
- Participants include an intervention group of older (12–16) children with spina bifida (n = 25) and cerebral palsy (n = 25) and a control group of healthy children (n = 50).
- Children receive a home computer and computer training to enable them to post notices, send e-mail messages, and 'chat' with other children in the group.
- Assess sources of stress, amount and function of peer support, satisfaction with support, and coping strategies to manage stress.
- Analyse discussions for emergence of leadership, patterns of support, and social learning and social comparison processes.
- Evaluate the impact of six-month intervention on loneliness and isolation.

Documentation of Processes and Outcomes

Quantitative

In a pre-intervention interview, all adolescents in the study will be interviewed in their home or clinic. Demographic information will be collected and three instruments will be administered: *The Children's Inventory of Social Support* (Wolchik, Sandler, & Braver, 1987b), which was also used in the assessment study; *The Loneliness and Social Dissatisfaction Scale* (Asher, Hymel, & Renshaw, 1984), a sixteen-item self-report measure for the assessment of adolescent satisfaction with peer relationships; and the 'seeking social support' subscale of *The Self-Report Coping Scale* (Causey & Dubow, 1992) (see appendix B), also used in the assessment study to assess support-seeking behaviours. These measures will be readministered at post-test and delayed post-test (three months). During the intervention, the number of minutes per day on line, the number of calls per day per child, and the use of communication options available on the network will be identified for the children in the intervention condition.

Qualitative

Interviews conducted with adolescents in the intervention condition at post-test and again three months later will be focused on continuing contacts with the other participants, the perceived impact of the intervention, and suggestions for improvements to the support program. The interviews will also explore whether the intervention focused on issues of concern to the adolescents, provided helpful information, influenced their behaviour and coping strategies for dealing with stress, and affected their relationships with people in their natural network. Discussions recorded in computer transcripts will be subjected to thematic content analysis of the adolescents' source of stress and support, coping strategies for managing stress, and appraisal of supporters. The transcripts will also be analysed for group process issues, including the emergence of leadership, types of support exchanged over time, patterns of support given and received, and social learning and social comparison among peers. (The research design is described in table 2.1.)

Implications for Policies and Programs

In studies of parents caring for children with chronic conditions, the lack of responsiveness of health and education ministries to their needs for information and support is documented (Edwards-Beckett & Cedargren, 1995; Gravelle, 1997). There is abundant evidence of the risks for psychological and social maladjustment associated with chronic childhood illness. Increasingly, however, there is also evidence to suggest that resilience (i.e., capacity to bounce back) in stressful life situations, such as chronic illness, is associated with the protective factor of social support (Bolig & Weddle, 1988; Brown, Doepke, & Kaslow, 1993; Lefebvre & McClure, 1996; Lord & Hutchison, 1996). Some intervention studies point to the need to invest in programs that foster resilient outcomes (Gortmaker et al., 1990; Stein & Jessop, 1984). The planned support intervention has the potential to foster resilience in children with chronic conditions through a system of dependable peer support that transcends physical and geographical barriers.

Rapid technological advances relevant to the support needs of persons with disabilities hold considerable promise for enhancing integration, independence, friendship, and accessibility. Little is known, however, about the mechanisms associated with the success of support programs that use technology. Most self-help groups that have developed on-line availability in recent years typically provide information rather than opportunities for interaction (Madara & White, 1997). Reports in the literature are optimistic but largely anecdotal (Garner & Campbell, 1987; Madara, 1992). Moreover, computer self-help groups for disabled persons rarely focus on children or adolescents. There are few published reports of publicly funded support programs for children with chronic illness that lead to positive social and emotional outcomes. The potential for programs for children of mutual aid, delivered through telephone and computer support groups, is just beginning to be examined.

The results of the intervention study will provide evidence of the capacity of computer-based support, delivered by peers and professionals, to influence the lives of children with disabilities in ways that diminish social isolation and enhance social integration. Furthermore, the intervention offers a foundation for planning programs that correspond to the support needs and wishes of children with chronic conditions. Equally important to these vulnerable children and their families are social and economic policies that lie beyond the range of conventional health promotion activities and accommodate their unique needs for healthy living. The National Forum on Health (1997) recommends a better balance between short-term economic needs and long-term health care needs of Canadians. This recommendation points to the importance of supportive programs and policies in health and health-related sectors (e.g., education, recreation, social services). The potential of children with chronic illness for meaningful and productive lives could be realized through sustainable, publicly funded programs of support that enhance coping, self-care, and capacity for independent living.

Acknowledgments

The assessment study reported in this chapter was funded by the IWK Grace Health Centre for Women, Children and Families.

Note

The assessment study is reported in Ellerton, Stewart, Ritchie, & Hirth (1996).

References

Appleton, P.L., Minchom, P.E., Ellis, N.C., Elliott, C.E., Ball, V., & Jones, P. (1994). The self-concept of young people with Spina Bifida: A population-based study. *Developmental Medicine and Child Neurology, 36*, 298–215.

Asher, S.R., Hymel, S., & Renshaw, P.D. (1984). Loneliness in children. *Child Development, 55*, 1456–1464.

Barnett., K, Darcie, G., Holland, C., & Kobasigawasa, A. (1982). Children's cognitions about effective helping. *Developmental Psychology, 18*, 267–277.

Baum, F., & Forehand, R. (1984). Social factors associated with adolescent obesity. *Journal of Pediatric Psychology, 9*, 293–302.

Belle, D. (1989). *Children's social networks and social supports.* New York: Wiley.

Belle, D., & Longfellow, C. (1983). Emotional support and children's well-being: An exploratory study of children's confidants. Paper presented at the biennial meeting of the Society for Research in Child Development, Detroit.

Belle, D., Dill, D., & Burr, R. (1991). Children's network orientations. *Journal of Community Psychology, 19,* 362–371.

Bolig, R., & Weddle, K. (1988). Resiliency and hospitalization of children. *Children's Health Care, 16,* 255–260.

Bradley, D.L. (1994). Moving into the mainstream. *Educational Forum, 59,* 81–91.

Breitmayer, B., Gallo, A., Knafl, K., & Zoeller, L. (1992). Social competence of school-aged children with chronic illness. *Journal of Pediatric Nursing, 71,* 181–187.

Breslau, N. (1985). Psychiatric disorder in children with physical disabilities. *Journal of the American Academy of Child Psychiatry, 24,* 87–94.

Brown , R.T., Doepke, K.J., & Kaslow, N.J. (1993). Risk-resistance-adaptation model for paediatric chronic illness: Sickle cell syndrome as an example. *Clinical Psychology Review, 13,* 119–132.

Bryant, B. (1985). The neighborhood walk: A study of sources of support in middle childhood from the child's perspective. *Monographs of the Society for Research in Child Development, (Serial No. 210), 50*(3)1–22.

Bryant, B. (1994). How does social support during childhood? In F. Nestmann & K. Hurrelmann (Eds), *Social networks and social support in childhood and adolescence* (23–35). Berlin: Walter de Gruyter.

Bull, B.A., & Drotar, R. (1991). Coping with cancer in remission: Stressors and strategies reported by children and adolescents. *Journal of Pediatric Psychology, 16,* 767–782.

Cadman, D., Boyle, M., Szatmari, P., & Offord, D.R. (1987). Chronic illness, disability, and mental and social well-being: Findings of the Ontario Child Health Study. *Pediatrics, 79,* 805–813.

Canadian Institute of Child Health (1994). *The health of Canada's children.* Ottawa: CICH.

Caplan, M., Weissberg, R., Grober, J.S., Sivo, P.J., Grady, K., & Jacoby, C. (1992). Social competence promotion with inner-city suburban young adolescents. Effects on social adjustment and alcohol use. *Journal of Consulting and Clinical Psychology, 60*(1), 56–63.

Cauce, A.M. (1986). Social networks and social competence: Exploring the effects of early adolescent friendships. *American Journal of Community Psychology, 14,* 607–628.

Cauce, A.M., Reid, M, Landesman, S., & Gonzales, N. (1990). Social support in young children: Management, structure, and behavioral impact. In B.R. Sarason,

I.G. Sarason, & G.R. Pierce (Eds), *Social support: An interactional view* (64–95). New York: Wiley.

Causey, D.L., & Dubow, E. (1992). Development of a self-report coping measure for elementary school children. *Journal of Clinical Child Psychology, 21*, 47–59.

Chiang, D. (1994). Navigate the net: Enabling the disadvantaged. *Medical References Quarterly, 13*, 69–74.

Compas, B.E., Malcarne, V.L., & Fondacara, K.M. (1988). Coping with stressful events in older children and young adolescents. *Journal of Consulting and Clinical Psychology, 56*, 405–411.

Compas, B.E., Slavin, L.A., Wagner, B.M., & Vannatta, K. (1986). Relationship of life events and social support with psychological dysfunction among adolescents. *Journal of Youth and Adolescence, 15*, 205–221.

Cowen, E.L., Pederson, A., Babigian, H., Izzo, L.D., & Trost, M.D. (1973). Long-term follow-up of early detected vulnerable children. *Journal of Consulting and Clinical Psychology, 41*, 438–446.

Cutrona, C. (1990). Stress and social support: In search of optimal matching. *Journal of Social and Clinical Psychology, 9*, 3–14.

Dakof, G.A., & Taylor, S.E. (1990). Victims' perceptions of social support: What is helpful from whom? *Journal of Personality and Social Psychology, 58*, 80–89.

Drotar, D. (1981). Psychological perspectives in chronic illness. *Journal of Pediatric Psychology, 6*, 211–228.

Drotar, D., & Bush, M. (1985). Mental health issues and services. In N. Hobbs & J.M. Perrin (Eds), *Issues in the care of children with chronic illness* (514–550). San Francisco: Jossey-Bass.

Dunham, P.J., Hurshman, A., Litwin, E., Gusella, J., Ellsworth, C., & Dodd, P. (1998). Computer mediated social support: Single young mothers as a model system. *American Journal of Community Psychology, 26,* 281–306.

Dunkel-Schetter, C., & Skokan, L. (1990). Determinants of social support provision in personal relationships. *Journal of Social and Personal Relationships, 7*, 437–450.

Edwards-Beckett, J., & Cedargren, D. (1995). The sociocultural context of families with a child with myelomeningocele. *Issues in Comprehensive Pediatric Nursing, 18*, 27–42.

Ellerton, M., Stewart, M., Ritchie, J., & Hirth, A. (1996). Social support in children with a chronic condition. *Canadian Journal of Nursing Research, 28*(4), 15–36.

Felner, R.D., & Adams, A.M. (1988). The school transition environment project: An ecological intervention and evaluation. In R.H. Price, E.L. Cowen, R.P. Lorion, & J. Ramos-McKay (Eds) *14 ounces of prevention: A casebook for practitioners.* (111–122). Washington, DC: American Psychological Association.

Ford, C., & Procidano, M. (1983). The relationship of self-actualization to social support, life stress, and adjustment. *Social Behavior and Personality, 18*, 41–51.

Fuhrman, W., & Buhrmester, D. (1985). Children's perceptions of the personal relationships in their social networks. *Developmental Psychology, 21*, 1016–1024.

Fullmer, S.L. & Walls, R.T. (1994). Interests and participation on disability-related computer bulletin boards. *Journal of Rehabilitation, 60*, 24–30.

Garmezy, N. (1991). Resiliency and vulnerability to adverse developmental outcomes associated with poverty. *American Behavioral Scientist, 34*, 416–430.

Garner, J.B., & Campbell, P.H. (1987). Technology for persons with severe disabilities: Practical and ethical considerations. *Journal of Special Education, 21*, 122–132.

Giangreco, M.F., Dennis, C., Cloninger, C., Edelman, S., & Schattman, R. (1993). I have counted John: Transformational experiences of teachers educating students with disabilities. *Exceptional Children, 59*, 359–372.

Gortmaker, S., Walker, D., Weitzman, M., & Sobol, A. (1990). Chronic conditions, socioeconomic risks, and behavioural problems in children and adolescents. *Pediatrics, 85*, 267–276.

Graetz, B., & Shute, R. (1995). Assessment of peer relationships in children with asthma. *Journal of Pediatric Psychology, 20*, 205–216.

Gravelle, A.M. (1997). Caring for a child with a progressive illness during the complex chronic phase: Parents' experience of facing adversity. *Journal of Advanced Nursing, 25*, 738–745.

Hassett, M., Lowder, & Rutan, D. (1992). Use of computer network bulletin board systems by disabled persons. *Proceedings – Annual Symposium on Computer Applications in Medical Care*, 151–155.

Hetherington, E.M., & Clingempeel, W.G., Anderson, E.R., Deal, J.E., Hagan, M.S., Hollier. E.A., & Lindner, M.S. (1992). Coping with marital transitions. *Monographs of the Society for Research in Child Development, 57*, (Serial No. 227), *59*(2–3), 1–242.

Holder-Brown, L., & Parette, H. (1992). Children with disabilities who use assistive technology: Ethical considerations. *Young Children, 47*, 73–77.

Hurtig, A.L., & White, L.S. (1986). Psychosocial adjustment in children and adolescents with sickle disease. *Journal of Pediatric Psychology, 11*, 411–427.

Jacobson, A.M., Hauser, S.T., Wertlieb, D., Wolfsdorf, J.I., Orleans, J., & Vieryra, M. (1986). Psychological adjustment of children with recently diagnosed diabetes mellitus. *Diabetes Care, 9*, 323–329.

Kaplan, H.B., Robbins, C., & Martin, S.S. (1983). Antecedents of psychological distress in young adults: Self-rejection, deprivation of social support, and life events. *Journal of Health and Social Behavior, 24*, 230–244.

King, G.A., Schultz, I.Z., Steel, K., Gilpin, M., & Cathers, T. (1993). Self-evaluation and self-concept of adolescents with physical disabilities. *American Journal of Occupational Therapy, 47*, 132–140.

Krappmann, L. (1992). On the social embedding of learning processes in the classroom. In R. Osler, T. Dick, & J.L. Patry (Eds), *Effective and responsible teaching* (173–186). San Francisco: Jossey-Bass.

La Greca, A. (1990). Social consequences of pediatric conditions: Fertile area for future investigation and intervention? *Journal of Pediatric Psychology, 15*, 285–307.

La Greca, A.M., & Hanna, N. (1983). Diabetes related health beliefs in children and their mothers: Implications for treatment. *Diabetes, 32* (Suppl. 1), 66.

Lefebvre, A. (1992). Ability-Online: Promoting social competence and computer literacy in adolescents with disabilities. *Rehabilitation Digest, 23*, 3–6.

Lefebvre, A., & McClure, M. (1996). Ability Online: Children in hospital now in touch with the world. *Leadership, 4*, 26–29.

Lord, J., & Hutchison, P. (1996). Living with a disability in Canada: Toward autonomy and integration. Position Paper No. 30 for the National Forum on Health.

Lyons, R. (1989). The effects of acquired illness and disability on friendships. In W.H. Jones & D. Perlman (Eds), *Advances in personal relationships*. Greenwich, CT: JAI Press.

MacLean, W.E., Perrin, J.M., Gortmaker, S., & Pierre, C.B. (1992). Psychological adjustment of children with asthma: Effects of illness severity and recent stressful life events. *Journal of Pediatric Psychology, 17*, 159–172.

Madara, E.J. (1992). Computerized self-help: The evolving communication. *Social Policy*, Fall-Winter, 32.

Madara, E.J., & White, B.J. (1997). On-line mutual support: The experience of a self-help clearinghouse. *Journal of the Alliance of Information and Referral Systems, 19*, 91–107.

Magyary, D., & Brandt, P. (1996), A school-based self-management program for youth with chronic health conditions and their parents. *Canadian Journal of Nursing Research, 28*(4), 57–77.

Melzer, S., S.M., Leadbeater, B., Reisman, L., Jaffe, L.R., & Lieberman, K.V. (1989). Characteristics of social networks in adolescents with end-stage renal disease treated with renal transplantation. *Journal of Adolescent Health Care, 10*, 308–312.

Meng, A. (1997). An asthma day camp. *American Journal of Maternal Child Nursing, 22*(3), 135–141.

Nassau, J.J., & Drotar, D. (1995). Social competence in children with IDDM and asthma: Child, teacher, and parent reports of children's social adjustment, social performance, and social skills. *Journal of Pediatric Psychology, 20*, 187–204.

National Forum on Health (1997). *Final Report*. Ottawa: Minister of Public Works and Government Services.

Nelson-Le Gall, S., & Gumerman, R. (1984). Children's perceptions of helpers and helper motivation. *Journal of Applied Developmental Psychology, 5*, 1–12.

Noll, R.B., Bukowski, W.M., Rogosch, F.A., LeRoy, S., & Kulkarni, R. (1990). Social interactions between children and their peers: Teacher ratings. *World Pediatric Psychology, 15*, 43–56.

Patterson, J.M., & Geber, G. (1991). Preventing mental health problems in children with chronic illness or disability. *Children's Health Care, 20*, 150–161.

Pearlin, L.J. (1989). The sociological study of stress. *Journal of Health and Social Behavior, 30*, 241–256.

Perrin, E.C., Ayoub, C.C., & Willett, J.B. (1993). In the eyes of the beholder: Family and maternal influences on perceptions of adjustment of children with chronic illness. *Developmental and Behavioral Pediatrics, 14*, 94–104.

Perrin, J.M., Stein, R.E.K., Walker, D.K., & Weitzman, M. (1993). Observations based on research about children with a chronic illness. *Journal of Pediatric Psychology, 16*, 411–421.

Pflederer, D. (1990). Using friends as a social support system for children. In M.J. Craft & J.A. Denehy (Eds), *Nursing interventions for infants and children*. Philadelphia: W.B. Saunders.

Pless, I.B. (1984). Clinical assessment: Physical and psychological functioning. *Pediatric Clinics of North America, 31*, 33–45.

Pless, I.B., & Pinkerton, P. (1975). *Chronic childhood disorder: Promoting patterns of adjustment*. London: H.O Klimpton.

Reid, M., Landesman, S., Treder, R., & Jaccard, J. (1989). My family and friends: Six-to twelve-year old children's perceptions of social support. *Child Development, 60*, 896–910.

Rook, K. (1990). Parallels in the study of social support and social strain. *Journal of Social and Clinical Psychology, 56*, 1266–1278.

Ross, D., & Ross, S. (1984). Teaching the child with leukemia to cope with teasing. *Issues in Comprehensive Nursing, 11*, 59–66.

Satterwhite, B. (1978). Impact of chronic illness on child and family: An interview based on five surveys. *International Journal of Rehabilitation Research, 1*, 7–15.

Simmons, R.J., Corey, M., Cowen, L., Keenan, N., Robertson, J., & Levinson, H. (1985). Emotional adjustment of early adolescents with cystic fibrosis. *Psychosomatic Medicine, 47*, 111–122.

Statistics Canada (1991). *The health and activity limitation survey (HALS)*. Ottawa: Statistics Canada.

Stein, R.E., & Jessop, D.L. (1984). Does pediatric home care make a difference for children with chronic illness: Findings from the pediatric ambulatory care treatment study. *Pediatrics, 73*, 845–853.

Stewart, M. (1993). *Integrating social support in nursing*. Newbury Park, CA: Sage.

Taylor, S. (1988). Caught in the continuum: A critical analysis of the principle of the least restrictive environment. *TASH, 13*, 41–53.

Thoits, P.A. (1985). Conceptual, methodological and theoretical problems in studying social support as a buffer against life stress. *Journal of Health and Social Behavior, 23*, 145–159.

Varni, J.W., Setoguchi, Y., Rappaport, L.R., & Talbot, D. (1992). Psychological adjustment and perceived social support in children with congenital/acquired limb deficiencies. *Journal of Behavioral Medicine, 15*, 31–44.

Walker, L.S., & Greene, J.W. (1987). Negative life events, psychological resources, and psychophysiological symptoms in adolescents. *Journal of Clinical Child Psychology, 16*, 29–36.

Wallander, J.L., & Thompson, R.J. (1995). Psychosocial adjustment of children with chronic physical conditions. In M.C. Roberts (Ed.), *Handbook of pediatric psychology* (2nd ed.) (124–141). New York: Guilford Press.

Wallander, J.L., & Varni, J.W. (1989). Social support and adjustment in chronically ill and handicapped children. *American Journal of Community Psychology, 17*, 185–201.

Wallander, J.,Varni, J., Babani, L., Banis, H., & Wilcox, K. (1988). Children with chronic physical disorders: Maternal reports of their psychological adjustment. *Journal of Pediatric Psychology, 3*, 197–212.

Weiss, R. (1974). The provisions of social relationships. In N.Z. Rubin (Ed.), *Doing unto others* (17–26). Englewood Cliffs, NJ: Prentice-Hall.

Wolchik, S.A., Beals, J., & Sandler, I.N. (1989). Mapping children's support networks. In D. Belle (Ed.), *Children's social networks and social supports* (191–220). New York: Wiley.

Wolchik, S.A., Sandler, I.N., & Braver, S.L. (1987a). Social support : Its assessment and relation to children's adjustment. In N. Eisenberg (Ed.), *Contemporary topics in developmental psychology*. New York: Wiley.

Wolchik, S.A., Sandler, I.N., & Braver, S.L. (1987b). *Children's Inventory of Social Support*. Tempe: Arizona State University.

Zelkowitz, P. (1981). Children's support networks: Their role in families under stress. Paper presented at the biennial meeting of the Society for Research in Child Development, Boston.

3

Parents of Children with a Chronic Condition: Fostering a Sense of Competence through Telephone Support Groups

Judith A. Ritchie, Miriam J. Stewart, Donna Thompson, Mary-Lou Ellerton, Michael Sullivan, and Sonia Salisbury

Abstract. Many families are dealing with a child or adolescent with some type of chronic condition. These parents experience wide-ranging demands and an increased risk of health problems. Social support serves as a protective resource and may help to moderate the health effects of stressful situations associated with caregiving. There is limited information about the social support that parents receive in relation to specific caregiving demands, however, and there have been few investigations of the impact of an intervention to enhance social support for parents. In this chapter we describe two studies: an initial assessment study that examined the caregiving demands and related social support that mothers experience in caring for their children with chronic conditions, and a follow-up intervention study that tested the impact of a twelve-week telephone support intervention for parents in a randomized control trial. The mothers of children with diabetes, cystic fibrosis, or spina bifida (n = 90) in the assessment study described a wide range of primary and secondary caregiving demands and support deficiencies related to each demand. Based on their expressed support needs and their desire for a peer support intervention and for partner support, we designed telephone support groups open to mothers (n = 103) and fathers (n = 11). The parents' responses on a series of questionnaires over nine months showed that the intervention effected some small improvements in quantitative measures of parents' perceptions of support satisfaction, resistance and susceptibility to illness, valuing and comfort aspects of parenting competence, and ego strength in their children. In qualitative data from weekly diaries and interviews over the six months following the intervention, the participants reported increased social support, enhanced coping, increased confidence, and changes in perspectives and in their behaviours in health care encounters. The vast majority were satisfied with the telephone support group experience.

Introduction

Although the rates of chronicity in childhood are lower than in any other age group, many families are dealing with a child or adolescent with some type of chronic condition (Hoffman, Rice & Sung, 1996). Differences in definitions and classifications of chronic conditions and in research methods lead to huge discrepancies in the reported rates of chronic illness (Jessop & Stein, 1995). As described in chapter 2, above, the Canadian Institute of Child Health reported that the prevalence of chronic conditions in children under twenty years of age is 7 per cent (Canadian Institute of Child Health, 1994). Earlier estimates from the Ontario Child Health Survey indicated that the provincial rate of childhood chronic conditions was 19.6 per cent (Cadman, Boyle, Offord, Szatmari, Rae Grant, Crawford, & Byles, 1986). In the United States, it is estimated that 31 per cent of children under eighteen years have one or more chronic conditions (Newacheck & Taylor, 1992). Although few children (5 per cent) have more than one chronic condition, in such circumstances there is dramatic impact on overall health indicators, such as emotional or behavioural problems, school absences, bed days, limitation in activity, use of health care services, and perceived poor or fair health (Newacheck & Stoddard, 1994).

While both parents share the emotional impact and demands of the child's condition, the impact of caregiving is greatest for mothers (Anderson & Elfert, 1989; Kazak & Marvin, 1984). There is evidence that these mothers are at increased risk for mental and physical health problems (Florian & Krulik, 1991; Miller, Gordon, Daniels & Diller, 1992; Quittner, DiGirolamo, Michel & Eigen, 1992). Hahn and Schone (1996) found that, while having a child with a chronic condition significantly increased mothers' psychological distress, mothers whose children had three or more acute conditions had even greater distress. They concluded that this was because of their inability to establish a routine, as mothers with children who have a chronic illness can. A recent meta-analysis of seventeen studies revealed that parents of children with disabilities experience social-psychological problems at twice the rate (30 per cent versus 15 per cent) of parents whose children do not have a disability (Singer & Yovanoff, cited in Patterson & Blum, 1996). Patterson and Blum attributed these problems to the 'increased set of long-term demands that are experienced by children with disabilities and their families' (693).

Some authors (e.g., Loebig, 1990) have pointed out both benefits and burdens of caring for children with demands related to their chronic condition. There is considerable discrepancy in the consistency with which researchers have described the burdens, however, and overall the full scope of demands or support pertaining to these demands has not been well documented.

Demands of Parenting Children with Chronic Conditions

Most researchers have focused on only a few types of caregiver burden, particularly those primary demands related to the care of children with chronic illness. These primary demands include the child's physical care or concerns about the child's physical condition, vigilance and monitoring of the child's day-to-day needs, and arranging and negotiating the health care encounters and illness episodes associated with the child's condition (Barbarin & Chesler, 1986; Burke, Kauffmann, Costello, Handley-Derry & Dillon, 1991; Ray & Ritchie, 1993; Thompson, Gustafson, Hamlett & Spock, 1992; Valentine, 1993). Only a few researchers (Burkhart, 1993; Cant, 1994; Loebig, 1990) have described primary demands related to the assistance the child may require in psychological, academic, and social adjustment.

The multiple secondary impacts of the child's condition on the child's family or the parent tend to be described in isolation in different studies. Several researchers have documented the considerable impact of childhood chronic illness on family dynamics or functioning (Drotar, Crawford, & Bush, 1984; Loebig, 1990; Quittner et al., 1992; Tomlinson & Mitchell, 1992; Williams, Lorenzo, & Borja, 1993). Others have reported the negative impact on maternal roles and socio-emotional burdens (Burkhart, 1993; Gottlieb & Wagner, 1991; Jessop & Stein, 1985; Stroller & Pugliese, 1989; Williams et al., 1993). Others (including LePontis, Moel, & Cohn, 1987; Williams et al., 1993) also have described the detrimental impact on maternal and family social roles.

There has been little documentation of the impact that having a child with a chronic condition has on the mother's attention to her own personal needs. Two groups of researchers, however, have found that maternal perceptions of burden are important predictors of psychological symptoms (Canning, Harris, & Kelleher, 1996; Jessop, Riessman, & Stein, 1988).

There is evidence that the demands that caregivers face may be mitigated by the type of support that they receive. For instance, in a study with mothers of children with cystic fibrosis ($n = 78$), good adjustment was associated with particular ways of coping and the family context, including family supportiveness (Thompson et al., 1992).

Social Support for Parents of Children with Chronic Conditions

Caregivers' needs for support have not been studied in depth. Researchers have concluded, however, that social support contributes positively to outcomes such as the child's behaviour (Hamlett, Pellegrini & Katz, 1992), management of the child's illness (Gibson, 1986), maternal satisfaction (Fagan & Schor, 1993), ability to manage other family responsibilities (Miller &

Diao, 1987), and parenting stress (Beckman, 1991). Hadadian (1994), in a study of thirty families (fifteen with children with special needs and fifteen whose children had no known handicapping condition), found that families with lower receipt of support from friends experienced higher stress.

Some parental coping strategies are dependent on interactions with family members, friends, health professionals, and other associates. Several researchers (e.g., Damrosh & Perry, 1989; Gibson, 1986; Ray & Ritchie, 1993) have reported patterns of support seeking, such as mothers seeking information, confiding in others, and seeking guidance, as well as attempts to maintain social support.

Despite parents' attempts to seek social support, their support networks and the availability of support within those networks are often inadequate. Parents may experience smaller or less available social networks (Cant, 1994; Kazak, 1989), or increasing strain in relationships with friends, neighbours, and relatives. While Valentine (1993) found that some families of children with developmental disabilities (n = 25) had a wide variety of important sources of support, parents in other studies have reported variation in the quality of support received from spouses and health professionals (e.g., Bailey, Blasco, & Simeonsson, 1992; Elliott, 1991; Fagan & Schor, 1993; Havermans & Eiser, 1991). A more recent study with mothers and fathers reveals that family members are the most common source of emotional and instrumental support, while health care providers are the usual source of informational support (Garwick, Patterson, Bennett, & Blum, 1998). Many of these parents, however, reported receiving some unhelpful support from family members and health care providers (Patterson, Garwick, Bennett, & Blum, 1998). Although spouses are a primary source of expected support (Konstantareas & Homatadis, 1989; VanCleve,1989), Gottlieb and Wagner (1991) found that parents of children with cystic fibrosis and diabetes had conflicts in their ways of coping that prevented them from gaining support from one another. Mothers of children with cystic fibrosis reported decreasing spousal support over time (Barbarin, Hughes, & Chesler, 1985), spouses' lack of helpfulness with child care, and spouses' absence (Quittner et al., 1992). Given this pattern of smaller or inadequate social networks, it is not surprising that mothers have reported wanting more support than they receive (Quittner, Glueckauf, & Jackson, 1990). Pelletier, Godin, Lepage, and Dussault (1994) concluded, from a survey of 213 mothers of children with asthma or juvenile diabetes, that mothers' levels of support were inadequate to meet their needs, and gaps were evident in emotional, affirmational, and informational support.

There is little research that identifies the specific gaps in support for mothers of children with chronic conditions. The needs for, use of, and appraisal of support received pertaining to particular burden domains have not been well investigated. Therefore, in the initial assessment study in this series of studies with families and their children with chronic conditions we investigated the demands and related social support that mothers receive in caring for their children who have chronic conditions.

Although there is evidence that social support serves as a protective resource and may help to moderate the health impact of stressful situations (Bloom, 1990; House, Umberson, & Landis, 1988) such as caregiving, there have been very few investigations of the impact of interventions designed to enhance social support available to parents. To illustrate, Hansell, Hughes, Caliandro, Russo, Budin, Hartman, and Hernandez (1998) attempted to 'boost' support for caregivers of children with HIV/AIDS by providing nursing visits once per month. They reported that there were improved levels of support for seronegative caregivers (foster parents and extended family members) but not for seropositive caregivers (parents). Two research teams have described important elements of dyadic peer support for parents of children who have chronic conditions. Although Ainbinder, Blanchard, Singer, Sullivan, Powers, Marquis, & Santelli (1998) did not report the effect of the intervention, they described the critical element for successful matches as the creation of a 'reliable ally,' characterized by comparability between partners in the dyad and mutuality of support. A small trial linking five 'mentors' (mothers whose children with juvenile rheumatoid arthritis were older) with five mothers of young children revealed tentative positive effects on maternal mental health and support (Ireys, Sills, Kolodner, & Walsh, 1996). However, we have found no careful evaluations of peer support groups. Peer support is typically encompassed in group-level interventions that either optimize support rendered by the existing network or graft on a set of new ties for target populations at risk due to social isolation, losses from the social network (Gottlieb, 1988), or deterioration of support in chronic stressful situations (Gottlieb, 1992). The support offered in groups composed of peers is based on experiential knowledge and is more specialized, therefore, than the general support provided by family and friends (Katz, 1993). In the intervention study, telephone support groups were designed to provide a network of peers that would enhance and supplement the limited natural networks of parents of children with chronic conditions.

Fit with Framework

These assessment and intervention studies were based on the framework (figure 3.1) that holds that social support, conveyed in personal relationships (Lyons, Sullivan, & Ritvo, 1995), influences adaptation to stressful situa-

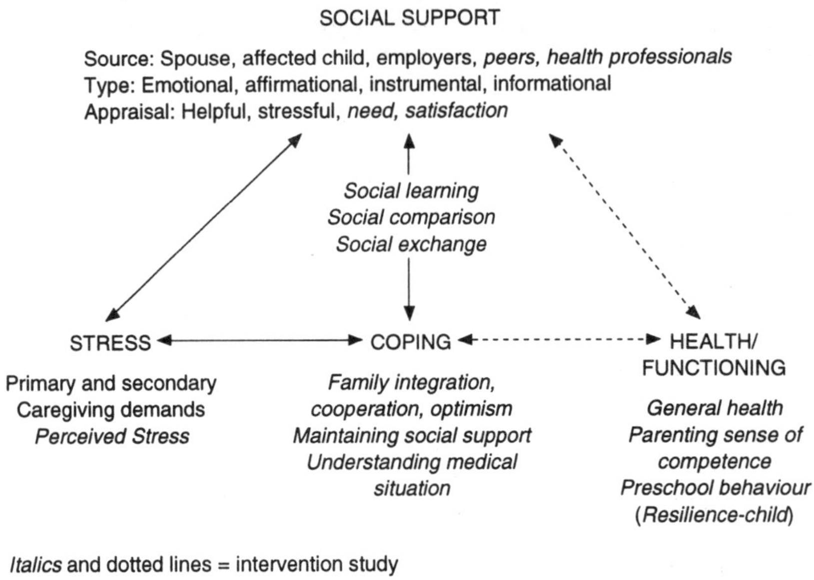

Figure 3.1 Framework for Assessment and Intervention Studies Involving Parents of Children with Chronic Conditions

tions; supportive persons can alter appraisal of stressors, sustain coping efforts, and influence the choice of coping strategies (Stewart, 1989). Social support was conceptualized as a coping resource or coping assistance (Folkman, Chesney, McKusick, Ironson, Johnson, & Coates, 1991; Thoits, 1986) with the stressful situations or demands associated with childhood chronic conditions and with caregiving. Both social support and coping moderate the effect of these stressful situations on the children's and parents' health and functioning outcomes.

The two-way arrow between support and coping indicates that they have bidirectional effects (Gottlieb & Wagner, 1991). The ways children or their parents cope provide clues to potential supporters about whether and what kind of support is needed (Silver, Wortman, & Crofton, 1990). For example, Gottlieb and Wagner (1991) found that conflicting parental coping behaviours preclude spousal support for mothers of children with chronic illness. The amount and type of support received could influence parents' choice of coping strategies.

Similarly, support and stress have bidirectional effects, as indicated by the arrow from stress to support. Appropriate support can result in lower stressful appraisals. Conversely, conflicted interactions, miscarried helping, and inadequate support can increase the stressfulness of the situation. Indeed, the costs of providing support include overinvolvement and burden for providers – in this case, parents (Albrecht & Adelman, 1987; Coyne, Wortman, & Lehman, 1988; Fisher, Goff, Nadler, & Chinsky, 1988; LaGaipa, 1990).

Social support is an important protective factor in the resilience process (Egeland, Carlson, & Sroufe, 1993; Fine, 1991; Garmezy, 1993). Social support shores up coping, esteem, and competence (Gottlieb, 1988). Social support has been described in relation to resilience in hospitalized children (Bolig & Weddle, 1988; Rodin, Striegel-Moore, & Silberstein, 1990), children with chronic illness, and families coping with illness (McCubbin & McCubbin, 1993). Bronfenbrenner (1986) points to the urgency of providing families with support to establish relationships and environments that foster resilience in children. The intervention study was focused on the resilience of parents of a child with a chronic condition, which in turn should affect the resilience of their children. Parental health and competence have been linked to their children's resilience (Alpern & Lyons-Ruth, 1993; Egeland et al., 1993; Garmezy, 1993; Werner, 1993).

We expected that during the telephone intervention the parents of children with chronic conditions in support groups would engage in three mediating processes: social comparison, social exchange, and social learning. In the process of social comparison with peers, parents could validate and normalize their experiences with their children, their children's health professionals, and their social networks (Gottlieb, 1988; 1992). Support groups are characterized by bidirectional exchanges (Antonucci & Jackson, 1990; Maton, 1987) and emphasize reciprocity and mutuality among equals (Gottlieb, 1992). Finally, social learning enhances the acquisition of new knowledge (e.g., new approaches to managing diabetes, strategies for coping with integration of children with cognitive or physical disabilities into the classroom, sources of support), since parents identify with peers who have shared a similar experience (Borkman, 1990).

Assessment Study: Caregiving Demands and Related Support

Almost all studies of demands related to caregiving for children with chronic conditions or the social support that parents received have been limited either in focus or in method. Most did not consider primary demands related to the child's cognitive, psychological, and/or social development, or secondary demands related to the impact on the primary caregiver or the family. Studies of social support in this population have not elucidated how support varies in relation to specific demands of caregiving. Many studies involved small sample sizes and insufficient attention was paid to issues of reliability and validity. Therefore, the assessment study pursued the following questions:

1. What are the primary and secondary demands that mothers face in caring for a child with a chronic condition?
2. What are the sources, types, and appropriateness of support that mothers receive in relation to specific types of caregiving demands?

Sample

Ninety mothers of children from three illness groups participated in the assessment study; there were equal numbers of children from each diagnostic group (diabetes, cystic fibrosis, or spina bifida). The children ranged in age from one to seventeen years. The children with diabetes were significantly older (M = 12 years) and had been diagnosed more recently (M = 5 years since diagnosis). The vast majority of mothers (85 per cent) were either married or cohabiting, and 67 per cent were employed at least part time outside the home.

Method

During an interview in their homes, the mothers described their current caregiving experience on a typical day, a recent acute illness experience, and the impact of the child's care and functional capacity on their own activities and those of the family. The investigators developed the interview guide for this study. As the mothers presented their stories, the interviewers probed to determine who in the mother's social network was involved in the situation, what they did, and whether those behaviours were helpful in managing each situation that was described. The interviewers elicited the mothers' appraisals of positive and negative interactions with their spouses/partners, family members, friends, and health professionals. The interviews averaged one hour in duration.

The interviewers were briefed on the research aims and design and received eight hours of specific training using interview simulation strategies. During the data collection period, the interviewers met routinely with members of the investigative team, and the investigators reviewed the interview transcripts at regular intervals to ensure maintenance of the interview standards.

The interview transcripts were subjected to content analysis using a category system that included types of caregiving demands, and types, sources, and appraisal of social support. The category system was based initially on

TABLE 3.1
Research Design

	Assessment Study	Intervention Study
Sample	Purposive Mothers of children with chronic conditions ($n = 90$)	Randomized Parents of children with chronic conditions ($n = 114$)
Design	Descriptive	Randomized Control Trial
Measures/instruments		
Stress	Interview Guide	*Perceived Stress Scale*
Coping	–	*Coping Health Inventory for Parents*
Social Support	Interview Guide	*Arizona Social Support Interview Schedule*
Health/Functioning	–	*Parenting Sense of Competence* *General Health Rating Index* *Preschool Child Behaviour Questionnaire*
Data Collection	One time only	Pre-test, post-test, delayed post-test (3 and 6 months)
Data Analysis		
Qualitative	Thematic content analysis of interviews	Thematic content analysis of interviews, participant diaries and facilitators' field notes
Quantitative		Repeated measures ANOVA

the full range of demands presented in the literature on caregiving and on social support and was revised later to ensure that it included all the information provided by the mothers. The coders achieved and maintained 80 per cent inter-rater and intra-rater reliability in designating units of analysis and coding of units. Once coded, the data were analysed using Ethnograph (Seidl, Kjolseth, & Seymour, 1988). The research design is summarized in table 3.1.

Key Findings

The mothers described a very wide range of both primary and secondary demands of caregiving. For the most part, the mothers characterized the child's care and family activities as routine. This picture of 'routineness' is consistent with the family management styles that Knafl, Breitmayer, Gallo, and Zoeller (1996) classify as 'thriving' and 'accommodating' and with Hahn and Schone's conclusions that 'mothers of children with disabilities know what to expect and can establish a routine' (1996, 70). These mothers clarified, however, that any unexpected event, including an illness event, resulted in rapid change to a state of chaos. Despite the mothers' perspectives of the 'routine' nature of caring for their child, related demands on mothers and their family life were pervasive.

All mothers reported primary demands of caregiving. These included physical care or concerns about the child's physical care or condition (100 per cent), negotiating health care encounters or illness episodes (92 per cent), fostering the child's psychological development and adjustment (89 per cent), and enabling the child's social development and participation in social activities (82 per cent). Fewer mothers discussed secondary demands that affected their own roles or those of the family. Nearly 95 per cent identified impacts on their ability to meet their own personal needs, and 90 per cent recounted the effect on family activity and roles. In contrast, only 50 per cent described any impact on their relationship with their partner or on their family's financial situation.

Although mothers' stories revealed the full range of types of social support and a wide range of people or organizations from whom support could be expected, the analysis of types, sources, and appraisal of social support in relation to specific demands revealed significant gaps. The most consistent type of support for primary demands was instrumental support (e.g., caring for the ill child) provided by the spouse/partner or family members. Less than 60 per cent of the mothers, however, described such support. Less than 35 per cent identified any specific type or source of helpful support in relation to health care situations or illness episodes or the child's psychological and/or cognitive development. In relation to the secondary demands of caring for a child with a chronic condition, the most consistent support was emotional support, in the form of their partners' listening (41.4 per cent). Only one-third of the mothers indicated that health professionals provided informational support related to the child's physical care or condition during the illness situation.

In addition to these deficiencies and gaps in available support, the mothers also described 'stressful support' from virtually all of their potential supporters. Most frequently the support was described as stressful because it was absent. A cross-tabulation of the types, sources, and appraisals of support in relation to specific types of demands revealed a pattern of low levels of helpful support and explicit appraisals of stressful support. For instance, 28 per cent of the mothers characterized their partners' lack of involvement in caring for the affected child as stressful. Their responses were similar both to Quittner et al.'s (1992) account of maternal distress due to lack of spousal helpfulness or spousal absence and to patterns of conflicting spousal coping observed by Gottlieb and Wagner (1991). In some instances, the mothers reported stressful support from health professionals, who either did not provide adequate care for the child when ill (13 per cent) or gave inadequate information (14 per cent). Mothers expressed concern about the lack of appropriate support from family members (13 per cent) and babysitters (21 per cent) for engaging in activities outside the home.

Overall, the mothers seemed to manage the demands related to having a child with a chronic condition in considerable isolation. They led extremely busy lives and experienced major gaps in their social networks. Fewer than 20 per cent described any support in relation to half of the demands faced. The range of caregiving demands and the inadequacy of support in relation to those demands could be major factors in negative health outcomes for parents of children with chronic conditions. Support interventions that bridge these gaps are needed. While a support group intervention of some type seemed appropriate, the challenge was to design an intervention that would be accessible and useful.

Key Findings from the Assessment Study

- The bidirectional relationship between stressful situations and social support affirmed.
- There is a direct relationship between coping responses and social support.
- Daily life is a busy 'routine' that rapidly changes to chaos with illness or other unexpected event.
- More than 80 per cent experienced all primary demands of caregiving; at least 50 per cent experienced all secondary demands of caregiving.
- There are significant gaps in support:
  - < 60 per cent described instrumental support (physical care of the child) from partners or family members
  - < 35 per cent described any type of support in relation to health care
  - 28 per cent described stressful (absent) instrumental support from partners in relation to caregiving.
- Stressful support from partners and professionals in particular was reported.
- The major need for support is at the time of diagnosis and during transitions.
- Peer support groups are preferred as support intervention.

Intervention Study: Telephone Support Intervention for Parents of Young Children

Most reports of social support interventions for parents of children with chronic conditions are descriptive and anecdotal. The impact of interventions on health outcomes is rarely tested. Telephone support interventions have been used with adults dealing with other types of stressful situations; they are particularly advantageous for caregivers whose participation in face-to-face groups would be hampered by distance or multiple demands on their time. However, this type of support intervention had not been tested with parents of children with chronic conditions. During the interviews in the assessment study, the mothers told us that their needs for support were paramount during the early years after diagnosis and at the time of major transitions such as school entry. Furthermore, the mothers contended that they were most interested in a peer support group. Therefore, we focused this intervention study on a peer support group strategy for parents whose children were seven years of age or younger. We hypothesized that parents in the intervention group would have lower perceived stress and greater gains in their perceived competence, psychological health, satisfaction with support, coping strategies, and in perceived child behaviour.

Intervention

A total of 114 parents from 104 families participated in the study and were randomly assigned to the intervention or control group . The parents lived in one of the four Atlantic provinces and had a child aged seven years or younger who had spina bifida ($n = 59$), diabetes ($n = 28$), or cystic fibrosis ($n = 27$). Fifty parents were in the control condition and sixty-four participated in telephone support groups (i.e., intervention condition), which were co-led by a peer (parent of a child with the same chronic condition) and a health professional. The participants in each group were drawn from similar disease categories so as to facilitate the sharing of common experiences as peers.

The groups were designed to address the needs that the mothers had identified in the assessment study; they had several characteristics of participatory research. Since many mothers in the assessment study described stressful spousal support, we offered an intervention that could enable both partners to participate. The parents could choose their preferred group structure, that is, mothers only, couples, or fathers only. The stressful situations delineated by the mothers in the assessment study were the basis for tentative themes identified for discussion during group sessions. One member of the team, the mother of two young adults with cystic fibrosis, contributed actively to the discussion of the design and content of the groups. During the initial meeting and at every subsequent session, the participants reviewed the proposed topics and reached a consensus about which topics the group would address.

As in most intervention studies in this program of research, the support groups met for one hour weekly for twelve weeks. The groups were designed to overcome the three most common barriers to face-to-face support group participation (Smith, Gabard, Dale, & Drucker, 1994): travel time, transportation, and choice of leader. The telephone support group format addressed the first two barriers. The third barrier was overcome by having both peers and health professionals as co-facilitators. The peer co-facilitators were mothers of older (seven to twelve years) children with the chronic condition. The professional co-facilitators had experience in working with families who were living with the chronic condition and were nominated by health professionals and organizations for diabetes, spina bifida, or cystic fibrosis. All co-facilitators participated in a full day's training session.

Each of the twelve groups had six to eight participants, including the co-facilitators. Consistent with the assessment study finding that mothers carry the majority of the caregiving burden, it was not surprising that most participants were mothers (n = 103) and that most mothers chose to participate in a support group for mothers only (i.e., peers). There were four mothers' groups and two couples' groups for twenty-nine families whose children had spina bifida; two mothers' groups and one couples' group for thirteen families of children with cystic fibrosis; and two mothers' groups and one couples' group for twelve families whose children had diabetes. The co-facilitators maintained contact with the participants in their groups and scheduled the group meetings at mutually agreeable times.

We designed the intervention to offer varied types of social support from peers in relation to specific types of caregiving demands and to enable the social support processes of social learning, social comparison, and social exchange. The participants received a draft outline of discussion topics for the twelve sessions, and the leaders had handbooks that provided background information on these themes. These topics represented the demands that mothers had identified in the assessment study and stressful situations that older children with a chronic condition had described in another study in our program (see chapter 2, above). The topics included the child's psychological, social and academic development, the child's physical care, coordinating the child's health care, impact on family routines and activities, parental personal needs and roles outside the caregiving role, and relationships with the partner/spouse and with the ill child. The handbook incorporated potential issues in each theme that parents might wish to discuss. For example, physical care encompassed equipment, time, tasks, vigilance, and scheduling, and parental roles outside the caregiving role included work for pay, friendships, volunteer activities, social activities, time for other family members, including other children, and housework. We encouraged each group to decide which topics they would discuss and when. The participants modified their plan for discussion topics throughout the twelve weeks.

The participants reported that the discussions were focused mainly on the primary demands of caring for a child with the specific condition and related coping strategies and support issues. They most commonly discussed the primary demands related to day-to-day management of the child's symptoms and deficits (83 per cent of parents), coordination of health care (79 per cent), facilitating the child's educational, social, and recreational activities (62 per cent), and managing illness-related crises (62 per cent). The most common secondary demands discussed were personal feelings and reactions (56 per cent), lack of time for oneself (54 per cent), and effect on family relationships (48 per cent). For some participants, the least frequently mentioned topics, such as spousal relationships, were a source of stress and conflict and difficult to discuss. Parents described a range of coping strategies, the majority of which they used to manage the day-to-day demands of caregiving, which one mother referred to as 'surviving.' These strategies included emotion-focused coping as well as behavioural and information-seeking strategies.

In every discussion, the co-facilitators invited the participants to explore their experience of the issue or stressful situation, and to discuss associated coping or management strategies and the support that was available, helpful, and/or needed. With our encouragement, the co-facilitators tried, not always successfully, to ensure that the group dynamics enabled each parent to participate and that no one parent dominated group sessions.

Key Features of the Telephone Support Group Intervention

- The groups had weekly one-hour sessions for twelve weeks.
- Both mothers and fathers were invited to participate.
- Groups were composed of parents of young children with the same diagnosis; group size = six to eight, including co-facilitators.
- Co-facilitators = mother of child over seven years with same condition and health professional experienced in care of children with chronic condition.
- Participants received a draft outline of discussion topics based on demands and stressful situations described by mothers in the assessment study and by older children with chronic conditions in related assess-

ment study (chapter 2, above). Participants modified the topics throughout the twelve weeks.
- The discussion focused on experiences, associated coping strategies, and support available, helpful, or needed.

Assessment of the Intervention Processes

We asked the participants to complete weekly diaries pertaining to the content and processes of the group session. The co-facilitators maintained field notes documenting the topics/issues discussed, the support processes (e.g., social comparison, reciprocity, social learning), member input, and leadership balance. In addition, we conducted interviews at the end of the twelve-week support group intervention, and at three months and six months following the termination of the group sessions.

There were some differences in response, depending on the child's medical diagnosis. All of the parents of children with cystic fibrosis expressed positive views about the support group's impact. Nearly 80 per cent of parents of children with spina bifida or diabetes expressed positive comments. They found the groups more useful when there were parents whose children had similar levels of involvement, were of similar ages, and were more recently diagnosed or facing similar transitions, such as starting school.

Group Processes

As planned, the group processes did include social learning, social comparison, social exchange, a participatory approach, and developmental dynamics. Social comparison was the major feature of the group discussions. When the parents perceived greater similarities, there was greater sharing and exchange of experiential knowledge and subsequently social learning. Participants compared their situations or problems and ways of solving or managing these situations with those of other group members. The diversity in age, severity of condition, or time since diagnosis within the groups, however, limited the potential of social comparison for some participants. For example, one mother said: '*My daughter has spina bifida, but related to the other kids, she was more severe and had more problems than what the other child had. So, I found it a little difficult there ... Because I just found the parents there didn't go through what I went through with my daughter, and it was hard to explain.*'

Social learning emerged as an exchange of information and experiential knowledge. One parent reported, '*I think the biggest thing ... whereas different people know about different things. So once you get all together, you know it all ... Like, I got a lot of information.*' Parents referred to learning things that they would use in the future: '*when situations arise, you remember. "Oh I remember so and so said ... or suggested." And that stuff is in your mind and you think of it. It's got to help in the long run.*' Parents also reported that they learned helpful hints and strategies for accomplishing the day-to-day demands they faced. As the parents reported, '*we bounced a lot of ideas off of one another. Like, "When I do this, this happens."*'

Participants perceived that they both gave something to and received something from the group discussions (i.e., social exchange). For instance, one parent said, '*I feel I just gave and got support. That seems to be the way this group is. We listen to each other and then we offer up a same situation or a potential solution.*' A few parents of older children felt they 'gave' more than they 'received.' Almost all appreciated the participatory approach and believed that they freely contributed to the selection of the discussion topics.

The data also reveal that the dynamics of the groups developed over time and that mutual respect for participants and co-facilitators was important. The support groups required more structure during their early sessions, but the process became more relaxed as the group developed. For example, one parent said, '*And the more we talked ... Like, each week, everybody would kind of open up a little bit more and talk more.*' While some groups increased their rapport and discussions over time and found they were just starting to 'roll' when the intervention ended, others felt they had completed their discussions by the eighth week. It seemed that issues such as homogeneity of situations, the nature of the interpersonal relationships, and the ability of participants to 'share air time' affected both group development and group processes.

Across groups there was a major focus on information and less discussion of personal emotion-laden issues, particularly spousal relationships. One leader reported, '*The group was really practically oriented. I mean, they wanted nuts and bolts. They did not want feelings and emotions.*' Another commented, '*They were willing to talk about the emotion, but only superficially.*'

Leadership

As we expected, the professional facilitators usually had the primary role of providing information about the condition, its treatment or management, and available services, and they supplemented the participants' experiential knowledge with expertise about the group process, the stressors members face, and germane coping strategies (Gottlieb, 1988). The participants saw the professional facilitators as the 'encyclopaedia' – the one to provide clinical insights. This was an expectation that increased the professional facilitators' preparation time. Also as anticipated, the peer facilitators offered experientially based coping strategies and informal help-seeking mechanisms. The peer leader was the 'seasoned veteran,' who could provide a great deal of information, since she had 'been through it.' The peer facilitators shared personal experiences and ideas about coping with a wide range of issues, including daily routines and the threat of death. One mother articulated the value of the peer leader's experiential knowledge as follows: '*she knew just what to say. I know a couple of times I was having difficulties when we were talking about certain subjects ... And when we were discussing that, she knew just what to say ... She just knew, as a parent, and someone so associated with the disease, she really knew what I was thinking and feeling and she knew what to say to get me out of it.*' We also expected and experienced some merging of domains and primary roles between the peer and professional facilitators.

Both the participants and the facilitators seemed to find the shared leadership effective and an important ingredient in the intervention. The participants believed that the facilitators 'kept each other in balance.' They believed that key leadership qualities entailed possessing current knowledge, experience working with children and families dealing with the condition, and a range of facilitation skills. The facilitators contended that the benefits of shared leadership included having a second perspective and shared responsibility for the group. One leader stated, '*It was less ... imposing. The job was easier to take knowing there was someone else there for you.*'

Assessment of the Impact of Intervention

The parents in the control and intervention conditions completed a series of questionnaires at baseline, immediately following the final support group session, and at three months and six months following the completion of the support groups. The questionnaires address the key elements in the framework (see table 3.1):

1. Stressful situation – measured by the *Perceived Stress Scale* (Cohen, Kamarck & Mermestein, 1983)
2. Social support – measured by the *Arizona Social Support Interview Schedule* (Barrera, 1980; Barrera, Sandler, & Ramsay, 1981)
3. Coping – measured by the *Coping Health Inventory for Parents* (CHIP) (McCubbin, McCubbin, Patterson, Cauble, Wilson, & Warwick, 1983) so as to address the specific issues faced by parents whose children have chronic conditions
4. Health in terms of parental perceived functioning – measured by the *Parenting Sense of Competence Scale* (Gibaud-Wallston & Wandersman, 1978; Johnston & Mash, 1989)

5. Health in terms of perceived limits in parental physical and role function due to poor health, acute symptoms, and mental health – measured by the *General Health Rating Index* (Davies & Ware, 1981)
6. Child resilience – measured by the *Swedish Revised Version of the Preschool Behavior Questionnaire* (Hagekull & Bohlin, 1996).

These measures are described in appendix B.

Key Findings

Over the study period, the parents in the intervention condition had greater gains in support satisfaction ($F(2,73) = 6.19$, $p = 0.002$), resistance and susceptibility in relation to their own health ($F(3,59) = 2.98$, $p = 0.03$), and perceived ego strength in their children ($F(3,59) = 2.06$, $p = 0.05$). Immediately following the intervention, parents in the intervention condition had enhanced perceptions in valuing and comfort aspects of parenting competence ($F(1,85) = 4.17$, $p = 0.04$). The parents in the control condition, however, had significantly decreased perceived stress over the study time periods ($F(3,57) = 3.02$, $p = 0.03$), while the intervention parents' perceived stress rose at the three-month post-test and then dropped again at the six-month interval. There were no statistically significant effects of the intervention on the parents' coping, support network size, support needs, or perceived conflict.

In their diaries and interviews, the participants described benefits and positive changes attributed to the support groups. All parents valued informational support from the groups. This included information about ways of coping with primary demands of the child's care. It seemed that comfort in parenting increased as parents learned from peers' helpful ideas about ways to organize the day or aspects of care, about the importance of some of the recommended treatments, or about ways to enhance the child's social experiences. Perhaps more important in view of the isolation that many parents describe, 98 per cent reported receiving affirmational support through normalizing and validating actions and feelings. Largely as a result of the processes of social comparison, parents discovered that they were not alone. For some parents, the groups provided their first opportunity to talk with other parents in the same situation. One mother said, '*What I got from this was a sense of belonging, being able to share experiences with people who have gone through the same type of problem.*' The groups helped parents to feel better about their reactions and to receive positive feedback and reassurance.

For instance, one mother said, '*I'm not alone. I don't feel so guilty for feeling the way I did and do now.*' Another said, '*Before I was worrying that maybe I'm not good at this, and I know I am because I am doing the best that I can do. And to have somebody tell you that is good.*' More than 80 per cent also reported receiving important forms of emotional support, such as sharing and empathy/understanding.

Just over 70 per cent of the parents described positive effects on their existing relationships with people in their network, and about half reported some form of enhanced coping, increased confidence, or change in perspective. Several commented that they had learned how important and beneficial for all involved it was to make time for themselves and their spouses without their child. Some parents also commented on what they had learned about their own reactions to each other. Two fathers realized that they needed to provide more help because '*It's too much for one parent to handle on their own.*' On the other hand, two mothers recognized the need to provide the fathers with some encouragement: '*I didn't realize that it was so important to tell my spouse what I was thinking about and to assure him from time to time how good he is doing caring for our child ... we never told each other how we are doing a good job with [the care]. It really makes a difference when you assure each other.*'

A large majority (84 per cent) took some action as a result of the intervention. Many parents (62 per cent) changed their use of health services. Most frequently, these changes resulted from learning about new options or services or from honing their ability to ask questions or express their needs. A few described less or different use of the health care system, such as not having to 'bug the doctors' or more confident decisions about going to the Emergency Department.

A few parents found that it was difficult to describe any positive impact. They could not say that the intervention met their needs, because they did not think of themselves as having 'needs.' Other parents found that they did not gain much from the group because they had already dealt with the issues that were discussed and no longer found such discussions useful.

The vast majority (85 per cent) were satisfied with the support group experience including group process and co-leadership by parents and professionals. More than half indicated that they missed the sessions when the intervention ended. One-third expressed dissatisfaction with some aspect of the support group process, in particular, with the amount of information available about the condition or treatment or the lack of similarity between their specific situation and that of the other parents.

Key Findings of the Intervention Study

- Parents prefer groups with other parents whose child's condition is similar in complexity and severity and who is very close in age.
- Group processes include social comparison, social learning, social exchange, participatory approach, and developmental dynamics.
- Peer leaders shared personal experiences, ideas about coping, and formal and informal resources.
- Professional leaders shared information about the condition, management, and resources/services.
- Participants and leaders found shared facilitatorship effective.
- There were small improvements in measures of support satisfaction, some aspects of health, parenting competence, and perceptions of the child's behaviour.
- Parents reported positive changes in support, coping, confidence, and perspectives.
- Eighty-five per cent were satisfied with the telephone support groups.

Lessons Learned

Adequacy of the Framework

The mothers' stories during the assessment study and the parents' interviews following the intervention confirmed several aspects of the social support framework (figure 3.1). These data show that the relationship between stressful situations and social support is clearly bidirectional and can be either positive or negative. For instance, one stressful situation for the mothers that changed pertained to the affected child's maturation in the course of development. That developmental change enabled the child to be less dependent on the mother and to assume more self-care. In relation to physical care, the mothers most frequently portrayed the affected child as a key source of support, which, in turn, diminished their demands and made life more manageable. They indicated that helpful support from any source decreased their caregiving demands, and stressful support increased the demands. The mothers also described direct relationships between their coping responses and their social support. For example, while mothers were sometimes critical of their partners' lack of support, they had rarely asked their partners for help or indicated to them that they required different support. After the support intervention, some partners acknowledged the need to communicate about needs and to provide feedback to each other and changed their relationship coping.

Other elements of the analysis, however, did not clearly confirm the framework. For example, although the qualitative data present a different picture, there was no change in measures of perceived stress or coping. The findings of the intervention study raise important questions about the outcome component of the framework and about suitable outcome measures. While there were time effects in parental perceptions of stress, coping, and social support networks, there was no intervention effect in these areas other than less perceived stress in the control group at the three-month measurement. Despite improvements in support satisfaction and widespread parental descriptions of positive changes in coping, confidence, and competence during interviews, there were limited improvements in the measures of parents' perceptions of health, competence, or child behaviour. The previous studies of professional or peer dyadic support also provide evidence of limited impact of a support intervention (Hansell et al., 1998; Ireys et al., 1996). These findings raise the usual questions about whether the particular measures, or indeed any quantitative measure, are sufficiently sensitive to detect changes in health outcomes. Perhaps more important, however, is the question of whether the types of outcome considered in the framework are too broad and too stable to be susceptible to the impact of a short-term intervention in the midst of chronic and complex life situations. Perhaps this type of structured short-term intervention can be expected to make only a small or temporary difference in the manageability of life and cannot be expected to affect the stable attributes assessed quantitatively in outcome measures of health, competence, or child behaviour. Or perhaps the parental reports of enhanced coping, confidence, competence and support and parental selected outcomes should be assigned greater value.

Design Issues

We had little difficulty in recruiting parents to participate in either the assessment or intervention study. Some health professionals in the clinics expressed concern about parents' being asked to participate in an interview (i.e., assessment study) that had no obvious benefit for them. Only ten mothers refused, however, and they gave reasons such as family stress, constraints of time, or lack of interest. Recruitment to the intervention study was greatly facilitated by health professionals in the clinics and by associations for the relevant chronic conditions. In some cases, these health professionals provided parents with information about the study. During the recruitment phase of the intervention study, the support of the health care personnel in the agency clinics was essential. These health professionals wanted to ensure that the professional facilitators had a current knowledge base.

Retention of participants over the full nine-month intervention study period was a greater challenge. Four parents withdrew from the study after attending one or two group sessions, and one parent in the control condition did not return any questionnaires. One parent in the intervention condition withdrew at the time of the first follow-up assessment. Despite attempts, as the study progressed, to try more 'user-friendly' strategies to increase parents' interest in returning diaries and questionnaires, the return rates did not change. The return rate varied with the questionnaire. Only 52 per cent of parents returned all four sets of the perceived stress questionnaire, but nearly 63 per cent completed the support satisfaction section of the ASSIS over all the time periods. Some parents were puzzled or even annoyed by the questions pertaining to their own health. From a research perspective these issues raise some difficult questions regarding the optimal extent of explanation to parents about the purpose of each measure, the usefulness of the standardized research 'instruments,' and the extent of demand added to the parents' lives. These parents lead extremely busy lives, and some simply did not have the time to complete the bank of questionnaires. The parents' reactions to some measures also raise questions about what outcomes parents would find most relevant. Ray (1997) puts forward important alternative perspectives in her report: parents' goals change with the fluctuation of their children's conditions; families' criteria for success can differ from those of professionals; and, while professionals seek particular changes in families, families may feel changes in health, education, or social services systems are more appropriate.

The vast majority of the participants completed all of the qualitative interviews, but one father refused to do any of the post-intervention interviews. Sixty-nine per cent of parents returned completed diaries. Many parents and facilitators commented negatively on the burden involved in completing the diaries, and some found the interviews repetitive. We did not tape and transcribe the group sessions for several reasons, including concern about invasion into the group process, the cost and difficulty of transcribing the group process from an audiotape, and the costs involved in data analysis relative to the merits of the detailed information obtained. Choice of the best strategies to document the nature of the group intervention, including the 'dose' of the social support mechanisms that unfold in the group, continues to be an issue of major debate (see chapter 12, below). Alternative approaches might include (1) random taping, (2) transcribing random sessions and retaining tapes of others for later secondary analysis, (3) random assignment of diary completion so that each participant completes a diary only for a small proportion of the group sessions, and (4) enhancing the visual appeal and diminishing the length of the diaries.

When asked for ways to improve the intervention, parents and facilitators focused on timing, frequency, and duration. They contended that the weekly sessions were preferable for the first four to six weeks to facilitate rapport building and group development, but that the frequency could then be reduced to biweekly. Although most believed that the duration of the intervention (i.e., twelve sessions) was reasonable, many parents felt a sense of loss when the sessions ended. Suitable duration of the intervention is difficult to determine. A better mechanism for follow-up, such as financial support for at least dyadic phone calls, should be an option for those participants who wish to pursue it.

At an early stage of the first wave of the intervention groups, we decided to add a 'booster session' for the co-facilitators. These sessions were held twice – once following the first few support group sessions and again prior to termination of the groups. The 'booster sessions' typically involved review of the groups' progress and strategies that worked, discussion of concerns, problem solving, and positive reinforcement about the quality of the facilitators' work. Although these sessions lasted longer than some facilitators found useful, overall they helped the facilitators to stay connected to each other and to the purpose and philosophy of the study, including its participatory elements, and they enabled the investigators to understand the issues facing the facilitators as the group processes unfolded. The facilitators found the first booster session particularly useful.

Lessons Learned

- Return rates for follow-up questionnaires were not improved by 'user-friendly' strategies.
- Parental perspectives on outcomes may yield more relevant outcome measures.
- Current outcome measures may assess too gross and stable constructs and miss important small changes that improve parents' quality of life.
- Parents need better explanations about the purpose of the questionnaires.
- Better strategies are needed to assess the 'dose' of social support in groups: complex, repetitive diaries are cumbersome for parents and

leaders to complete; taping and transcribing all sessions for detailed analysis is expensive and time intensive.
- 'Booster sessions' for co-facilitators mobilize peer support among the facilitators, problem solving, and positive reinforcement.
- The need for support is greatest at the time of diagnosis and at major life transitions.
- Groups need to be weekly early in the process and then spaced more widely.
- The duration of support interventions should ensure sufficient dose for the chronic stressful situation and for sustaining impact over time.

Implications for Future Intervention Research, Programs, and Policies

The support needs that emerged in the assessment study and the readiness of these busy mothers and nearly 10 per cent of the fathers to be involved in such an intensive intervention study provides considerable evidence of the needs of this population for more support than is currently provided. It is important to note that all these families were living with children whose conditions were quite stable at the time of the study. The numbers of families facing extremely stressful demands are increasing as more children with complex, severe, and multiple medical conditions are surviving to be discharged to their family homes and as health care delivery patterns shift from institution-based and professional care to community-based and family caregivers. Most often these caregivers are women (Gottlieb, 1998). Given the pattern of women's participation in the workforce, there is considerable impact of caregiving on women's capacities to participate fully in work and in the nation's productivity. These facts raise serious questions about the nature of the support that society should provide for families caring for children with chronic conditions. Programs like the social support groups tested in this study may improve the day-to-day quality of life for parents. If designed in a way that meets parents' needs, support programs may provide an important buffer to the increased risk of long-term negative health effects of caregiving. Such programs, however, are expensive, and families may not have the financial resources to access them. Moreover, it is likely that to be meaningful and to have any major impact the support groups must be available over a much longer term than twelve weeks and perhaps, for some, for more than twelve sessions. The group meetings need to be spaced differently than those in this study were, and they need to be sufficiently flexible for parents to gain access to the groups when they need the support (e.g., early periods after diagnosis, times of transitions, or stressful situations).

The sustainability of innovative support strategies like telephone support groups is challenging. Do the small changes demonstrated in this study provide a sufficient reason to invest in the sustainability? If we assume that such strategies are effective in meeting parental needs for accessible peer support, we are compelled to find ways to support such interventions on an ongoing basis. The telephone support group is an extremely expensive approach because of the long-distance and teleconference bridge charges. Given the worldwide constraints in health care spending, a timely strategy may involve approaching the private sector to develop special programs that would foster social linkages.

It is clear from our studies that not all parents are interested in being members of support groups and that maintaining involvement is variable for some parents. The parents in these studies, however, and those described in virtually every other investigation with families living with chronic caregiving situations reveal major needs for support. What are the alternatives?

In health care and educational systems, families face the reality that programs and decisions are system driven rather than family centred. Health professionals frequently are seen as sources of stressful support because of their lack of sensitivity to the individual family situation and their unwillingness to view the family as partners in the care of the child (Ainbinder et al., 1998; Stewart et al., 1994). In the United States, such problems experienced by families whose children had severe developmental delay and needed early intervention to optimize their development led the surgeon general to articulate the elements of family-centred care (U.S. Department of Health and Human Services, 1987). Johnson, Jeppson, and Redburn note that family-centred approaches were legislated subsequently in 'the Maternal and Child Health Block Grant Amendments in the Omnibus Budget Reconciliation Act of 1989 (P.L. 101-239), the Individuals with Disabilities Assistance and Bill of Rights Act (P.L. 101-496), and the Mental Health Amendments of 1990 (P.L. 101-639)' (992, xiii). We hope that such change will not require legislation in Canada, but it will necessitate a much greater emphasis, both in educational programs for health professionals and in health, social, and education agencies, on the knowledge and skills required for partnerships with families and communities. Similarly, provision of adequate funding and resources to enable both health professionals and teachers to work in partnership with parents is crucial.

Given Bronfenbrenner's (1986) call for providing these families with the support that enables them to foster the development of resilient children, however, additional broad social policies and programs are required to address adequately the support needs of parents as caregivers in chronic illness situations. For instance, programs like the 'Family Support Clusters' described by Lord and Hutchison (1998) are effective means of mobilizing support for families living with a relative who has a developmental or mental health disability. It is time that society acknowledged the contribution that parents of children with chronic conditions are making to the social fabric of Canada. The National Forum on Health (1997a, b) recognized the need for broader social action through its recommendations for an increase in publicly funded home care programs and for workplace policies and programs that support families through strategies such as flexibility in job structures and leave policies.

Acknowledgments

The assessment study was supported by Grant No. XG92-024 from the Hospital for Sick Children Foundation, Toronto, and the Spina Bifida Association of Canada. The intervention study was funded by Grant No. 6070-10-3/9507 from Health Canada.

Note

A partial but more detailed report of the findings of the assessment study appears in an earlier publication: Stewart, Ritchie, McGrath, Thompson, & Bruce (1994).

References

Ainbinder, J.G., Blanchard, L.W., Singer, G.H., Sullivan, M.E., Powers, L.K., Marquis, J.G., & Santelli, B. (1998). A qualitative study of parent to parent support for parents of children with special needs. *Journal of Pediatric Psychology, 23*, 99–109.

Albrecht, S.A., & Adelman, M. (1987). Communication networks as structures of social support. In T. Albrect & M. Adelman (Eds), *Communicating social support* (40–61). Newbury Park, CA: Sage.

Alpern, L., & Lyons-Ruth, L. (1993). Preschool children at social risk: Chronicity and timing of maternal depressive symptoms and child behavior problems at school and at home. *Development and Psychopathology, 5*, 371–387.

Anderson, J.M., & Elfert, H.(1989). Managing chronic illness in the family: Women as caretakers. *Journal of Advanced Nursing, 14*, 735–743.

Antonucci, T.C., & Jackson, J.S. (1990). The role of reciprocity in social support. In B.R.Sarason, I.G. Sarason, & G.R. Pierce (Eds), *Social support: An interactional view* (173–198). New York: Wiley.

Bailey, D.B., Blasco, P.M., & Simeonsson, R.J. (1992). Needs expressed by mothers and fathers of young children with disabilities. *American Journal of Mental Retardation, 97*, 1–10.

Barbarin, O.A., & Chesler, M. (1986). The medical context of parental coping with childhood cancer. *American Journal of Community Psychology, 14*, 221–235.

Barbarin, O.A., Hughes, D., & Chesler, M. (1985). Stress, coping, and marital functioning among parents of children with cancer. *Journal of Marriage and the Family, 47*, 473–480.

Barrera, M., Jr (1980). A method for the assessment of social support networks in community survey research. *Connections, 3*, 8–13.

Barrera, M., Jr, Sandler, I., & Ramsay, T. (1981). Preliminary development of a scale of social support: Studies of college students. *American Journal of Community Psychology, 20*, 435–447.

Beckman, P.J. (1991). Comparison of mothers' and fathers' perceptions of the effect of young children with and without disabilities. *American Journal of Mental Retardation, 95*, 585–595.

Black, M.M., Nair, P., & Harrington, D. (1994). Maternal HIV infection: Parenting and early child development. *Journal of Pediatric Psychology, 19*, 595–616.

Bloom, J.R. (1990). The relationship of social support and health. *Social Science and Medicine, 39*, 635–637.

Bolig, R., & Weddle, K.D. (1988). Resiliency and hospitalization of children. *Children's Health Care, 16*, 255–260.

Borkman, T. (1990). Self-help groups at the turning point. Emerging egalitarian alliances with the formal care system. *American Journal of Community Psychology, 18*, 321–332.

Bronfenbrenner, U. (1986). Ecology of the family as a context for human development. *Developmental Psychology, 22*, 723–742.

Burke, S.O., Kauffmann, E., Costello, E.A., Handley-Derry, M., & Dillon, M.C. (1991). A trial of stress-point preparation for parents of repeatedly hospitalized children with chronic conditions. *Developmental Medicine & Child Neurology, 33*, 13.

Burkhart, P.V. (1993). Health perceptions of mothers of children with chronic conditions. *Maternal-Child Nursing Journal, 21*, 122–129.

Cadman, D., Boyle, M.H., Offord, D.R., Szatmari, P., Rae Grant, N.I., Crawford, J., & Byles, J. (1986). Chronic illness and functional limitations in Ontario children: Findings of the Ontario child health study. *Canadian Medical Association Journal, 135*, 761–767.

Canadian Institute of Child Health (1994). *The health of Canada's children: A CICH profile.* (2nd ed.). Ottawa:

Canning, R.D., Harris, E.S., & Kelleher, K.J. (1996). Factors predicting distress among caregivers with chronic medical conditions. *Journal of Pediatric Psychology, 21*, 735–749.

Cant, R.V. (1994). An analysis of caregiving work. *Australian Journal of Marriage and Family, 15*(2), 66–75.

Cohen, S., Kamarck, T., & Mermelstein, R. (1983). A global measure of perceived stress. *Journal of Health and Social Behavior, 24*, 385–396.

Coyne, J.C., Wortman, C.B., & Lehman, D.R. (1988). The other side of support: What is helpful from whom? *Journal of Personality and Social Psychology, 58*, 80–89.

Damrosh, S.P., & Perry, L.A. (1989). Self reported adjustment, chronic sorrow, and coping of parents of children with Down's Syndrome. *Nursing Research, 38*, 25–30.

Davies, A.R., & Ware, J.E. (1981). *Measuring health perceptions in the Health Insurance Experiment (R-2711-HHS)*. Santa Monica, CA: Rand.

Drotar, D., Crawford, P., & Bush, M. (1984). The family context of childhood chronic illness: Implications for psychosocial intervention. In M.G. Eisenburg, L.C. Sutkin, & A. Jansen (Eds), *Chronic illness and disability through the life span: Effects on self and family* (103–129). New York: Springer.

Egeland, B.R., Carlson, E., & Sroufe, L.A. (1993). Resilience as process. *Development and Psychopathology, 5*, 517–528.

Elliott, K.A. (1991). Testing a specificity model of social support available to parents of chronically ill children. *Dissertation Abstracts International: The Humanities and Social Sciences*. Ann Arbor: University of Michigan.

Fagan, J., & Schor, D. (1993). Mothers of children with spina bifida: Factors related to maternal psychosocial functioning. *American Journal of Orthopsychiatry, 63*, 146–152.

Fine, S.B. (1991). Resilience and human adaptability: Who rises above adversity? *American Journal of Occupational Therapy, 45*, 493–503.

Fisher, J.D., Goff, B.A., Nadler, A., & Chinsky J.M. (1988). Social psychological influences on help seeking and support from peers. In B.H. Gottlieb (Ed.), *Marshaling social support: Formats, processes, and effects* (267–304). Newbury Park, CA: Sage.

Florian, V., & Krulik, T. (1991). Loneliness and social support of mothers of chronically ill children. *Social Science and Medicine, 32*, 1291–1296.

Folkman, S., Chesney, M., McKusick, L., Ironson, G., Johnson, D.S., & Coates, T.J. (1991). Translating coping theory into an intervention. In J. Eckenrode (Ed.), *The social context of coping* (240–260). New York: Plenum Press.

Garmezy, N. (1993). Children and poverty: Resilience despite the risk. *Psychiatry – Interpersonal and Biological Processes, 56*, 127–136.

Garwick, A.W., Patterson, J.M., Bennett, F.C., & Blum, R.W. (1998). Parents' perceptions of helpful vs unhelpful types of support in managing the care of preadolescents with chronic conditions. *Archives of Pediatrics & Adolescent Medicine, 152,* 665–71.

Gibaud-Wallston, J., & Wandersman, L.P. (1978). Development and utility of the Parenting Sense of Competence Scale. Paper presented at the meeting of the American Psychological Association, Toronto, Canada.

Gibson, C.H. (1986). How parents cope with a child with cystic fibrosis. *Nursing Papers, 18*(3), 31–45.

Gottlieb, B.H. (1988). Marshaling social support: The state of the art in research and practice. In B.H. Gottlieb (Ed.), *Marshaling social support: Formats, processes, and effects* (11–52). Newbury Park, CA: Sage.

Gottlieb, B.H. (1992). Quandries in translating support concepts to intervention. In H. Veiel & H. Baumann (Eds), *The meaning and measurement of social support* (293–309). New York: Hemisphere.

Gottlieb, B. (1996). Summary of protecting and promoting the well-being of family caregivers. In National Forum on Health (Ed.), *What determines health?* (115–118). Ottawa: National Forum on Health.

Gottlieb, B.H., & Wagner, F. (1991). Stress and social support processes in close relationships. In J. Eckenrode (Ed.), *The social context of coping* (165–187). New York: Plenum Press.

Hadadian, A. (1994). Stress and social support in fathers and mothers of children with and without disabilities. *Early Education and Development, 5,* 226–235.

Hagekull, B., & Bohlin, G. (1996). The Swedish revised version of the Preschool Behavior Questionnaire. Uppsaala, Sweden: Uppsaala University.

Hahn, B.A. & Schone, B.S. (1996). Maternal psychological distress: The role of children's health. *Women & Health, 24,* 59–75.

Hamlett, K.W., Pellegrini, D.S., & Katz, K.S. (1992). Chronic childhood illness as a family stressor. *Journal of Pediatric Psychology, 17,* 33–47.

Hansell, P.S., Hughes, C.B., Caliandro, G., Russo, P., Budin, W.C., Hartman, B., & Hernandez, O.C. (1998).The effect of a social support boosting intervention on stress, coping, and social support in caregivers of children with HIV/AIDS. *Nursing Research, 47,* 79–86.

Havermans, T., & Eiser, C. (1991). Mothers' perceptions of parenting a child with spina bifida. *Child: Care, Health and Development, 17,* 259–273.

Hoffman, C., Rice, D., & Sung, H.Y. (1996). Persons with chronic conditions: Their prevalence and costs. *Journal of the American Medical Association, 276,* 1478–1479.

House, J.S., Umberson, D., & Landis, K. (1988). Structures and processes of social support. *Annual Review of Sociology, 14,* 293–318.

Ireys, H.T., Sills, E.M., Kolodner, K.B., & Walsh, B.B. (1996). A social support intervention for parents of children with juvenile rheumatoid arthritis: Results of a randomized trial. *Journal of Pediatric Psychology, 21*, 633–641.

Jessop, D.J., & Stein, R.E.K. (1985). Uncertainty and its relation to the psychological and social correlates of chronic illness in children. *Social Science and Medicine, 20*, 993–999.

Jessop, D.J., & Stein, R.E.K. (1995). Consistent but not the same: Effect of method on chronic condition rates. *Archives of Pediatric and Adolescent Medicine, 149*, 1105–1110.

Jessop, D.J., Riessman, C.K., Stein, R.E. (1988). Chronic childhood illness and maternal mental health. *Journal of Developmental and Behavioral Pediatrics, 9*, 147–156.

Johnson, B.H., Jeppson, E.S., & Redburn, L. (1992). *Caring for children and families: Guidelines for hospitals*. Bethesda, MD: Association for the Care of Children's Health.

Johnston, C., & Mash, E.J. (1989). A measure of parenting satisfaction and efficacy. *Journal of Clinical Child Psychology, 18*, 491–502.

Katz, A.H. (1993). *Self-help in America: A social movement perspective*. New York: Twayne.

Kazak, A.E. (1989). Families of chronically ill children: A systems and social-ecological model of adaptation and challenge. *Journal of Consulting and Clinical Psychology, 57*, 25–30.

Kazak, A.E., & Marvin, R.S. (1984). Differences, difficulties, and adaptation: Stress and social networks in families with a handicapped child. *Family Relations, 33*, 67–77.

Knafl, K., Breitmayer, B., Gallo, A., & Zoeller, L. (1996). Family response to childhood chronic illness: Description of management styles. *Journal of Pediatric Nursing, 11*, 315–326.

Konstantareas, M.M., & Homatadis, S. (1989). Assessing child symptom severity and stress in parents of autistic children. *Journal of Clinical Psychology and Psychiatry, 30*, 459–470.

LaGaipa, J.J. (1990). The negative effects of informal support systems. In S. Duck (Ed.), *Personal relationships and social support* (122–139). London: Sage.

LePontis, J., Moel, D.I., & Cohn, R.A. (1987). Family adjustment to pediatric ambulatory dialysis. *American Journal of Orthopsychiatry, 57*, 78–83.

Loebig, M. (1990). Mothers' assessment of the impact of children with spina bifida on the family. *Maternal-Child Nursing Journal, 19*, 251–264.

Lord, J., & Hutchison, P. (1998). Living with a disability in Canada: Toward autonomy and integration. In *Canada health action: Building on the legacy.*

Papers commissioned by the National Forum on Health. Vol. 3, *Determinants of health: Settings and issues* (375–431). Sainte-Foy, QC: Editions MultiMondes.

Lyons, R., Sullivan, M., & Ritvo, P. (Eds). (1995). *Relationships, chronic illness and disability.* Thousand Oaks, CA: Sage.

Maton, K.I. (1987). Patterns and psychological correlates of material support within a religious setting: The bidirectional support hypothesis. *American Journal of Community Psychology, 15,* 185–207.

McCubbin, H.I., McCubbin, M.A., Patterson, J.M., Cauble, A.E., Wilson, L.R., & Warwick, W. (1983). CHIP: Coping Health Inventory for Parents: An assessment of parental coping patterns in the care of the chronically ill child. *Journal of Marriage and the Family, 45,* 359–370.

McCubbin, M.A., & McCubbin, H.I. (1993). Families coping with illness: The resiliency model of family stress, adjustment, and adaptation. In C.B. Danielson, B. Hamel-Bissell, & P. Winstead-Fry (Eds), *Families, health, & illness* (21–63). St Louis, MO: Mosby.

Miller, M., & Diao, J. (1987). Family friends: New resources for psychosocial care of chronically ill children in families. *Children's Health Care, 15,* 259–264.

Miller, A.C., Gordon, R.M., Daniels, R.J., & Diller, L. (1992). Stress, appraisal, and coping in mothers of disabled and nondisabled children. *Journal of Pediatric Psychology, 17,* 587–605.

National Forum on Health. (1996a). *Canada health action: Building on the legacy.* Vol. 1, *Final report of the National Forum on Health.* Ottawa: Minister of Public Works and Government Services.

National Forum on Health. (1996b). *Canada health action: Building on the legacy.* Vol. 2, *Synthesis reports and issues papers.* Ottawa: Minister of Public Works and Government Services.

Newacheck, P.W., & Taylor, W.R. (1992). Chronic childhood illness: Prevalence, severity, and impact. *American Journal of Public Health, 82,* 364–371.

Newacheck, P.W., & Stoddard, J.J. (1994). Prevalence and impact of multiple childhood chronic illnesses. *Journal of Pediatrics, 124,* 40–48.

Patterson, J., & Blum, R.W. (1996). Risk and resilience among children and youth with disabilities. *Archives of Pediatric and Adolescent Medicine, 150,* 692–698.

Patterson, J.M., Garwick, A.W., Bennett, F.C., & Blum, R.W. (1998). Social support in families of children with chronic conditions: Supportive and nonsupportive behaviors. *Journal of Developmental & Behavioral Pediatrics, 18,* 383–91.

Pelletier, L., Godin, G., Lepage, L., & Dussault, G. (1994). Social support received by mothers of chronically ill children. *Child: Care, health and development, 20,* 115–131.

Quittner, A., DiGirolamo, A.M., Michel, M., & Eigen, H. (1992). Parental response to cystic fibrosis: A contextual analysis of the diagnosis phase. *Journal of Pediatric Psychology, 17*, 683–704.

Quittner, A.L., Glueckauf, R.L., & Jackson, D.N. (1990). Chronic parenting stress: Moderating and mediating effects of social support. *Journal of Personality and Social Psychology, 59*, 1266–1278.

Ray, L. (1997). Designing research with families of children with chronic conditions. *Communicating Nursing Research, 30*, 117.

Ray, L. & Ritchie, J.A. (1993). Caring for chronically ill children: Factors that influence parents' coping. *Journal of Pediatric Nursing, 8*, 217–226.

Rodin, J., Striegel-Moore, R.H., & Silberstein, L.R. (1990). Vulnerability and resilience in the age of eating disorders: Risk and protective factors for bulemia nervosa. In J.E. Rolf, A.S. Masten et al. (Eds), *Risk and protective factors in the development of psychopathology* (361–383). New York: Cambridge University Press.

Seidl, J., Kjolseth, R., & Seymour, E. (1988). *The Ethnograph. A users' guide* (computer program). Littleton, CO: Qualis Research Associates.

Silver, R.C., Wortman, C.B., & Crofton, C. (1990). The role of coping in support provision: The self-presentational dilemma of victims of life crisis. In B. Sarason, I. Sarason, & G. Pierce (Eds), *Social support: An interactional view* (397–426). New York: Wiley.

Smith, K., Gabard, D., Dale, D., & Drucker, A. (1994). Parental opinions about attending parent support groups. *Children's Health Care, 23*, 127–136.

Stewart, M.J. (1989). Social support: Diverse theoretical perspectives. *Social Science and Medicine, 28*, 1275–1282.

Stewart, M.J., Ritchie, J.A., McGrath, P., Thompson, D., & Bruce, B. (1994). Mothers of children with chronic conditions: Supportive and stressful interactions with partners and professionals regarding caregiving burdens. *Canadian Journal of Nursing Research, 26*(4), 61–82.

Stroller, E., & Pugliese, K. (1989). Other roles of caregivers: Competing responsibilities or supportive resources. *Journal of Gerontology, 44*(6), S231–S238.

Thoits, P.A. (1986). Social support as coping assistance. *Journal of Consulting and Clinical Psychology, 54*, 416–423.

Thompson, R.J., Gustafson, K.E., Hamlett, K.W., & Spock, A. (1992). Stress, coping and family functioning in the psychosocial adjustment of mothers of children with cystic fibrosis. *Journal of Pediatric Psychology, 17*, 573–585.

Tomlinson, P., & Mitchell, K.E. (1992). On the nature of social support for families of critically ill children. *Journal of Pediatric Nursing, 7*, 386–394.

U.S. Department of Health and Human Services. (1987). *Surgeon General's report: Children with special health care needs*. DHHS Publication No. HRS/D/MC87-2. Rockville, MD: DHHS.

Van Cleve, L. (1989). Parental coping in response to their child's spina bifida. *Journal of Pediatric Nursing, 4*, 172–176.

Valentine, D.P. (1993). Children with special needs: Sources of support and stress for families. *Journal of Social Work and Human Sexuality, 8*, 107–121.

Werner, E.E. (1993). Risk, resilience, and recovery: Perspectives from the Kauai longitudinal study. *Development and Psychopathology, 5*, 503–515.

Williams, P.D., Lorenzo, F.D., & Borja, M. (1993). Pediatric chronic illness: Effects on siblings and mothers. *Maternal-Child Nursing Journal, 21*, 111–121.

4

Mobilizing Spousal Support for Coping with Cardiac Conditions

Miriam J. Stewart, Karina Davidson, Gerald Klassen, Lydia Makrides, and Hermann Wolf

Abstract. Ischaemic heart disease (IHD) generates the highest percentage of all hospitalization costs and lost earnings. The aim of the assessment study was to identify psychological and social factors associated with early readmission to hospital of persons admitted with a diagnosis of IHD. Forty participants had experienced their first hospital admission and sixty had a history of prior admissions. The two most frequently identified coping strategies were 'seeking social support' and 'positive reappraisal.' Readmitted participants used the coping strategy 'accepting responsibility' significantly less than those not readmitted. Support scores for all participants were lower than reported normative scores. Individuals with a prior history of admissions received more support from health professionals and less support from neighbours than first-time admissions did. Spouses were primary sources of support. Despite the importance of spousal support for readjustment, there were no reports of support interventions for couples coping with cardiac conditions.

Accordingly, the aim of the second study was to design, implement, and evaluate a face-to-face support group intervention, involving peer and professional supporters, for persons with first-time myocardial infarction and their spouses. The groups were co-facilitated by peer (affected couple) and professional leaders. Twenty-eight persons participated. The key types of support provided by the group were informational, affirmational, and emotional. There was a significant decrease in guidance support need and a corresponding increase in guidance support satisfaction. The significant reduction in perceived network size can be interpreted in part by reduced network conflict and in part by changes in social network composition. Participants referred to the positive impact of the intervention on their coping, confidence, and spousal relationship.

Introduction

Cardiovascular disease (CVD) remains the leading cause of mortality and premature death in Canada (Labonté, 1992). CVD accounts for 37 per cent of all deaths and one form – ischaemic heart disease (IHD) – for the most mortality (21 per cent). In Atlantic Canada, the site of the two studies described in this chapter, consistently higher CVD mortality rates are reported than in other regions. Premature death from CVD is associated with an estimated 294,000 years of life lost. In 1995 the total days in hospital for a diagnosis of CVD were 6,522,117; IHD was responsible for 1.5 million hospital days. Indeed, hospital care is the most expensive direct cost of CVD ($4.8 billion annually). Indirect costs associated with cardiac conditions include lost productivity due to illness or disability and the loss of future earnings from premature death ($12.3 billion) (Heart and Stroke Foundation of Canada, 1997).

Persons who have myocardial infarction (MI) – one form of IHD - represent the highest percentage of all hospitalization costs and loss of earnings (Beach, Maloney, Plocica, Sherry, Weaver, Luthringer, & Utz, 1992). In one investigation, 43 per cent of MI survivors had one or more subsequent hospitalizations for cardiac-related reasons within four months (Rost & Smith, 1992). Over the six years preceding the initial assessment study reported in this chapter, we observed a readmission rate of 20 per cent during the first year following initial hospitalization with IHD; 80 per cent of these readmissions occurred within the first four months (Stewart, Hirth, Klassen, Makrides, & Wolf, 1997).

Diverse factors have been linked to readmission of persons with cardiac diseases. Although earlier studies were focused on pathophysiological abnormalities as major predictors of readmissions (Krakauer & Jacoby, 1993), social-psychological factors are beginning to be implicated (Frasure-Smith, 1991). For example, when disease severity was controlled for, depression associated with MI had a significant direct effect on rehospitalization. Potential cost savings associated with decreasing depression could equate to six to nine days of hospitalization (Levine, Covino, Slack, Safran, Boro, Davis, Buchanan, & Gervino, 1996). The influence of social support and of coping strategies for managing stress associated with cardiac disease on readmissions had not been studied prior to our initial investigation. Therefore, the aim of the assessment study was to identify psychological and social factors (e.g., stress, coping, social support) associated with early readmission to hospital of persons admitted with a diagnosis of IHD.

Stress of Cardiac Conditions

Numerous stressors are experienced by persons with cardiac conditions, such as family tensions, financial problems, self-care obstacles, and work difficulties (Lesperance, Frasure-Smith, & Talajic, 1996). Indeed, anxiety and depression are common among MI survivors (Conn, Taylor, & Abele, 1991). Persons with continued anxiety and uncertainty post-MI are less likely to return to work and have higher hospital readmission and mortality rates (Webster & Christman, 1988).

The ongoing need for support in chronic cardiac illness can burden family caregivers (Coyne & Fiske, 1992). The spouse, in particular, can be profoundly affected by the stress of the MI (Coyne & Smith, 1991). Spouses often experience anxiety, depression (Thompson & Cordle, 1988), and distress (Hilbert, 1996), which can hamper the recovery of survivors (Beach et al., 1992).

Coping with Cardiac Conditions

Survivors employ varied strategies to regain control and reduce the uncertainties associated with an MI, including seeking reassurance and information from health professionals (Johnson & Morse, 1990). Post-MI survivors who perceived a loss of control had greater adjustment problems (McCauley, 1990). The use of passive coping strategies (Martin & Lee, 1992) has been linked to delays in seeking medical assistance for cardiac symptoms (Nolan & Wielgosz, 1991) and to poor social-psychological (Keckeisen & Nyamathi, 1990; Terry, 1992) and physiological (Faller, 1990) recovery from an MI. Survivors also use optimism, confrontation, self-reliance, support seeking (Scherck, 1992), venting, and 'thinking things through' (Miller, McMahon, Garrett, & Ringel, 1989) to cope with MI.

Communication of anxiety and tension within close relationships (i.e., active engagement coping strategies) has been found to alleviate survivor stress (Moser, 1994; Thompson, Ersser, & Webster, 1995). In this context, some studies revealed links between spousal coping and the coping of the MI survivor (Beach et al., 1992; Coyne & Smith, 1991).

Social Support and Cardiac Conditions

Coping and social support are significant predictors of survival of heart transplant patients (Clarke, Walker, & Cuddy, 1996). Moreover, social support has a direct effect on recovery from MI (Conn et al., 1991). For example, support has been linked with self-esteem, mastery (Ben-Sira & Eliezer, 1990), readjustment (Fontana, Kerns, Rosenberg, & Colenese, 1989), and stress reduction (Helgeson, 1993). Further, social support predicted personal control (Markle-Reid, 1989), interpersonal dependence, and health outlook (Riegel & Dracup, 1992) in first-time MI survivors.

The presence of a spouse/confidante influences later mortality from MI, after medical prognostic factors are controlled for (Williams, Barefoot, Califf, Haney, Saunders, Pryor, Hlatky, Siegler, & Mark, 1992; Gorkin, Schron, Brooks, Wiklund, Kelen, Verter, Schoenberger, Pawitan, Morris, & Shumaker, 1993). Spousal support has been related to reduced stress (Frasure-Smith, 1991), and to readjustment, self-esteem, mastery, coping with physical restrictions (Ben-Sira & Eliezer, 1990), and adherence to risk-reduction behaviours (Helgeson, 1991) in MI survivors. Despite evidence that spouses play an important role in survivors' recovery, there have been few studies (cf. Beach et al., 1992; Coyne & Smith, 1991) that include the spouse in cardiac rehabilitation or support interventions.

Social support interventions may help MI survivors to adopt healthy behaviours (Moser, 1994; Alonzo & Reynolds, 1995; Rodeman, Conn, & Rose, 1995). Moreover, support interventions by health professionals have been linked to enhanced knowledge, life satisfaction, and perceived health, and to reduced anxiety, depression, MI recurrence, and cardiac mortality (Frasure-Smith, 1991; Thompson & Meddis, 1990; Thompson, Webster, & Meddis, 1990). Health professional phone calls or visits increased survivors' confidence, adjustment (Keeling & Dennison, 1995), and satisfaction with health care (Linden, 1995) and reduced their stress and mortality (Frasure-Smith & Prince, 1989). Although this evidence is encouraging, supportive interventions following an MI have involved health professionals only (Thompson, 1991; Thompson & Meddis, 1990; Frasure-Smith, 1991) and typically have focused solely on the survivor.

Despite the importance of spousal support for the MI survivor's readjustment, there are no reports of interventions that test the efficacy of support from professional *and* peer sources for both survivors *and* spouses. Accordingly, the aim of the second study was to design, implement, and evaluate a face-to-face support group, involving peer and professional supporters, for persons with a first-time MI and their spouse.

Fit with Framework

The assessment and intervention studies were based on a conceptualization of social support as a coping resource or assistance in coping with stresses associated with IHD and MI (see figure 4.1). Social support, like other coping resources, can moderate negative effects of stressful conditions such as MI and enhance health outcomes and physical recovery (Bloom, 1990; Kaplan & Toshima, 1990). Conversely, chronic illnesses, such as cardiac conditions, may drain support resources and lead to estrangement from the social net-

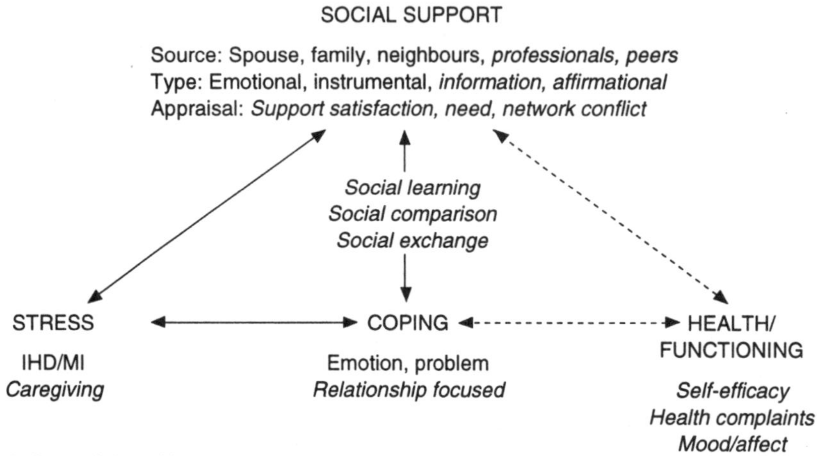

Italics and dotted lines = intervention study

Figure 4.1 Framework for Assessment and Intervention Studies Focused on Adults with Cardiac Conditions

work. The negative costs of support may include over-involvement and burden for providers (e.g., spouse/partner) and diminished self-esteem for recipients (e.g., person with MI) (LaGaipa, 1990).

Both MI survivors and their spouses/partners have to cope with the disruptions imposed on their lives as they strive to adjust to new routines and restrictions. The ways survivors and spouses cope provide clues to each other about whether support is needed and the types of support needed (Silver, Wortman, & Crofton, 1990). Coping with an MI can be conceptualized as managing distress (emotion focused), completing instrumental tasks (problem focused), and attending to each other's needs (relationship focused) (Coyne & Smith, 1991).

In the intervention study, a network of peers was created to enhance and supplement the depleted networks of persons with MI and their partners by providing emotional, affirmational, and informational support. Three mediating processes were anticipated within the support groups. *Social comparison* with peers (MI survivors and spouses) can validate and normalize adjustment post MI. Mutual aid / support groups of peers are characterized by *social exchange* and equitable, bidirectional exchange. According to *social learning* theory, peers as role models can elicit and enhance experiential knowledge of MI survivors and spouses.

Assessment Study: Support Needs and Support Seeking

No published investigations were located that examined whether social support, stress appraisal, and coping varied, as risk factors for readmission to hospital, between persons with first-time or prior admissions for IHD. The research questions used to guide the study were as follows: Are there differences between persons with a first admission for IHD and persons with previous admissions for IHD in: (1) types, sources and duration of social support? (2) appraisal of stressors associated with IHD? (3) coping strategies used to manage the stressors associated with IHD? and (4) social-psychological factors associated with readmission?

Sample

Forty participants had experienced their first hospital admission for IHD; six of them were readmitted during the four-month study period. Sixty participants had a history of prior admissions for IHD; eighteen were readmitted during the study period.

Significant differences in gender and functional class (i.e., severity of IHD) emerged. Compared with persons with a first admission for IHD, the group with a history of multiple admissions had a significantly higher representation of men and more functional disability due to IHD.

Methodology

Participants completed a sociodemographic data sheet (age, sex, living arrangements) and three study instruments in a private room in the hospital. They required approximately one hour to complete these three measures – *Stress Appraisal Measure*, *Ways of Coping Checklist*, and *Norbeck Social Support Questionnaire* (see appendix B). The coping measure was prefaced by the question, 'How have you dealt with / managed your heart disease since being in hospital?' The stress measure was used to determine how participants appraised the stressfulness of their heart disease. Participants' physicians provided information regarding the number of visits for cardiac problems over the study period. At the end of four months, participants were contacted by mail to determine whether they had been readmitted to hospital. Readmission for a primary diagnosis of IHD was confirmed, using the MONICA database.

Chi square analysis was used to examine the ordinal level sociodemographic and clinical data. Data elicited by study instruments, participants' age, and

TABLE 4.1
Research Design

	Assessment Study	Intervention Study
Sample	Convenience Adults admitted to hospital for IHD/MI (*n* = 100)	Convenience First time MI survivors and partners (*n* = 28)
Design	Descriptive, correlational	Pre-test-post-test within subjects
Measures		
Stress	*Stress Appraisal Measure*	
Coping	*Ways of Coping Checklist*	*Michigan Family Heart Questionnaire*
Support	*Norbeck Social Support Questionnaire*	*Arizona Social Support Interview Schedule*
Health	Functional Status (MONICA)	*Positive and Negative Affect Schedule* *Health Complaints Scale* *Information to Manage Health Behaviour Change* (*Michigan Questionnaire*)
Data collection	T_1 (in hospital) T_2 (4 months later)	T_1 Pre-test T_2 Post-test (following 3 month intervention)
Data analyses		
Quantitative	Chi square *T*-Tests	Paired *t*-tests
Qualitative		Content analysis (using Ethnograph) of weekly participant diaries, weekly facilitator fieldnotes, and post-intervention interviews of participants and leaders

number of visits to physicians were analysed as interval level data, and *t*-tests were employed to explore for significant differences ($p < 0.05$). The research design is summarized in table 4.1.

Key Findings and Interpretations

There were significant differences in *stress appraisal.* Participants who were readmitted to hospital appraised their cardiac condition as less under the control of others and more uncontrollable than those who were not readmitted during the study period. Moreover, multiple readmitted persons appraised their IHD as more threatening and central than first-time readmitted persons.

The two most frequently identified *coping* strategies were 'seeking social support' and 'positive reappraisal' (i.e., problem-focused coping). There was a significant difference in use of the coping strategy 'seeking social support': persons who were readmitted used this coping strategy more than persons who were not readmitted. Indeed, the key variable associated with readmission of persons admitted for the first time with IHD at the beginning of the study was greater use of 'seeking social support.' Readmitted participants used the coping strategy 'accepting responsibility' significantly less than those not readmitted to hospital. In this context, readmission of persons with a history of multiple admissions for IHD was associated with decreased use of the coping strategy 'accepting responsibility.'

Spouses/partners and family members were the predominant sources of *social support* for both first-time and multiple admitted participants. Individuals with a prior history of admissions for IHD received more support from health professionals and less support from neighbours than those with first-time admissions. Further, participants who had experienced previous admissions for IHD reported more total support, as well as more emotional and affirmational support, from health professionals. Mean total support scores as well as scores for all three types of support – affect, affirmation, and aid – were lower than reported normative scores (Norbeck, Lindsey, & Carrier, 1983).

As illness can involve loss of independence, capacity to work, and relationships (Coyne & Fiske, 1992), the lower support scores are not surprising. In other investigations, spouses were also the key supporters of persons with MI (Coyne & Smith, 1991; Krikevold, Gortner, Berg, & Saltvold, 1996; Riegal & Gocka, 1995), and family members and close friends were named most frequently as sources of support (Conn et al., 1991; Winefield & Katsikitis, 1987). The ties of kinship and marriage may create commitment to the support recipient. Intimates, such as a spouse/partner, are valued for emotional and affirmational support (Dakof & Taylor, 1990) that may not materialize in interactions with health professionals. It is noteworthy that participants with multiple admissions received more support from professionals. For persons not previously hospitalized, members of the natural network are likely still providing support, and the family caregiver burden has probably not yet accumulated to the point of requiring supplementary support from professionals.

Seeking social support was the most common coping strategy in our investigation (Stewart et al., 1997) and in a study of first-time admissions for MI (Hudson, 1994). Similarly, in other studies, MI survivors reported frequent use of 'supportive' coping strategies (Scherck, 1992) and discussed symptoms with others (Nolan & Wielgosz, 1991). Support seeking is used in stressful encounters in which the outcome is appraised as changeable (Lazarus & Folkman, 1984). Individuals with IHD must contend with major life transitions and may seek informational support concerning requisite lifestyle changes.

Implications for Interventions

Participants with a first admission for IHD who were readmitted during the study period may be struggling to manage their illness. Greater use of the coping strategy 'seeking social support' seems to reflect their need for assistance. The lower scores for social support also reveal a need for supplementary support. Consequently, first-time MI survivors who reported less support from health professionals may benefit from additional support not only from professionals but also from peers to help them manage this life-threatening illness. Reported interventions have emphasized health professional rather than peer support. Given that support from peers with experiential (i.e., first-hand) knowledge of cardiac illness may enhance recovery, peer support interventions should be tested. Spouses/partners as key support providers should be included in interventions.

Salient Findings from the Assessment Study

- Most support for IHD survivors came from spouse/partner and family.
- All types of support reported by persons with IHD were lower than norms.
- The key coping strategy was 'seeking social support.'
- Readmission was linked to less 'acceptance of responsibility.'
- Persons with prior admissions experienced:
  - more support from health professionals
  - less support from neighbours.
- First-time-admitted people and their spouses/partners may need more support from health professionals and peers.

Intervention Study: Support Group for Survivors and Spouses

Rationale

The literature revealed no support-education interventions designed for couples coping with MI, and no support interventions involving both professionals and peers. To determine preferred supportive interventions, a survey was conducted of participants (*n* = 26) in cardiac rehabilitation programs. The two top-ranked interventions were support groups for persons with cardiac disease and support groups for couples in which one partner has cardiac disease. An intervention was designed to accommodate these support-intervention preferences.

Intervention Design

The MI survivors and their spouses participated in a support group intervention that involved professional and peer supporters. The intervention was time limited (approximately one hour weekly for twelve weeks) to ensure comparability of intervention dose among the different support groups. The face-to-face groups were designed to convey emotional, informational, and affirmational support specific to stressful situations encountered by persons who had suffered an MI and by their spouse/partner. Group discussions were augmented by a variety of techniques and resources (e.g., role playing, invited consultant or guest speaker, focused group discussion, guided group exercises). (Note: The research design for the intervention study is summarized in table 4.1.)

Peer and Professional Facilitators

The face-to-face support groups were co-facilitated by peer and professional leaders. Peer facilitators (i.e., couples in which one spouse was at least one year post-MI) were assessed for their insight into requisite adjustments, interpersonal skills, and potential for leadership. All survivor facilitators were men who had extensive involvement with various community organizations, and many spouse facilitators had experience with non-profit organizations. The professional facilitators, representing nursing, social work, psychology, and health education disciplines, had worked with persons who had cardiac illness and with community-based groups.

Facilitator Handbook

The facilitator handbook outlined the responsibilities of the group facilitators and the project goals. In the initial week, proposed topics and group members' commitment and expectations were discussed. The outlines for the subsequent sessions were focused on common stresses experienced by MI survivors and spouses (e.g., hospitalization, lifestyle changes, health care, routines, recovery, caregiving roles, return to work, economic constraints, intimacy, conflict, dependence), coping/managing strategies, and support needed/available. Information about these topics was based on relevant literature and on feedback from a focus group of couples who had experience in coping with MI. Case study scenarios were created for each weekly theme.

The support group participants were consulted during the initial session regarding content foci and timing of sessions and topics. Furthermore, members were invited to alter and add topics in subsequent sessions. A review of the facilitators' field notes revealed that the themes and ordering of topics discussed by groups during initial meetings closely resembled the proposed outline in the facilitator's handbook. In later sessions, participants emphasized emotional impact, food selection and preparation, exercise, stress management, avoiding burn-out, and communication to a greater extent than projected in the original outline.

Data Collection and Analysis

The professional and peer facilitators recorded field notes following each session, in which particular attention was paid to the discussion topics, the coping strategies suggested, the sources of support identified, the support processes within the group, and factors that affected discussions. Participants completed weekly diaries about the perceived importance of the topics, their contribution to the discussion, group processes, and facilitator roles and co-leadership. Group members also participated in individual post-intervention interviews focused on continuing contacts with other members, reciprocity of supportive interactions, social comparison, social learning, the impact of the intervention, and their satisfaction with the intervention. Peer and professional facilitators were interviewed jointly about the facilitator training session, leadership issues, group processes, interactions with group members following the intervention, and the advantages, disadvantages and impact of the intervention.

The diaries, field notes, and interview data were subjected to content analysis, using a category system of key concepts and themes that the investigators and research assistant developed inductively from the data. A computer-based program, the Ethnograph, was employed to sort the qualitative data by codes and to conduct frequency counts.

Sample

This intervention was limited to first-time MI in order to enhance the homogeneity of the group and to focus on a time of uncertainty and transition for survivors and their spouses. The project was open to men or women recently discharged from hospital (less than six months) with an uncomplicated first-time MI who were living with a spouse/partner. Potential participants with spouses who also had cardiac conditions were excluded.

Twenty-eight persons participated in the intervention. Only one of the MI survivors was female. All participants were Caucasian. The survivors ranged in age from forty-two to seventy-one years (mean = 57 years), while spouses were forty to sixty-six years old (mean = 56.1 years). Although some participants (36 per cent) were employed, the majority (64 per cent) were either not currently employed or retired. Fifty per cent of the support group participants had an income of greater than $40,000; 40 per cent had incomes under $30,000.

Measurement of Outcomes

All survivors and their spouses completed pre- and post-intervention questionnaires. Demographic data and 'pre-marital adjustment' and 'functional disability' scores were collected once at baseline. The pre- and post-test questionnaires comprised items from several scales within four measures used to assess the following outcomes: support need and satisfaction (*Arizona Social Support Interview Schedule*): affect (*Positive and Negative Affect Schedule*), adequacy of information for managing health behaviour changes post-MI, coping with MI, self-efficacy (*Michigan Family Heart Questionnaire*), and perceived health status (*Health Complaints Scale*) (MI survivors only) (see appendix B). Paired *t*-tests were conducted to determine if the differences in pre-and post-test responses were statistically significant for the various outcome measures. Separate analyses were performed for spouse, survivor, and couples.

Key Features of the Intervention

- Face-to-face support group intervention was for MI survivors and spouses.
- Groups met weekly over a twelve-week period.
- Emotional, informational, and affirmational support specific to stressful situations was conveyed in groups.
- Groups were co-facilitated by peer (affected couple) and professional leaders.
- A facilitator handbook incorporated information on common stresses, coping strategies, and support needed/available, along with case studies.
- Participants could change topics and timing/sequencing of topics.

- Facilitators recorded field notes.
- Participants completed weekly diaries.
- Participants and facilitators were interviewed post-intervention.
- Impact on affect, self-efficacy, relationship-focused coping, and perceived health was evaluated.

Support Group Discussion Themes

Stress of Living with MI

Primary Demands of Caregiving: Spouses identified four demands directly related to caring for the MI survivor: monitoring lifestyle changes, dealing with survivor's reactions, interacting with the health system, and maintaining vigilance. These caregivers expressed frustration with the lack of specific, concrete information available to them. Spouses felt excluded, alone, and overwhelmed, particularly during the time of acute care and diagnosis. Some participants found interactions with health professionals stressful and lacking in empathy. Interacting with survivors whose emotional reactions were different following the MI and negotiating their caregiving role with their ill spouse also generated strain.

Secondary Demands of Caregiving: Spouses eloquently articulated the impact of the MI on themselves and their families. They experienced anger, frustration, and resentment in the early stages of rehabilitation. The MI had a significant impact on their family and marital relationships. In another study, spouses of persons who had experienced cardiac surgery were dissatisfied with sexual relations (Monahan et al., 1996). Social life and relationships with friends of the family are often based on shared activities, which changed dramatically following the cardiac episode.

Some older couples had retired earlier than expected. Several spouses returned to work to manage financial constraint and assumed responsibility for income generation. Caregiving responsibilities forced others to terminate paid employment. In another study, working spouses of MI survivors perceived more stresses related to responsibility and economics than non-working spouses did (Collins, White-Williams, & Jalowiec, 1996).

Stress of Illness for MI Survivor: The emotional impact of heart disease on survivors ranged from denial and confusion at the outset to subsequent frustration and irritability. Fear and uncertainty emerged from their perceived loss of control. Adjustment to MI necessitated radical changes in survivors' self-care and lifestyle in our study.

Survivors found it difficult to access appropriate information. To illustrate, inadequate or conflicting information about resumption of sexual relations and related side-effects of medications created concerns. Lack of emotional support from health professionals also generated stress for some survivors.

The need to modify normal activities and tasks created conflict between spouses and survivors. Overprotectiveness by the spouse was another key stressor for survivors. In another study, perceived spousal overprotectiveness was positively associated with survivors' anxiety and depression and negatively correlated with their quality of life (Clarke et al., 1996). In our study, withdrawal and negative reactions by friends had a detrimental impact on social routines.

The prospect of returning to work raised survivors' concerns about their energy levels and their ability to concentrate and manage pressure. Financial constraint was a related worry.

Strategies Used by Participants to Cope with MI

Emotion-focused coping strategies included personal time out and adjustment of expectations following the MI. Seeking informational support was a key problem-focused coping strategy. Couples endorsed 'active engagement' (i.e., mutual problem solving and communication) as a relationship-focused coping strategy. Some caregiving spouses spoke of protecting their partner from stressful information and from parenting demands. 'Protective buffering' was also evident among some survivors, who kept threatening information from their spouses.

Social Support and Support Needs

During group meetings, although members described salient support from their social network and health professionals, they also reported stressful interactions and absent support in these relationships. Physicians were the main source of informational support about the MI. Participants received empathy and understanding from family, friends, and colleagues. Family, friends, and faith in God generated comfort (i.e., emotional support). Two survivors socialized with other 'heart attack victims' (peers). Instrumental (i.e., practical) support was rarely mentioned.

Some survivors exhibited negative reactions, such as resentment and frustration, to their spouses' caregiving. These helping efforts were construed as overprotectiveness or misplaced concern. Participants often perceived interactions with health professionals as non-supportive, and relationships with friends sometimes became stressful following the MI. Moreover, support for spouses was absent or inadequate.

In summary, the stress incurred by uncontrollable situations, the predominant use of seeking support and positive reappraisal as coping strategies, and inadequate support from professionals for these first-time-admitted survivors reinforced the findings of the prior assessment study.

Support Intervention Processes

Social Comparison

Group members compared coping strategies for dealing with health professionals, dietary changes, emotional reactions, and modifications in activity. Social comparison reassured spouses and survivors that they were managing well, that others encountered the same situations, and that they were 'normal.' '*I think [I compared] my feelings of anger ... I was so relieved to see this coming out in them [other participants] because nowhere had I read that you could be angry*' (survivor). Peer leaders often described situations similar to those experienced by members.

Downward social comparison led participants to perceive that their stressful situations (e.g., symptoms, difficulties with children, finances) were 'not so bad.' Positive framing, in turn, fostered beliefs that they were managing these situations effectively. Moreover, comparison helped participants to understand and accept their own situation and to appreciate the circumstances of others.

Social Learning

Participants gained insight into their behaviour through members' role modelling and exchange of experiential knowledge regarding coping strategies and lifestyle management. A few participants learned more from peers than from professionals because of the common experience and user-friendly information available from members and peer leaders. Some participants learned about themselves by observing the behaviour of group members and peer leaders (vicarious learning). Survivors and family caregivers gained a new appreciation for their spouse's point of view. '*I guess I suddenly realized how much care and concern I have been to my spouse and am relieved that I have returned to a normal routine part time and alleviated some of his concerns and worry*' (survivor).

Reciprocity/Social Exchange

Participants shared information, common concerns, and potential solutions, and exchanged support within the group. There was a strong sense of mutuality and equality. '*I think there was equality actually involved in everything. That we grew to respect each others views, which is good*' (spouse).

Social Support Provided by Group Intervention

According to the participants, the key types of support provided by the group were informational support, affirmational support, and emotional support.

Informational Support

Scientific explanations focused on causes of MI, prognosis, diet, side-effects of medications, exercise, and so forth, seemed to be received more favourably when delivered by a professional. Peer leaders and group members, however, were other important sources of informational support. Peer leaders provided understandable and realistic information about dealing with conflict and intimacy, relaxing, dieting, and returning to work. '*I got a lot of information that I was unaware of. It really educated me ... I didn't know half or even one-quarter of what I learned there*' (spouse).

Affirmational Support

Positive feedback emanated from group members, peer leaders, and guest speakers. Affirmation helped to decrease survivors' uncertainty regarding resumption of activities and reassured spouses that the negative reactions of the survivor were not their fault. All participants were relieved that they were not alone in their experiences. '*We have felt the emotional upheaval and it's good to hear that other couples have as well; it's normal or typical*' (spouse).

Emotional Support

Peer facilitators offered reassurance and hope, and members demonstrated concern for others' difficulties. Some participants identified friendship with members as a key benefit of the intervention. Furthermore, survivors and spouses felt understood by group members. '*The verbal sharing of the experience of dealing with my husband's heart attack, how it affected me, my fears, my frustrations, the impact on my family and their reaction. This was good support in realizing others shared a similar experience and understood'* (spouse).

Instrumental Support

This type of support was rarely mentioned. On one occasion transportation was arranged for a participant.

Perceived Impact of the Intervention (Qualitative)

During the post-intervention interviews, all participants indicated that they were satisfied with the face-to-face support groups for couples. Participants referred to the positive impact of the intervention on their coping, spousal relationship, confidence, and outlook.

Enhanced Coping

All groups discussed different ways of managing negative feelings. Almost 50 per cent of participants indicated that they had changed their coping strategics as a direct result of information gained through the support groups. Moreover, the intervention enabled participants to seek more information from their health care providers (i.e., support seeking). Members also learned to manage lifestyle adjustments, such as returning to work and ensuring a balance between pre-MI existence and health maintenance. This study reinforces previous research that revealed that support groups for persons living with cardiac conditions can enhance coping ability (Hildingh, Fridlunch, & Segesten, 1995). *'I am actively trying with my wife and other people to tell them how I feel when they ask. And I find it makes life better for me and hopefully those around me'* (survivor). *'I am coping with a decrease in productivity, decreased level of excellence, and the ability to say "no" to many requests ... One other member returned to a stressful position on a part time basis, and has encouraged me to take my time returning to normal hours and workload'* (survivor).

Improved Relationship with Spouse

The relationship between MI survivor and spouse benefited from the survivor's assuming increased responsibility for his/her health and self-care. (This fact is significant, given the association between diminished acceptance of responsibility and MI survivors' readmission to hospital found in our earlier assessment study.) The support group expanded participants' awareness that their spouses were also affected by the MI. Clearly, relational adjustments were needed. The opportunity to hear the spouse's perspective greatly enhanced communication, understanding, and acceptance within the dyad. '*Because of the fear, between the two of us, there has been a great lack of communication. The program has ... brought us together. It has taught the two of us to understand each other a bit better*' (spouse).

Increased Confidence

Following the intervention, participants expressed more confidence about making suitable nutrition choices, maintaining an exercise program, dealing with the health care system, and managing day-to-day life. '*You just felt that you had more information, and so you felt more comfortable with what you were doing, based on the information received*' (survivor).

Change in Perspectives and Priorities

The intervention altered the survivors' and spouses' outlook on life and perspectives on managing the MI. '*Through the meetings, we have learned that ... is the human thing [reaction] after a heart attack. And you deal with it, like your life ... It [the support group] made a lot of difference in our lives*' (spouse).

The quantitative data elicited by the standardized measures revealed changes in support need and satisfaction, network size, negative affect, and protective buffering coping.

Impact of the Intervention (Quantitative)

Spouse and Survivor Combined

Overall, spouses' and survivors' scores revealed changes in the expected direction for self-efficacy, perceived adequacy of information, negative affect, and support need and satisfaction. It is noteworthy that there was a significant decrease in guidance support need and a corresponding increase in guidance support satisfaction. A significant reduction in perceived network size was observed. Although unexpected, this finding is potentially explained by the significant decrease in network conflict and in actual network size. In addition, there were notable changes in the composition of social networks, in particular, an increase in friends and a decrease in physicians and family members identified as supporters.

Spouses

There was a significant reduction in spouses' actual network size from pre-test to post-test. This reduction was supported by an associated (albeit non-significant) decrease in perceived network size and network conflict. Spouses reported a significant increase in total support satisfaction and guidance support satisfaction and a significant reduction in feedback support need. As hypothesized, there was a significant decrease in negative affect ($p = 0.05$) and protective buffering coping ($p = 0.01$) among spouses following the intervention.

Survivors

The impact of the intervention on MI survivors was less clear. Although changes in outcome measures were generally in the anticipated direction, only two factors were statistically significant. A significant decrease in guidance support need was observed. Survivors also reported a significant decrease in actual network size. This change may be explained, in part, by another study, which revealed that the match between social support wanted and received diminished and support satisfaction decreased over time in males following MI (Riegel & Gocka, 1995).

Summary

There were significant differences from pre- to post-test: satisfaction with guidance support increased; need for guidance support decreased; perceived and actual network size decreased; and actual conflict in the network decreased. The fact that spouses reported decreased protective buffering following the intervention is important, because protective buffering has been linked to negative outcomes for survivors in other research. For example, low self-efficacy in MI survivors was attributed to excessive protective buffering (overprotection) by spouses (Coyne & Smith, 1991). In another study, perceived overprotectiveness was positively correlated with survivors' anxiety and depression and negatively correlated with their quality of life, adaptation, and functional recovery (Clarke et al., 1996). During the post-intervention interview, many participants maintained that the program had had a positive impact on their relationship with their spouse.

The diminished network size following the intervention can be interpreted in part by reduction in conflict in the network and in part by changes in social network composition. In another study, spousal overprotectiveness was linked to MI survivors' perceptions of criticism by spouses (i.e., conflicted interaction) and dissatisfaction with family relationships (Clarke et al., 1996). Family, neighbour, and physician support decreased, while support from friends increased following the termination of the support groups. During the interviews, participants identified friendship as a benefit of the intervention. It is noteworthy that health professionals rarely were spontaneously named as supporters; this is a common finding in other research (Dakof & Taylor, 1990; Norbeck, 1988). Our earlier assessment study revealed increased professional support only for those who had repeat admissions to hospital for cardiac illness. The support groups may have offered substitute sources of support, particularly since these participants, living with a first MI, often recounted inadequate or stressful interactions with health professionals. Alternatively, the need for professional support may have diminished as physical recovery progressed. Finally, survivors and spouses may have dropped from their network people who were sources of conflict and miscarried helping efforts.

Clearly, the intervention met spouses' and survivors' needs for guidance and feedback support, as indicated by decreased need for these two support functions and increased satisfaction with guidance support. Thus, the informational and affirmational support provided by both professionals and peers seemed to be particularly effective. Group members, peer facilitators, and guest speakers provided positive feedback, and peer facilitators, offered guidance on dealing with conflict and intimacy, relaxing, dieting, and returning to work.

Key Findings from the Intervention Study

Qualitative

- Impact on the relationship with the spouse:
  - improved communication
  - enhanced comprehension of spouse's perspective
  - increased understanding and acceptance
- Expanded coping repertoire
- Increased confidence

- Change in perspective and priorities
- Skills learned

Quantitative
- Support need ↓
- Support satisfaction ↑
- Social network size ↓
- Conflict in network ↓
- Negative affect ↓
- Protective buffering coping ↓

Lessons Learned

While most participants were satisfied with the informational support provided by groups, some wanted more information about diet, exercise, stress, communication skills, and sexual intimacy. In this context, those support groups that invited professional resource people (e.g., dietitians, pharmacists) to some sessions received particularly positive feedback during post-intervention interviews.

The success of this group intervention can be attributed, in part, to the fact that the content of discussions could be controlled by participants. One professional facilitator said: '*I know I sort of relaxed after the first three or four sessions and kind of almost instinctively knew the next session is going to go okay ... I relaxed and allowed the group to work the process themselves.*'

Leadership was another critical factor in the optimum functioning of these support groups. Participants expressed considerable satisfaction with co-peer and professional leadership. The leadership typically fluctuated between the peers and the professionals. On occasions when some groups relied more on the professional leaders, however, social comparison, learning, and exchange seemed to be inhibited. The joint interview of peer and professional facilitators revealed a consensus concerning the benefits of balanced leadership and an egalitarian relationship. '*I think that it's like anything in life; if you've had some experience with the problem, you bring a different perspective to it in some ways*' (professional facilitator).

The similarity of group members also influenced the impact of the intervention. Some participants believed that members of their group were too different in background and experience to permit exchange of experiential knowledge. The size of the group was another important ingredient in success; the smallest group had difficulty in maintaining the momentum of discussion. Finally, several leaders and participants contended that the groups could have continued beyond the pre-specified twelve weeks. '*These people ... were so anxious to see something continued, and whether we could take some initiative to continue meeting like we had been doing. Every time I see them they're saying "Can we start something? Can we meet?" They're ... very keenly interested to continue*' (professional facilitator).

Lessons Learned

- Increased information is desirable in support interventions.
- Similarity in age and circumstances is important.
- Consistent balance between peer and professional facilitators is needed.

Implications for Policy and Programs

Age is a major risk factor for coronary artery disease. This has important implications because of Canada's ageing population and decreasing resources available for support. There is clear evidence that the clinical treatment of coronary disease events is effective in reducing mortality. Consequently, while there is no real change in incidence, the prevalence of the disease is rapidly accelerating, in association with the ageing population. As people get older, however, their peers disappear and their capacity to obtain help is impaired. Coupled with the demographics of the baby boomers and the predictability of support deficits, the need for support systems is clear.

According to the ICONS study in Nova Scotia and other studies, women caregivers who have a coronary event experience delayed admission to hospital and increased mortality, perhaps because social support systems for caregivers and for the elderly are deteriorating. In this context, important gender factors need to be addressed. As the disease is increasing in prevalence in the female population, particularly among the elderly, unique support strategies for older women should be created. Undoubtedly, the kind of support that a young working male needs is vastly different from that required by an eighty-five-year-old female.

The traditional term 'risk factors for cardiovascular disease' suggests that people have made bad choices. This negative connotation not only neglects support deficiencies as a determinant but is an important deterrent to treatment.

Finally, it should be emphasized that although the prognosis in cardiac illness has improved, attributable primarily to advances in clinical therapy, support systems for MI survivors and their spouses have not improved. With the marked increase of prevalence, government policies should reflect the fact that preventive programs do not make the disease disappear; they simply delay its onset. For all these reasons, support programs and supportive policies for survivors and family caregivers are essential.

Acknowledgments

The assessment study was funded by the Nova Scotia Heart and Stroke Foundation, and the intervention study was supported through a grant from the Cardiac Prevention Research Centre.

Note

Results of the initial assessment investigation were partially reported in a peer-reviewed publication: Stewart, Hirth, Klassen, Makrides, & Wolf (1997).

References

Alonzo, A., & Reynolds, N. (1995). Responding to symptoms and signs of acute myocardial infarction, how do you educate the public? A social psychological approach to intervention. Paper presented at the Annual Meeting of the Pacific Sociological Association, 6–9 April, San Francisco, CA.

Beach, E., Maloney, B., Plocica, A., Sherry, S., Weaver, M., Luthringer, L., & Utz, S. (1992). The spouse: A factor in recovery after acute myocardial infarction. *Heart & Lung, 21*(1), 30–38.

Ben-Sira, Z., & Eliezer, R. (1990). The structure of readjustment after heart attack. *Social Science & Medicine, 30*, 523–536.

Bloom, J. (1990). The relationship of social support and health. *Social Science & Medicine, 39*(5), 635–637.

Clarke, D., Walker, J., & Cuddy, T. (1996). The role of perceived overprotectiveness in recovery 3 months after myocardial infarction. *Journal of Cardiopulmonary Rehabilitation, 16*(6), 372–377.

Collins, E.G., White-Williams, C., & Jalowiec, A. (1996). Spouse stressors while awaiting heart transplantation. *Journal of Acute and Critical Care, 25*(1), 4–13.

Conn, V., Taylor, S., & Abele, P. (1991). Myocardial infarction survivors: Age and gender differences in physical health, psychosocial state and regimen adherence. *Journal of Advanced Nursing, 16*, 1026–1034.

Coyne, J., & Fiske, V. (1992). Couples coping with chronic illness. In T.J. Akamatsu, J.C. Crowther, S.C. Hobfoll, & M.A.P. Stevens (Eds), *Family health psychology*. Washington, DC: Hemisphere.

Coyne, J., & Smith, D. (1991). Couples coping with a myocardial infarction: A contextual perspective on wives' distress. *Journal of Perspectives on Social Psychology, 61*(3), 404–412.

Dakof, G., & Taylor, S. (1990). Victims' perceptions of social support: What is helpful from whom? *Journal of Personality and Social Psychology, 58*(1), 80–89.

Faller, H. (1990). Coping with myocardial infarction: A cognitive-emotional perspective. *Psychotherapy Psychosomatic, 54*(1), 8–17.

Fontana, A., Kerns, R., Rosenberg, R., & Colenese, K. (1989). Support, stress and recovery from coronary heart disease: A longitudinal causal model. *Health Psychology, 8*(2), 175–193.

Frasure-Smith, N. (1991). In-hospital symptoms of psychological stress as predictors of long-term outcome after acute myocardial infarction in men. *American Journal of Cardiology, 67*(1), 121–127.

Frasure-Smith, N., & Prince, R. (1989). Long-term follow-up of the ischemic heart disease life stress monitoring program. *Psychosomatic Medicine, 51*, 485–513.

Gorkin, L, Schron, E., Brooks, M., Wiklund, I., Kelen, J., Verter, J., Schoenberger, J., Pawitan, Y., Morris, M., & Shumaker, S. (1993). Psychosocial predictors of mortality in the cardiac arrythmia suppression trial-1 (CAST-1). *American Journal of Cardiology, 71*, 263–267.

Heart and Stroke Foundation of Canada (1997). *Heart disease and stroke in Canada.* Ottawa: HDSC.

Helgeson V. (1991). The effects of masculinity and social support on recovery from myocardial infarction. *Psychosomatic Medicine, 53*, 621–633.

Helgeson, V. (1993). Two important distinctions in social support: Kind of support and perceived versus received. *Journal of Applied Social Psychology, 23*(10), 825–845.

Hilbert, G. (1996). Cardiac couples at hospitalization and 3 months later. *Journal of Family Nursing, 2*(1), 76–91.

Hildingh, C., Fridlund, B., & Segesten, K. (1995). Social support in self-help groups, as experienced by persons having coronary disease and their next of kind. *International Journal of Nursing Studies, 32*(3), 224–232.

Hudson, C. (1994). The relationship between coping responses and social support post-myocardial ischemic event: A comparison of males and females. Unpublished MN thesis, Dalhousie University.

Johnson, J., & Morse, J. (1990). Regaining control: The process of adjustment after myocardial infarction. *Heart & Lung, 19*(2), 126–135.

Kaplan R., & Toshima T. (1990). The functional effects of social relationships on chronic illnesses and disability. In B. Sarason, I. Sarason, & G. Pierce (Eds) *Social support: An interactional view* (421–453). New York: Wiley.

Keckeisen, M., & Nyamathi, A. (1990). Coping and adjustment to illness in the acute myocardial infarction patient. *Journal of Cardiovascular Nursing, 5*(1), 25–33.

Keeling, A.W., & Dennison, P.D. (1995). Nurse-initiated telephone follow-up after acute myocardial infarction: A pilot study. *Heart & Lung, 24*(1), 45–49.

Krakauer, H. & Jacoby, I. (1993). Predicting the course of disease. *Inquiry, 30*(2), 115–127.

Krikevold, M., Gortner, S.R., Berg, K., & Saltvold, S. (1996). Patterns of recovery among Norwegian heart surgery patients. *Journal of Advanced Nursing, 24*(5), 943–951.

LaGaipa, J. (1990). The negative effects of informal support systems. In S. Duck (Ed.), *Personal relationships and social support* (122–139). London: Sage.

Lazarus, R., & Folkman, S. (1984). *Stress appraisal and coping.* New York: Springer.

Lesperance, F., Frasure-Smith, N., & Talajic, M. (1996). Major depression before and after myocardial infarction: Its nature and consequences. *Psychosomatic Medicine, 58*, 99–110.

Levine, J., Covino, N., Slack, C., Safran, D., Boro, J., Davis, R., Buchanan, M., & Gervino, E. (1996). Psychological predictors of subsequent medical care among patients hospitalized with cardiac disease. *Journal of Cardiopulmonary Rehabilitation, 16*(2), 109–16.

Linden, B. (1995). Evaluation of a home-based rehabilitation programme for patients recovering from acute myocardial infarction. *Intensive and Critical Care Nursing, 11*(1), 10–19.

Markle-Reid, M. (1989). Social support and perception of illness in the early discharge phase for the MI patient. *Canadian Journal of Cardiovascular Nursing, 1*(2), 9–18.

Martin, D., & Lee, H. (1992). Indicators of active and passive coping in myocardial infarction victims. *Journal of Gerontology, 47*(4), 238–241.

McCauley, K. (1990). The relationship between causal attributions and adjustment and coping in patients following a myocardial infarction. PhD thesis, University of Pennsylvania.

Miller, P., McMahon, M., Garrett, M., & Ringel, K. (1989). A content analysis of life adjustments post-infarction. *Western Journal of Nursing Research, 11*, 559–560.

Monahan, D., Kohman, L., & Coleman, M. (1996). Heart surgery: Consequences for caregivers. *Journal of Gerontological Social Work, 25*(3), 53–70.

Moser, D.K. (1994). Social support and cardiac recovery. *Journal of Cardiovascular Nursing, 9*(1), 27–36.

Nolan, R., & Wielgosz, A. (1991). Assessing adaptive and maladaptive coping in the early phase of acute myocardial infarction. *Journal of Behavioral Medicine, 14*(2), 111–124.

Norbeck, J.S. (1988). Social support. *Annual Review of Nursing Research, 6*, 85–109.

Norbeck, J., Lindsey, A., & Carrier, V. (1983). The development of an instrument to measure social support. *Nursing Research, 30*, 264–169.

Riegel, B., & Dracup, K. (1992). Social support and cardiac invalidism following acute myocardial infarction. *National Critical Care Nursing Research Conference Research Abstracts, 21*(3), 298.

Riegel, B., & Gocka, I. (1995). Gender differences in adjustment to acute myocardial infarction. *Heart and Lung: Journal of Critical Care, 24*(6), 457–466.

Rodeman, B., Conn, V., & Rose, S. (1995). Myocardial infarction survivors: Social support and self-care behaviors. *Rehabilitation Nursing Research, 4*(2), 58–71.

Rost, K., & Smith, R. (1992). Return to work after an initial myocardial infarction and subsequent emotional distress. *Archives of International Medicine, 152*, 381–385.

Scherck, K. (1992). Coping with acute myocardial infarction. *Heart and Lung, 21*(4), 327–334.

Silver, R., Wortman, C., & Crofton, C. (1990). The role of coping in support provision: The self presentational dilemma of victims of life crises. In B. Sarason, I. Sarason, & G. Pierce (Eds), *Social support: An interactional view* (397–426). New York: Wiley.

Stewart, M., Hirth, A., Klassen, G., Makrides, L. & Wolf, H. (1997). Stress, coping and social support as factors in readmissions for ischemic heart disease. *International Journal of Nursing Studies, 34*(2), 151–163.

Terry D. (1992). Stress, coping and coping resources as correlates of adaptation in myocardial infarction patients. *British Journal of Clinical Psychology, 31*, 215–225.

Thompson, D. (1991). Effects of in-hospital counselling on knowledge in myocardial infarction patients and spouses. *Patient Education and Counselling, 18*(2), 1171–1177.

Thompson, D., & Cordle C.J. (1988). Support of wives of myocardial infarction patients. *Journal of Advanced Nursing, 13*, 223–228.

Thompson, D., & Meddis, R. (1990). A prospective evaluation of in-hospital counselling for first-time myocardial infarction men. *Journal of Psychosomatic Research, 34*(3), 237–248.

Thompson, D., Webster, R., & Meddis, R. (1990). In-hospital counselling for first-time myocardial infarction patients and spouses: Effects on satisfaction. *Journal of Advanced Nursing, 15*(9), 1064–1069.

Thompson, D., Ersser, S., & Webster, R. (1995). The experiences of patients and their partners one month after a heart attack. *Journal of Advanced Nursing, 22*, 707–714.

Webster, K., & Christman, N. (1988). Perceived uncertainty and coping post myocardial infarction. *Western Journal of Nursing Research, 10*(4), 384–440.

Williams, R., Barefoot, J., Califf, R., Haney, T., Saunders, W., Pryor, D., Hlatky, M., Siegler, I., & Mark, D. (1992). Prognostic importance of social and economic resources among medically treated patients with angiographically documented coronary artery disease. *Journal of the American Medical Association, 267*(4), 520–524.

Winefield, H., & Katsikitis, M. (1987). Medical professional support and cardiac rehabilitation of males and females. *Journal of Psychosomatic Research, 31*(5), 567–573.

5

Overcoming the Loneliness of Hemophiliacs with AIDS and Their Caregivers through Telephone Support

Miriam J. Stewart, Geraldine Hart, and Karen Mann

Abstract. The support needs of persons with hemophilia and HIV/AIDS and their family caregivers have been neglected in research, despite the fact that almost one-half of hemophiliacs in the United States and Canada were infected with HIV. Therefore, we conducted an assessment study of the AIDS-related stresses, coping strategies, support, and support needs of HIV-infected hemophiliacs (n = 30), family caregivers (n = 23), and bereaved family caregivers (n = 17). This study revealed that participants experienced loneliness because of prejudice, insensitivity, avoidance, and isolating behaviours by family, friends, and professionals. Furthermore, the fear of stigma and the perceived need to preserve confidentiality diminished their willingness to seek support. Although participants expressed a preference for support groups composed of peers, their geographic dispersion limited the accessibility of face-to-face support interventions. Participants also recommended shared peer-professional leadership. Accordingly, we created telephone support groups co-led by a professional and a peer in the follow-up intervention study.

The telephone intervention provided emotional, informational, and affirmational support. Participants expressed great satisfaction with the telephone support groups and wanted them to continue beyond the originally prescribed twelve weeks. Sessions lasted up to two hours, rather than the planned forty-five minutes. There were statistically significant changes in the desired direction in support satisfaction and support needs. Furthermore, caregivers reported enhanced confidence and coping and diminished loneliness and isolation, and affected men described changes in coping behaviours and reduced emotional isolation. These trends, although statistically non-significant because of the small sample, were reinforced in the qualitative results. Future telephone support groups for people with AIDS and their family caregivers should be longer in duration.

Introduction

The World Health Organization predicts that by the year 2000 the number of adults and children infected with human immunodeficiency virus (HIV) will triple from the current 9–11 million to 30–40 million (World Health Organization, 1991). In 1995 Health Canada reported 11,377 cases of AIDS and 8,204 deaths related to AIDS. The number of reported new AIDS cases for clotting factor recipients (n = 117) and for blood transfusion recipients (n = 585) represented 3 per cent of the total population of adult males with AIDS. Children and adult males with hemophilia who were infected by tainted blood products prior to 1985 are now HIV positive or have developed or died from AIDS.

The prevalence of HIV infection increases with the severity of hemophilia. Fifty per cent of persons with hemophilia in the United States were infected with HIV (Hall, 1994), while in Canada, HIV/AIDS affected at least 40 per cent of the country's estimated 2,300 hemophiliacs (Canadian Hemophilia Clinic Directors Group, 1993; Dunn, 1993). At the time of the assessment study reported here, approximately 1,000 Canadians with hemophilia had been infected with HIV; approximately 100 had developed AIDS or HIV-related symptoms; and 200 had died from AIDS. This group of boys and men is supported predominantly by family caregivers and lives in traditional nuclear families. Two Canadian studies of persons with hemophilia and AIDS, including the assessment study described in this chapter (Hart, Mann, & Stewart, 1991; Lamping, 1991), revealed the loneliness and social isolation that persons with AIDS (PWA) and hemophilia and their family caregivers experience. The prevalence of loneliness reflects their needs for support.

Support Needs of Persons with AIDS and Family Caregivers

The literature illuminates both the importance of social support for persons living with AIDS and also their support deficits. Most PWA in one study had less than two sources of close support, and men at risk for HIV via heterosexual contact relied on traditional family sources of support (Smith & Rapkin, 1996). Barriers to support for PWA include interpersonal costs, negative interactions, fear of disclosure, and inadequate access, acceptance, and intimacy (Smith & Rapkin, 1996); social stigma, isolation, family members' health problems, and survivors' emotional exhaustion, and removal from non-supportive relations (Johnston, Stall, & Smith, 1995). Clearly, PWA have substantial unmet needs for support (Wight, LeBlanc, & Aneshensel, 1995). This deficit is problematic because persons with life-threatening illnesses such as AIDS, who are less satisfied with social support, are less hopeful, and experience more severe stressors, are more vulnerable to emotional distress (Servellen, Sarna, Padilla, & Brecht, 1996).

AIDS also has a devastating impact on the supportive resources and social network structure of confidants and caregivers of PWA (Jankowski, Videka-Sherman, & Laquidara-Dickinson, 1996). Caregivers of children with HIV/AIDS reported low support. Furthermore, social support, along with hostility, predicted 37 per cent of the variance in caregiving impact, and social support predicted 17.5 per cent of the variance in their perceived caregiving competence (Hughes & Caliandro, 1996). Bereaved caregivers of PWA reported lower levels of social support than cancer-bereaved individuals and a greater number of bereavements. Furthermore, they were more likely to conceal the cause of death from significant others, and they perceived greater rejection from others (Kelly, Lawrence, Smith, Hood, & Cook, 1987). Clearly, caregivers of PWA also have major needs for support (Wight et al., 1995).

A review of the literature on social support and HIV/AIDS from 1985 to 1995 indicated that no articles were focused on hemophiliacs with HIV/AIDS or their family caregivers, with the exception of our assessment study of the support needs of persons with hemophilia and HIV/AIDS, family caregivers, and bereaved family caregivers (Stewart, Hart, & Mann, 1995). This study revealed the need for a support group intervention.

Support Group Interventions for Persons with AIDS and Caregivers

Support interventions can decrease conflict, create new sources of support (Barrera, 1991), or alleviate social isolation (Maguire, 1991) and loneliness. Although support groups for PWA and their families had been reported at the time of our intervention study (Fawzy, Namir, & Wolcott, 1989; Frierson, Lippman, & Johnson, 1987; Getzel & Mahoney, 1989; Kelly & Sykes, 1989; Levy, Tendler, Van Devanter, & Cleary, 1990; Posey, 1988; Wong & Forrister, 1989), they were face-to-face groups, which were not accessible for geographically and socially isolated persons, and they emphasized the needs of homosexuals and illegal drug users. Four more recent support group interventions pertinent to PWA were focused on health professional caregivers (Lego, 1994), bereaved caregivers (Sikkema, Kalichman, Kelly, & Koob, 1995), people in institutional settings or half-way houses (Daniolos, 1994), and HIV donors (Cleary, Van Devanter, Steilen, Stuart, Shipton-Levy, McMullen, Rogers, Singer, Avorn, & Pindyck, 1995). The latter emphasized changes in sexual behaviour solely.

The few reported support group interventions for PWA point to their potential impact on coping and health outcomes. For instance, one short-term support group enabled HIV-infected persons and PWA to cope with psychological, social, and medical hardships and resulted in better adherence to treatment and improved psychological symptoms (Weishut, 1996). A support group for bereaved caregivers of PWA led to reduced depression, grief reactions, intrusive experiences, demoralization, and psychological distress (Sikkema et al., 1995). Another study pointed to the factors influencing impact. Gay men with HIV/AIDS who participated in support groups on a long-term basis had less access to other social networks and more interest in emotional support; those who participated for a short time had greater access to alternative support networks and more interest in illness-related information and coping strategies (Sandstrom, 1996).

All support group interventions for PWA were facilitated by professionals alone, and none was designed for hemophiliacs with HIV/AIDS and their family caregivers. We therefore tested a telephone support group intervention that was predicted to lower their risk of loneliness and social isolation and enhance their ability to cope with stresses.

Fit with Framework

The assessment study was based on a conceptualization of social support as a coping resource or source of assistance in coping with stressful situations (Folkman, Chesney, McKusick, Ironson, Johnson, & Coates, 1991) associated with hemophilia and HIV/AIDS, and caregiving (see figure 5.1). Social support and coping are mediators of the stress process involved in AIDS (Pearlin, Semple, & Turner, 1988). Coping strategies, both problem focused and emotion focused, can influence the type and quality of support received and the maintenance of social relationships (Pearlin, 1991).

Drawbacks of support, such as conflicted interactions, miscarried helping (Coyne, Ellard, & Smith, 1990), and inadequate support, can be stressful for persons with HIV/AIDS and their family caregivers. The costs of support include over-involvement and burden for providers (e.g., family caregivers), and diminished self-esteem for recipients (La Gaipa, 1990), such as men with hemophilia and HIV/AIDS. AIDS can be a major chronic stressor, involving loss of social contacts, depleted support resources, and estrangement of affected men or family caregivers from their social networks (Hobfoll & Freedy, 1990).

In the intervention study, social support was conceptualized as interactions with family members, friends, health professionals, and peers that can improve coping, moderate the impact of stressors associated with HIV/AIDS, and alleviate loneliness and isolation. *Loneliness* is a subjective, unpleasant experience resulting from a perceived deficiency in social relationships or relational provisions. Rook (1984) claims that loneliness is 'an enduring con-

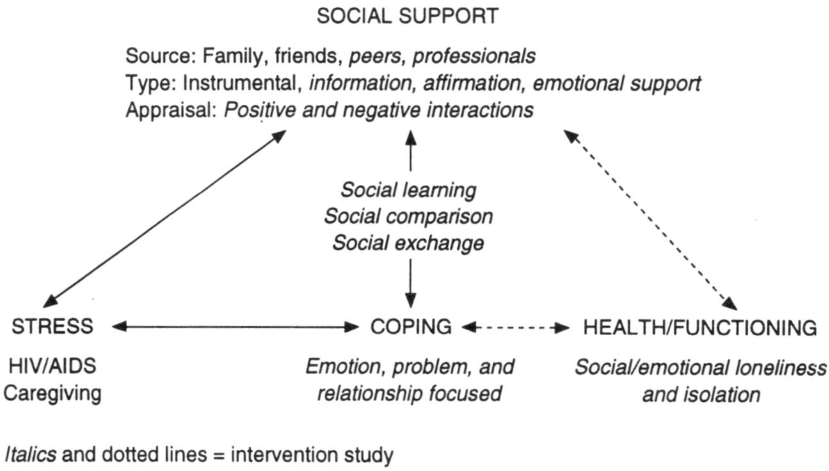

Figure 5.1 Framework for Assessment and Intervention Studies Focused on Adults with AIDS

dition of emotional distress that arises when a person feels estranged from, misunderstood, or rejected by others and/or lacks appropriate social partners for desired activities, particularly activities that provide a sense of social integration and opportunities for emotional intimacy.' Weiss (1974) distinguishes between the loneliness of emotional isolation and social isolation. Social support can prevent and redress both forms of loneliness and isolation.

In the intervention study, a telephone support group was created to enhance and supplement the depleted, strained natural networks of persons with hemophilia and HIV/AIDS and those of their family caregivers, and to alleviate their loneliness. Solomon, Waysman, & Mikulincer (1990) concluded that perceived support promoted mental health indirectly through its impact on loneliness. We predicted that loneliness, conceived as an indicator of mental health, should be decreased by the indirect impact of the telephone support group on the stress associated with HIV/AIDS and caregiving.

Three mediating processes were anticipated within the telephone support groups. The process of *social comparison* occurs in mutual aid groups. Feedback from peers can validate and normalize, particularly important effects in conditions evoking stigma (e.g., HIV/AIDS). Norms of *social exchange* suggest that support should be bidirectional (Tilden & Gaylen, 1987). However, ill persons and family caregivers frequently encounter non-egalitarian, nonreciprocal relationships (Stewart, 1993). Support reciprocity has been associated with diminished loneliness (Rook, 1987) in self-help group members (Maton, 1987). *Social-learning* theory can interpret behaviour and cognitive change mechanisms and influences on coping in support groups. Peers, viewed as role models, elicit and enhance experiential knowledge, based on first-hand experience (Borkman, 1976, 1982), which can be distinguished from information relayed by professionals. In the intervention study, support groups of peers were created, co-led by a peer and professional.

Assessment Study: Support Needs

Research Questions

The five research questions focused on (1) AIDS-related stresses, (2) coping strategies, (3) types and sources of support, (4) evaluation of support, and (5) support needs of HIV-infected hemophiliacs and their family caregivers.

Sample

Those eligible to participate were male hemophiliacs over eighteen years of age who were in the later stages of HIV infection (i.e., they had experienced symptoms) or who had developed AIDS and family caregivers and bereaved family caregivers of males with hemophilia and HIV/AIDS.

There were seventy participants in the first phase of this study. Thirty persons with hemophilia and AIDS or HIV-related illness were interviewed (mean age = 32.4 years, range = 19–56 years). Seventeen were married. Twenty-three family caregivers participated (mean age = 38.5 years, range = 27–67 years). Sixteen caregivers were spouses of the person with hemophilia and seven were parents. Seventeen bereaved family caregivers were interviewed (mean age = 47.8 years, range = 24–71). Over one-third (35 per cent) of affected men and family caregivers lived in rural areas. Of the original seventy interviewees, fifty-six persons participated in the second phase of the study, yielding a response rate of 80 per cent – affected persons (n = 21), family caregivers (n = 19), and bereaved family caregivers (n = 16). (Two persons with AIDS had died during the interval between the first and second stages.)

Methodology

The study was conducted in two phases: phase 1 comprised individual interviews; phase 2 involved mailed questionnaires.

Phase 1

The individual interviews were focused on specific needs for support pertaining to AIDS-related stressors, particular sources and types of support, and appraisal of support received. Although similar interview guides were developed by the researchers for affected persons, family caregivers, and bereaved caregivers to enhance consistency, they were modified to reflect the different stressors likely to be experienced by each group. A panel of professional and lay consultants from the Canadian Hemophilia Society reviewed and revised the guides, which were then pilot tested and further modified. The semi-structured interview guides elicited information about (1) the most stressful AIDS-related situation experienced by participants; (2) coping strategies used to manage this stressful situation; (3) availability of informational, practical, emotional, and affirmational support; (4) sources of each type of support; (5) satisfaction with support received; (6) negative interactions; and (7) needs for support. The investigators reviewed the recorded qualitative data from the interviews, identified emergent themes, and developed a category system inductively from the data. Inter-rater reliability for selecting units and coding data was required to be 80 per cent or higher.

Phase 2

In the second stage, a questionnaire was developed, based on the themes found in the interview data and mailed to respondents from phase 1. The thirty items in the questionnaire elicited information about the frequency with which the respondent used specific coping strategies; the impact of managing a pre-existing chronic illness (hemophilia) on the respondent's ability to cope with this new illness; types and sources of support, negative experiences related to support, problems in seeking support (e.g., concerns about confidentiality), satisfaction with each type of support, preferred sources of varied types of support, and needs for specific types and sources of support (e.g., support groups). This questionnaire asked respondents to indicate their level of agreement with the interpretations of the interview data, thereby yielding a clearer understanding of the consensus of this sample regarding support experiences and needs as well as coping strategies.

Frequency distributions and proportions of responses were examined, as were means and standard deviations. Responses and rankings by PWA, caregivers, and bereaved caregivers were compared. Statistical techniques included analyses of variance, Students' *t*-test and chi square analyses. The research design is summarized in table 5.1.

TABLE 5.1
Research Design

	Assessment Study			Intervention Study
		Phase 1	*Phase 2*	
Sample	Hemophiliacs with HIV/AIDS	($n = 30$)	($n = 21$)	Hemophiliacs with HIV/AIDS ($n = 3$)
	Family caregivers	($n = 23$)	($n = 19$)	Family caregivers ($n = 4$)
	Bereaved caregivers	($n = 17$)	($n = 16$)	
Design	Descriptive, correlational Delphi technique – 2 phases			Pre-test–post-test within subjects design
Measures				
Stress	Interview schedule and questionnaire			
Coping	Interview schedule and questionnaire			*Ways of Coping Checklist*
Support	Interview schedule and questionnaire			*Arizona Social Support Interview Schedule*
Health				*Emotional/Social Loneliness Inventory*
Data collection	Phase 1 – Interview schedule Phase 2 – Questionnaire			Pre-test Post-test following 3-month intervention
Data analyses				
Quantitative	Phase 2 – Analyses of variance, students' *t*-test, chi square analysis			Descriptive statistics
Qualitative	Thematic content analysis, inductive from interview data			Thematic content analysis of facilitators' field notes and post-intervention interviews of participants and facilitators

Support Needs and Satisfaction

In this study, the spouse and close relatives were primary sources of *emotional* support for HIV-infected hemophiliacs and their family caregivers. In contrast, support from family members for homosexuals with AIDS may be inadequate (Hays, Chauncay, & Tobey, 1990; Namir, Wolcott, & Fawzy, 1989; Zich & Temoshok, 1987).

This study confirmed that *informational* support for hemophiliacs with AIDS and their family caregivers was typically provided by health professionals. Respondents selected four types of information as particularly important: current state of the disease, likely course of the disease, symptom management, and available treatments with relative risks and benefits. Participants also assigned high priority to information about rights and responsibilities, sources of support, managing AIDS in themselves or a family member, and prevention of spread of the disease. They reported, however, that information was not always current, valid, honest, or sensitively communicated. Clearly, the uncertainty of AIDS seems to evoke needs for informational and emotional support (Hays, Turner, & Coates, 1992).

Participants experienced *affirmational* support through validation of the realities of their lives and actions from two sources: others who were in the same situation and some health professionals who had worked with persons with HIV/AIDS. Many participants were inhibited from sharing their experiences with like others, however, because of their need for confidentiality, and they reported more unhelpful than affirming responses from health professionals.

Practical aid was usually provided by relatives. Family caregivers were less satisfied with *instrumental* support than the hemophilia group, a finding consistent with the physical burdens associated with AIDS caregiving (McCann & Wadsworth, 1992; Ward & Brown, 1994). Almost half identified a need for respite from caregiving. Instrumental support was most frequently needed to care for their loved one's physical needs, to keep him at home, and to protect his rights.

Both affected men and family caregivers confirmed a high need for all types of support.

Negative Interactions

Many participants in both the hemophilia and caregiver groups reported negative interactions with people who they had anticipated might support them. Others experienced problems with support they had given or received. Physicians were perceived to be insensitive significantly more often than others, whereas friends were cited most frequently in incidents involving isolation/avoidance. Prejudice was experienced equally from health professionals and friends. Negative attitudes about AIDS had interfered with the assistance participants received from health professionals and community services. Family caregivers reported experiencing more negative reactions from relatives than bereaved caregivers reported.

The costs of support associated with insensitivity and prejudice from professionals and non-professionals and with avoidance and isolation by friends and family illustrate the 'victimization model,' whereby victims of negative events encounter conflicting reactions (Sarason, Sarason, & Pierce, 1990). The physically ill are subjected frequently to strained relationships and insensitive, uncaring behaviour. Victim blaming and avoidance can be experienced because others attribute responsibility for the cause of the problem to the victim. In another study, PWA encountered hardships in the health system associated with ensuring privacy, provision of information, sensitivity to emotional needs, and communication with physicians (Weishut, 1996). Avoidance is considered the most unhelpful action of friends (Malone, 1988); yet in this study friends most frequently engaged in isolation or avoidance tactics. Fear of social contagion, social strain, and uncertainty about intruding on privacy (La Gaipa, 1990; Rook, 1990) may have been factors in the avoidance of these hemophiliacs with HIV/AIDS and their family caregivers.

Coping Strategies

In close relationships, one partner's coping influences the coping behaviours used by the other (Coyne & Smith, 1991). These hemophiliacs with AIDS and their family caregivers, who were typically in close spousal or parent-child relationships, primarily used coping strategies aimed at 'keeping their personal relationships normal.' These caregivers and persons with hemophilia may have been attempting to reduce the stigma and victim blaming associated with AIDS. This coping strategy can enhance available support and expand social networks. The second most frequent coping strategy was 'seeking informational support.' Informational support from laypersons and professionals could provide suggestions about appropriate or alternative coping strategies. By seeking informational support, affected men and family caregivers may have been striving to reduce their uncertainty (Adelman, Parks, & Albrecht, 1987) concerning the effects of AIDS. Participants who actively sought support perceived the need to enhance or extend their natural network, which had been depleted by the stresses associated with AIDS.

In contrast, hemophiliacs with AIDS who coped by withdrawing from others did so because of fear of negative reactions and associated reluctance to seek support. Perceptions of stigma may have also inhibited family caregivers from confiding in others and seeking support. The effects of confiding depend in part on the nature of the relationship and the source of support (La Gaipa, 1990). Almost two-thirds of respondents indicated that concern for confidentiality had prevented them from seeking support. Anticipated rejection and lack of trust were cited most commonly as reasons for not confiding in others. This pattern could have serious consequences, given that self-disclosure has been associated with improved immune function (Kennedy, Kiecolt-Glaser, & Glaser, 1990), an important issue in HIV/AIDS.

Summary

Themes that emerged in both phases of the assessment study included the conflicting interrelationships among needs for confidentiality, for confiding the diagnosis, and for seeking support; discriminatory and demeaning interactions with some health professionals and the detrimental impact on support; and professional and public stigmatization and resultant social isolation and loneliness. Both negative (conflicted) and positive support were expressed towards hemophiliacs and their caregivers by professionals, family members, and friends. Consequently, multiple types of support (e.g., emotional, affirmational, informational) were needed.

Support Intervention Preferences

Participants in hemophilia and caregiver groups experienced deficiencies in affirmational support, preferring feedback from 'peers' in similar stressful situations. Indeed, respondents wished to have support groups composed of their peers. The least preferred option for intervention was support groups for anyone with AIDS, reflecting the unique support needs and stressors experienced by persons with hemophilia and HIV/AIDS and their family caregivers and the stigmatizing nature of AIDS acquired from drug use or homosexual activity. In other studies, peer support was also preferred by homosexual men with AIDS (e.g., Hays et al., 1990). Social comparison with peers in groups, linked with affirmational support, can enhance self-esteem, self- and collective efficacy, and empowerment of PWA (Ribble, 1989); diminish stigma; and augment coping strategies. Participants in our assessment study indicated that peers were needed for emotional and affirmational support and that professionals were needed for informational support. They also preferred a group led jointly by a peer and a professional.

At the time of the intervention study, support groups for PWA (Ribble 1989) and family caregivers of PWA (Kelly & Sykes, 1989) had been described but not tested. The impact of these support groups on social-psychological health and functioning (e.g., loneliness) and on satisfaction with support received from professional and peer sources had not been evaluated. Furthermore, no support groups had been created for persons with hemophilia and HIV/AIDS and their family caregivers. Following the assessment study, we conducted a survey of hemophilia clinics across Canada that confirmed the need for both face-to-face and telephone support groups.

Key Findings from the Assessment Study

Stress
- Illness interfered with participants' ability to fulfil work, education, and community responsibilities.
- AIDS had a stressful impact on their sexual intimacy.

Coping
- They normalized personal relationships.
- They sought informational support.

Support
- Informational support was provided by health professionals.
- Practical aid was provided by family members.
- There were gaps in emotional, informational, and affirmational support.

Prejudice, isolation, insensitivity, avoidance, loss of confidentiality in relationships
- Loneliness ↑
- Self esteem ↓
- Social contact ↓

Fear of stigma of AIDS and perceived need to preserve confidentiality
- Support seeking ↓

Needs for support intervention
- They did not identify with predominant groups of persons with AIDS.
- Geographic dispersion limited accessibility to face-to-face support groups.
- The preferred support group was support intervention.
- They preferred joint professional-peer leadership of support groups.

Intervention Study: Telephone Support Group

The purpose of the intervention study was to design, implement, and evaluate telephone support groups directed at the assessed support needs of persons with hemophilia and HIV/AIDS and family caregivers who could not access face-to-face groups because of illness, geographic isolation, and need for confidentiality. As this was a complex intervention, a pilot study was considered necessary.

Objectives of the Pilot Study

The objectives of the pilot study were as follows:

1. to test the feasibility of the planned support intervention, including accessibility for participants, mode of support intervention, frequency of telephone contacts, and model of shared peer-professional leadership;
2. to develop a facilitator guide for themes/topics for teleconference discussion;
3. to test the effectiveness of a training session for peer and professional leaders;
4. to assess the acceptability and appropriateness of the interview guide and standardized measures.

Hypotheses

We hypothesized that the telephone support group intervention for men with hemophilia and HIV/AIDS and family caregivers would accomplish the following:

1. decrease feelings of isolation/loneliness;
2. increase support satisfaction and decrease support needs;
3. increase social network size; and
4. enhance coping with stresses of hemophilia and HIV/AIDS.

Intervention Design

The pilot intervention involved separate telephone support groups for persons with hemophilia and HIV/AIDS and for family caregivers in order to enhance similarity of stressful situations experienced by members in each group. Each group was co-led by a professional and a peer, as recommended by participants in our assessment study. The predetermined maximum group membership was six, including group facilitators, because telephone support groups do not readily accommodate more people. Including the peer and professional facilitators, there were four people in the group for men with hemophilia and five in the group for family caregivers. (Note: The research design for this intervention study is summarized in table 5.1.)

Participants met weekly, by telephone. The intervention was twelve weeks long, to overcome problems associated with the brevity of previous telephone support interventions reported in the literature. Although teleconference sessions were originally scheduled to last 45 minutes, the sessions for the men with hemophilia ranged from 76 to 122 minutes (mean = 102 minutes) and the caregiver group sessions ranged from 79 to 153 minutes (mean = 105 minutes).

A background document was developed for facilitators, using input from the hemophilia clinics, needs expressed in the earlier assessment study, and the literature. Topics included the disease, treatment options, the health care system, preventing contagion, coping with illness stressors, managing negative interactions, disclosure versus confidentiality, disrupted family functioning/communication, practical support needs, support seeking, and social isolation/loneliness. This document was sent to experts in HIV/AIDS and hemophilia in Canada and was revised according to feedback received. During the first support group teleconference meeting, members were invited to comment on the suggested content and format and to recommend further additions and amendments. Members were encouraged to discuss the topics of their choice in all sessions. At the conclusion of the intervention, the facilitator's guide was revised to incorporate more recent literature and additional topics raised by group members during the teleconference sessions. The major addition pertained to bereavement.

To prepare leaders for facilitating the support groups, an orientation session was conducted via teleconference between Halifax and Montreal. During training particular attention was given to how beliefs might influence the facilitators' ability to interact with group participants and strategies for using personal strengths to assist others and to build capacity. The purpose and intended outcomes of the telephone support groups, the use of telephone technology, communication processes, responsibilities of participants, and the nature, scope, and sequencing of content were discussed.

Both professional and peer leaders encouraged group members to voice their experiences and concerns. The professional leader contacted participants to determine a mutually agreeable time for each meeting and collaborated with the teleconference operator to initiate each teleconference session. Group members received written information about teleconferencing and instructions for rejoining the teleconference if they had to leave for part of a meeting or were disconnected accidently. The peer and professional leaders contacted group members individually between sessions if there were any issues requiring monitoring or if a member missed a session. Any unintended factors or unanticipated crises were recorded.

Key Features of the Intervention

- Weekly telephone support group sessions over twelve-week period
- Separate telephone support groups for men with hemophilia and HIV/AIDS and for family caregivers
- Maximum group membership was six
- Groups co-led by a professional and a peer
- Telephone sessions originally scheduled for forty-five minutes
- Facilitator guide focused on prominent themes in assessment study and literature
- Facilitator training by teleconference
- Telephone support group discussions taped and transcribed
- Follow-up telephone interviews of participants and facilitators
- Measurement of outcomes (e.g., loneliness) pre- and post-intervention

Documentation of Support Processes

The telephone support group discussions were taped and transcribed. The professional and peer facilitators recorded field notes, which paid particular attention to social comparison, social learning, social exchange, collaboration in leadership, key topics/issues discussed, and factors influencing the discussion. After the twelve-week intervention, group members participated in follow-up telephone interviews, which emphasized continuing contacts with support group member(s), shared leadership, social comparison, reciprocity of supportive interactions, social learning, satisfaction with the intervention, and impact on relationships and coping. Following the intervention, the peer and professional facilitators were interviewed jointly about leadership issues and the advantages and disadvantages of the support groups. The data derived from the interaction record of the transcribed sessions, the facilitators' field notes, and the interviews of members and facilitators were subjected to content analysis using projected themes in a framework. These themes included sources, types and appraisal of support, stressful situations, coping strategies, support group processes, impact of intervention, leadership, and so on.

Measurement of Outcomes

Measurement of outcomes was conducted prior to (pre-test) and following (post-test) the intervention using standardized instruments (see table 5.1.). Instruments were sent to each participant by mail to be completed and returned. The impact of the telephone support intervention on social support, loneliness, and coping strategies was measured by three questionnaires: the *Emotional/Social Loneliness Inventory*, the *Arizona Social Support Interview Schedule*, and the *Ways of Coping Checklist* (appendix B).

Profile of Participants

All three men with hemophilia and AIDS were in their early thirties and lived in three different rural areas. One was single, two had a spouse/partner, and one had children. They were infected with HIV in the mid-1980s. Severity of reported symptoms varied.

In the caregivers' support group, three members were female and one was male. All caregivers were in conjugal relationships: three were married and one was in a common-law relationship. Two caregivers were a married couple who had two children other than the HIV-infected boy. Caregivers had known for nine to ten years that their spouse or child was infected with HIV.

Topics Discussed in Support Groups

Stressful Situations

Men with HIV/AIDS: The men faced the stresses of public stigma, fear, ignorance, and avoidance. These group members were activists who attempted to reduce ignorance about HIV, to promote public awareness, to redress injury, and to increase financial support. There was little organizational support for their efforts. The system's failure to accept responsibility lay at the heart of their quest for justice. They were dedicated to following the issues and actions surrounding the Krever Inquiry into the transmission of HIV and other infections via contaminated blood products.

The hemophiliacs infected with HIV bore the stress of multiple illnesses and treatments and their suppressed immune systems rendered them vulnerable to infection. The serious and complex nature of their illness dictated a need for information about their condition and the products and medications with which it was treated. They reported an urgent need to keep abreast of developments in research, and they viewed the inaccessibility of information as stressful. The cost of information contributed to its inaccessibility. Moreover, available information was frequently inadequate and inaccurate.

Negative experiences with the system were prevalent. The participants experienced rejection and lack of respect, and they dealt with different layers of a complex and bureaucratic system. The men identified cutbacks and inadequate financial support and compensation as key sources of government-induced stress. The participants also decried the provincial Hemophilia Society's uncaring treatment, inappropriate use of funds, and lack of recognition or voice within the system.

Isolation and loneliness were pervasive. Within the organizations intended to help hemophiliacs or persons with AIDS, their cause was considered marginal (*organizational isolation*). The participants experienced different situations than the majority of people in both the HIV/AIDS and the hemophiliac populations did. The population of HIV-infected hemophiliacs is very small and is decreasing (*demographic isolation*). With so few voices, it was difficult to attract attention to their cause. The lifestyle changes and restrictions that accompanied their illness created *social isolation*. They could no longer participate in some sports or work activities and found formation of new relationships difficult. Infected hemophiliacs were distributed across the province and most could not afford long-distance phone calls (*geographical isolation*).

Caregivers: Caregivers monitored the health of their family members with hemophilia and HIV. Discussions of physical health focused on treatment for hemophilia, treatment for HIV, side-effects of treatment, monitoring of symptoms, and susceptibility to other illnesses.

A frequently recurring theme was their ill relatives' reluctance to communicate about their illness with other family members and friends. Consequently, caregivers were constrained from discussing the illness and its related injustices openly in public and within their families.

Caregivers were concerned about the effects of the HIV infection on other family members and family relationships. They worried about their other children's feelings of neglect, and about their relatives' reactions.

Caregivers expressed anger at the circumstances surrounding the infection of their family members and at the continuing inattention to their needs. They recounted stressful experiences involving bad blood products and product recalls. Caregivers' anger at the health care system was sometimes directed towards specific health professionals, such as physicians. One of the greatest sources of anger and frustration was the inadequacy and unreliability of information. In the face of these perceived injustices, caregivers often felt powerless to obtain the care they believed their ill relatives needed.

Caregivers expressed concern that although PWA were encouraged by the potential benefit of medications, the government refused to pay for these medications. Caregivers also shared their scepticism regarding the support they received from the Canadian Hemophilia Society, given its links to government. They feared further marginalization arising from this society's support of people who contracted other illnesses through the blood system and the diminishing number of people with hemophilia and HIV/AIDS.

Caregivers found themselves in vulnerable positions with respect to public knowledge and attitudes about HIV/AIDS and the insensitivity and ignorance of others. While caregivers' concern for their families and ill relatives was the most prominent focus of support group discussions, they also talked about their own feelings of isolation.

Coping with Stressful Situations

Affected Men: The affected men coped with the emotional stresses of isolation and injustice by speaking out against injustice, providing support to others, and writing a book about their lives and experiences. Most transcripts included references to laughter among the participants. Indeed, laughter was a coping strategy. There were more references to 'talking about it' than to other coping behaviours. Information gathering, lobbying, and contributing to public education were more problem-focused ways of coping. The participants expended considerable time and energy trying to access current information related to their illness. One man discussed how he handled the stress that his public profile created for his wife (i.e., relationship-focused coping).

Caregivers: Caregivers maintained a positive attitude and lived '*one day at a time*,' as strategies for managing the combined stresses of hemophilia and HIV/AIDS. Other emotion-focused strategies for coping included discussing the reactions of various family members to the illness and talking to others who were experiencing similar circumstances. Problem-focused coping was reflected in caregivers' advocacy efforts and their support for their relative's advocacy. Relationship-focused coping was evident in the couple who shared caregiving tasks and the emotional stresses of caring (i.e., active engagement). Caregivers tried to protect their affected relative with HIV/AIDS and the family from 'outsiders' who might express negative attitudes about HIV infection ('protective buffering').

Summary

The discussion themes reinforced the findings from the initial assessment study. The stressfulness of the disease process, need for information, negative interactions with the health care system and with others in the community, stigma, isolation and loneliness, and attempts to manage by normalizing personal relationships and by seeking informational support were prevalent themes in both assessment and intervention studies.

Support Provided by the Intervention

Affected Men

During the post-intervention interviews, the men referred to explanations about the illness and its treatment, and to information on interacting with the system (*informational support*). They reported that they learned things they did not know before the intervention. The men also frequently referred to *emotional* and *affirmational support* received from the telephone group (e.g., listening, sharing feelings, solidarity, trust, encouragement).

The men praised the professional leader as a source of informational and instrumental support. To illustrate, she found and communicated information from the health care community back to the group and edited a letter written by the men to a daily newspaper. Three guest speakers included a prominent AIDS activist, an activist peer and friend of the participants, and a writer. The teleconferences provided a forum for giving and receiving informational support (i.e., reciprocity). The participants regularly shared their knowledge about AIDS, treatments, and resources in the community (i.e., social learning), and the peer leader provided informational support.

Towards the end of the intervention, the two support groups combined for one teleconference session during which the men provided informational support to the caregivers.

Caregivers

Informational support focused on the management of illness symptoms, treatments, side-effects of treatments, and dealing with the health care system. Often, the information obtained in the support groups was not available elsewhere. The professional leader provided the group members with written materials that explained medical treatments for HIV/AIDS. Members were also important sources of informational support for each other regarding hemophilia, HIV, health and social welfare systems, and community resources. Caregivers exchanged information about the genetic basis of hemophilia, the quality of blood products, strategies for obtaining medications and financial support for medications, alternative coping strategies, and the health status of their family members. Thus, the support in the teleconferences was reciprocal.

The emotional support received by caregivers addressed demands related to the emotional reactions of their family members with hemophilia and HIV/AIDS, negative social attitudes, and their own emotional needs and isolation. Caregivers shared family histories, their ways of coping with serious illness in the family, and their experiences with the various 'systems.' Sharing their feelings and experiences, talking with others who understood and empathized, and having the opportunity to laugh were important ingredients in the emotional support received in the support groups.

Caregivers encouraged one another in their caregiving and advocacy efforts (i.e., affirmational support). Positive feedback and guidance were exchanged.

Evaluation of the Intervention

As the intervention was nearing termination, caregivers were profuse in their commendations of 'the project.' All participants expressed a desire to continue communicating and were disappointed that the intervention was terminating. Group members exchanged telephone numbers and hoped to arrange a face-to-face meeting. During the post-intervention interviews, caregivers reported very high levels of satisfaction with the support group. They were '*very thankful*' for the opportunity provided by the intervention and emphasized the value of informational, affirmational, and emotional support from both group members and leaders. Caregivers found that there were other people who understood their situations and who were willing to provide support, even outside the group context. In their view, the reciprocity of sharing information and experiences with peers and their reciprocal interactions with the professional were influential in the success of the group.

Similarly, the men with hemophilia were impressed with the informational and emotional support received from members and peer leaders and the informational and instrumental support provided by the professional leader. They were very disappointed when the telephone support group intervention finished and wanted to find some means to continue their telephone discussions. The following quotations illustrate participants' positive perceptions of the intervention. '*... that there were resources available, that people were there for us. There were people we could trust. [We] didn't believe in it at the beginning.*' '*Someone can understand you only if someone has the same thing* *as you. There was a lot of sharing. Everybody took the time to listen to everybody else. It can't get any better than that with regard to meeting one's needs. You know that there are people there that will take the time to listen to what you have to say.'*

Impact of the Intervention on Health and Functioning Outcomes

Support

During the post-intervention interviews, participants in both groups reported that the intervention had had a positive impact on meeting their support needs and had increased their support satisfaction. Moreover, caregivers identified some positive impact on their relationships with others (e.g., family members). The small sample size notwithstanding, the intervention had a statistically significant positive effect on caregivers' perceived support satisfaction. Specifically, total support satisfaction scores increased from pre- to post-test, while total perceived support need decreased.

The affected men reported that the intervention enhanced their contact time in relationships and quality of support. They maintained regular contact between teleconferences. There were no statistically significant differences in the pre- and post-test scores for social network size, however, or in satisfaction with and need for support. The largest changes were increased perceived and actual support network size and increased total support satisfaction.

Coping

Caregivers reported that their confidence in their knowledge and skills increased through their participation in the support groups and that they had undertaken problem-solving strategies based on what they had learned in the group. One had engaged in extensive research, another had attended a Hemophilia Society function, and others had changed their approach to the health care system. No statistically significant changes, however, were reported on the coping measure.

The men also reported an impact on coping actions, such as seeking information and writing a book about their experiences, although there were no significant changes on the coping measure from pre-test to post-test.

Loneliness/Isolation

The caregivers believed that the support groups had decreased their feelings of isolation. Their scores on social and emotional loneliness and social and emotional isolation decreased following the intervention. As expected with this small sample, no statistically significant differences were found.

The emotional support provided during the teleconferences was effective, in the men's view, in reducing the stress of isolation. In this context, there was a mean decrease in their emotional isolation at post-test.

The key findings from the intervention study are summarized in table 5.2.

Lessons Learned

The greatest challenges faced by the research team pertained to recruitment of participants and to translation. Although the study started in Atlantic Canada, the small population in these four provinces and the difficulties inherent in recruitment strategies that did not permit direct access to potential participants necessitated a move to Quebec. Specifically, professionals in clinics exhibited protective, somewhat patronizing behaviours that inhibited access. The shift in locale because of the larger target population generated the need to (1) translate the measures, consent forms, and information letter from English to French; (2) engage a bilingual site coordinator and a bilingual professional group facilitator; (3) add a bilingual Quebec-based investigator to the team; (4) translate diaries, field notes, interview responses, and transcripts of taped group discussions from French to English; and (5) translate a summary of the results for participants from English to French. These strategies were successful and the study was completed.

All the group sessions lasted much longer than the originally scheduled forty-five minutes, reflecting the members' need for support and discussion with others in similar circumstances. Participants wanted the support group to continue beyond the predetermined twelve weeks, reinforcing their support needs and their positive perceptions of the intervention.

The model of shared peer and professional facilitation and the facilitator guide were viewed as successful. The outcome measure on loneliness and isolation appeared to be sensitive to change, and changes in all measures were in the desired direction.

In general, participants indicated that the support group intervention did not require revision. One caregiver suggested that a few topics could be explored in greater depth (e.g., death and bereavement). The intervention may have rekindled hope and raised expectations that an ongoing telephone network for HIV-infected hemophiliacs might be supported. Nevertheless, the men feared that the study might not produce results in time to address the urgency of their situation.

TABLE 5.2
Key Findings from the Intervention Study

	Affected Men	Family Caregivers
Stressful situations	*Negative social attitudes* *Inadequate, inaccessible information* *Dealing with health/social systems* *Isolation* Illness treatment Financial strain Injustice Advocacy	*Negative social attitudes* *Inadequate, inaccessible information* *Dealing with health/social systems* *Isolation* Managing and monitoring relative's health Dealing with relative's reactions Impact on family Personal needs
Coping strategies	*Talking with others who understand (EF)* *Advocacy (PF)* Positive attitude (EF) Seeking information (PF)	*Talking with others who understand (EF)* *Advocacy (PF)* Protective buffering (RF) Expressing anger (EF) Naming emotions/concerns (EF) Sharing caregiving and stresses (RF)
Sources of support	*Support group members* *Support group leaders* *Family*	*Support group members* *Support group leaders* *Family*
Types of support	*Affirmational* *Informational* *Emotional*	*Affirmational* *Informational* *Emotional*
Impact of intervention	*Satisfaction of emotional support needs* *Satisfaction of informational support needs* *Actions taken* *Reciprocity* *Reduced emotional isolation* Enhanced communication	*Satisfaction of emotional support needs* *Satisfaction of informational support needs* *Actions taken* *Reciprocity* *Reduced emotional isolation* Enhanced confidence Improved interactions with natural network

Notes
Italics denote common themes in the discussions of both groups.
EP = emotion focused; PF = problem focused; RF = relationship focused.

Lessons Learned

- There are recruitment challenges with small populations.
- Telephone mode is appropriate for participants in rural settings.
- The interview guide elicited important information about supportive processes and satisfaction with intervention.
- The standardized measures are appropriate and sensitive to change.
- The facilitator guide is helpful; it was updated and modified for future use.
- The training session anticipated issues that arose during support group sessions.
- Both individual sessions and support groups should be of longer duration.
- There were similarities in receptiveness of men and women to telephone support intervention.

Future Directions in Research, Programs, and Policy

Participants believed that the intervention enhanced their support and diminished their isolation and loneliness. These qualitative data were reinforced by the quantitative findings. Several future directions are suggested.

The assessment and intervention studies illuminate the pervasive loneliness and isolation experienced by persons living with AIDS and their family caregivers and their paramount need for supplementary support from peers and professionals. Given the increasing incidence of AIDS in traditional families and the continuing stigma surrounding this chronic condition, support interventions that protect confidentiality and enhance accessibility are timely. Telephone support groups proved to be successful strategies from the perspective of both confidentiality and accessibility. However, such interventions are costly. Indeed, financial barriers persist that should be addressed through policy changes. Health system policy could foster these innovative forms of social-psychological interventions through amended insurance schemes. Furthermore, financial support or reduced conference-call rates should be sought from telephone competitors such as Unitel, Sprint, and provincial companies. These companies could be assured of public relations benefits and their contributions would be acknowledged.

As many family caregivers were forced to leave work because of the demands of caring for those in our assessment study experiencing AIDS symptomatology, some of the policy recommendations in Gottlieb's paper on caregiving for the National Forum on Health (e.g., legislation for unlimited periods of unpaid leave, tax relief, family care credits under Canada's Employment Insurance program, family responsibility leave legislation, full benefits for part-time employment) could be implemented (National Forum on Health, 1997).

This intervention yielded unique insights about the suitability of telephone support groups for stigmatized groups of ill persons and caregivers who have experienced negative interactions with social networks and societies. Confidentiality was crucial in such circumstances. Participants in both studies wanted to exchange support with peers, but they worried that other support vehicles might not protect confidentiality or be facilitated by positively disposed persons. Telephone support provided a mechanism that fostered mutual aid among persons in similar circumstances and avoided negative reactions of and interactions with others. Trust building among peers and professionals was an essential element in the success of this strategy. Similar support vehicles for people with chronic conditions who suffer stigma and social isolation deserve recognition in programs and policies integrated into health and health-related sectors.

Future support programs should take into consideration the lessons learned about intervention dose in this pilot. It was clear from the length of the discussions and from participants' recommendations that the duration of individual sessions and of the intervention itself should be extended. Consequently, future group sessions should be scheduled for up to a maximum of two hours. Furthermore, intervention trials of long-term support groups (e.g., one year) should be launched, and measures of social support, loneliness, and other outcomes (e.g., confidence) should be administered every three months to determine the most effective duration of these groups.

Our studies emphasized a population that typically lives in traditional nuclear families. There is evidence that a growing number of Canadians, including women, children, heterosexual men, and persons infected through 'health care' interventions such as surgery and infusions, have been affected by HIV and AIDS either through illness or caregiving. McDonald (1996) speculates that HIV-infected women are diagnosed later than men and experience discrimination in research, treatment, and society. Yet assessment and intervention research to date has been focused on the needs of homosexual men with HIV/AIDS. This discrepancy has implications for the design of support programs and intervention research. The effectiveness of telephone support group programs for persons infected with HIV through treatment of other health conditions and for their family caregivers could be evaluated through a randomized controlled trial. Furthermore, other intervention modalities, such as computer mutual aid, could be designed and tested.

Our studies uncovered the perceived importance of support from peers in similar, if not the same, circumstances. According to participants, dyadic or group support from anyone with AIDS was neither sufficient nor appropriate. Nevertheless, it is difficult to create accessible groups for persons in identical situations, particularly for Canadians living with AIDS in rural sites. Therefore, telephone and computer mutual aid programs, co-facilitated by peers and professionals, should be launched for persons in similar situations (e.g., women infected with HIV by their marital partners).

Acknowledgments

The assessment study was funded through a grant from NHRDP and the intervention study was supported by grants from NHRDP and the Canadian Foundation for AIDS Research.

Note

Some results from the assessment study were published in Stewart, Hart, & Mann (1995).

References

Adelman, M., Parks, M., & Albrecht, T. (1987). Supporting friends in need. *Communicating social support.* Newbury Park, CA: Sage.

Barrera, M. (1991). Social support interventions and the third law of ecology. *American Journal of Community Psychology, 19*(1), 133–138.

Borkman, T. (1976). Experiential knowledge: A new concept for the analysis of self-help groups. *Social Service Review, 50*, 445–454.

Borkman, T. (1982). *A social experiential model in programs for alcoholism recovery.* Rockville, MD: U.S. Department of Health and Human Services.

Canadian Hemophilia Clinic Directors Group. (1993). Effect of using safer blood products on prevalence of HIV infection in haemophilic Canadians. *British Medical Journal, 306*, 306–307.

Cleary, P., Van Devanter, N., Steilen, M., Stuart, A., Shipton-Levy, R., McMullen, W., Rogers, T., Singer, E., Avorn, J., & Pindyck, J. (1995). A randomized trial of an education and support program for HIV-infected individuals. *AIDS, 9*, 1271–1278.

Coyne, J., & Smith, D. (1991). Couples coping with a myocardial infarction: A contextual perspective on wives' distress. *Journal of Personality and Social Psychology, 61*(3), 404–412.

Coyne, J., Ellard, J., & Smith, D. (1990). Social support, interdependence, and the dilemmas of helping. In B.R. Sarason, I.G. Sarason, & G.R. Pierce (Eds), *Social support: An interactional view* (129–149). New York: Wiley.

Daniolos, P. (1994). House calls: A support group for individuals with AIDS in a community residential setting. *International Journal of Group Psychotherapy, 44*(2), 133–152.

Dunn, K. (1993). HIV and Canada's hemophiliacs: Looking back at a tragedy. *Canadian Medical Association Journal, 148*(4), 609–612.

Fawzy, I., Namir, S., & Wolcott, D. (1989). Structured group intervention model for AIDS patients. *Psychiatric Medicine, 7*, 35–45.

Folkman, S., Chesney, M., McKusick, L., Ironson, G., Johnson, D., & Coates, T. (1991). Translating coping theory into an intervention. In J. Eckenrode (Ed.), *The social context of coping* (239–260). New York: Plenum Press.

Frierson, R., Lippmann, S., & Johnson, J. (1987). AIDS: Psychological stresses on the family. *Psychosomatics, 28*, 65–68.

Getzel, G., & Mahoney, K. (1989). Confronting human finitude: Groupwork with people with AIDS. *Groupwork, 2*, 95–107.

Hall, C.S. (1994). The experience of children with hemophilia and HIV infection. *Journal of School Health, 64*(1), 16–17.

Hays, R., Chauncay, S., & Tobey, L. (1990). The social support networks of gay men with AIDS. *Journal of Community Psychology, 18*(4), 374–385.

Hays, R., Turner, H., & Coates, T. (1992). Social support, AIDS-related symptoms, and depression among gay men. *Journal of Consultations in Clinical Psychology, 60*(3), 463–469.

Hobfoll, S., & Freedy, J. (1990). The availability and effective use of social support. *Journal of Social and Clinical Psychology, 9*(1), 91–103.

Hughes, C., & Caliandro, G. (1996). Effects of social support, stress, and level of illness on caregiving of children with AIDS. *Journal of Pediatric Nursing, 11*(6), 347–58.

Jankowski, S., Videka-Sherman, L., & Laquidara-Dickinson, K. (1996). Social support networks of confidants to people with AIDS. *Journal of the National Association of Social Workers, 41*(2), 206–213.

Johnston, D., Stall, R., & Smith, K. (1995). Reliance by gay men and intravenous drug users on friends and family for AIDS-related care. *AIDS Care, 7*(3), 307–319.

Kelly, J. & Sykes, P. (1989). Helping the helpers: A support group for family members of persons with AIDS. *Social Work, 34*, 239–242.

Kelly, J.A., Lawrence, J.S., Smith, S., Hood, H., & Cook, D. (1987). Stigmatization of AIDS patients by physicians. *American Journal of Public Health, 77*(7), 789–791.

Kennedy, S., Kiecolt-Glaser, J., & Glaser, R. (1990). Social support, stress and the immune system. In B.R. Sarason, I.B. Sarason, & G.R. Pierce (Eds), *Social support: An interactional view* (253–266). New York: John Wiley.

La Gaipa, J.J. (1990). The negative effects of informal support systems. In S. Duck (Ed.), *Personal relationships and social support* (122–139). London: Sage.

Lamping, D. (1991). The impact of a social support intervention for persons with symptomatic HIV infection: Psychosocial, clinical and economic outcomes. In *Directory of current HIV/AIDS research in Canada*. Montreal: Centre for AIDS Studies, Department of Community Health, Montreal General Hospital.

Lego, S. (1994). AIDS-related anxiety and coping methods in a support group for caregivers. *Archives of Psychiatric Nursing, 8*(3), 200–207.

Levy, R., Tendler, C., VanDevanter, N., & Cleary, P. (1990). A group intervention model for individuals testing positive for HIV antibody. *American Journal of Orthopsychiatry, 60*, 452–459.

Maguire, L. (1991). *Social support systems in practice.* Silver Spring, MD: National Association of Social Workers Press.

Malone, J. (1988). The social support-social dissupport continuum. *Journal of Psychosocial Nursing and Mental Health Services, 26*(12), 18–22.

Maton, K.I. (1987). Patterns and psychological correlates of material support within a religious setting: The bidirectional support hypothesis. *American Journal of Community Psychology, 15*, 185–207.

McCann, K., & Wadsworth, E. (1992). The role of informal carers in supporting gay men who have HIV related illness: What do they do and what are their needs? *AIDS Care, 4*(1), 25–34.

McDonald, K. (1996). Sexual and reproductive health and rights in Canada. Paper presented to the Canada-USA Forum on Women's Health. Ottawa: Health Canada.

Namir, S., Wolcott, D., & Fawzy, F. (1989). Social support and HIV spectrum disease: Clinical and research perspectives. *Psychiatric Medicine, 7*(2), 97–105.

National Forum on Health. (1997). *Who determines health?* Ottawa: National Forum on Health.

Pearlin, L. (1991). The study of coping: An overview of problems and directions. In J. Eckenrode (Ed.), *The social context of coping* (261–276). New York: Plenum Press.

Pearlin, L., Semple, S., & Turner, H. (1988). Stress of AIDS caregiving: A preliminary overview of the issues. *Death Studies, 12*(5-6), 501–517.

Posey, C.E. (1988). Confidentiality in an AIDS support group. *Journal of Counselling and Development, 66*, 226–227.

Ribble, D. (1989). Psychosocial support groups for people with HIV infection and AIDS. *Holistic Nursing Practice, 3*(4), 52–62.

Rook, K. (1984). Promoting social bonding strategies for helping the lonely and socially isolated. *American Psychology, 39*, 1389–1407.

Rook, K. (1987). Reciprocity of social exchange and social satisfaction among older women. *Journal of Personality and Social Psychology, 52*, 145–154.

Rook, K. (1990). Parallels in the study of social support and social strain. *Journal of Social and Clinical Psychology, 9*(1), 118–132.

Sandstrom, K. (1996). Searching for information, understanding, and self-value: The utilization of peer support groups by gay men with HIV/AIDS. *Social Work in Health Care, 23*(4), 51–74.

Sarason, B.R., Sarason, I.G., & Pierce, G.R. (1990). *Social support: An interactional view*. New York: Wiley.

Servellen, G., Sarna, L., Padilla, G., & Brecht, M. (1996). Emotional distress in men with life-threatening illness. *International Journal of Nursing Studies, 33*(5), 551–565.

Sikkema, K., Kalichman, S., Kelly, J., & Koob, J. (1995). Group intervention to improve coping with AIDS-related bereavement: Model development and an illustrative clinical example. *AIDS Care, 7*(4), 463–475.

Smith, M., & Rapkin, B. (1996). Social support and barriers to family involvement in caregiving for persons with AIDS: Implications for patient education. *Patient Education and Counselling, 27*(1), 85–94.

Solomon, Z., Waysman, M., & Mikulincer, M. (1990). Family functioning, perceived social support, and combat-related psychopathology: The moderating role of loneliness. *Journal of Social and Clinical Psychology, 9*(4), 456–472.

Stewart, M. (1993). *Integrating social support in nursing*. Newbury Park, CA: Sage.

Stewart, M., Hart, G. & Mann, K. (1995). Living with haemophilia and HIV/AIDS: Support and coping. *Journal of Advanced Nursing, 22*, 1101–1111.

Tilden, V., & Gaylen, R. (1987). Cost and conflict: The darker side of social support. *Western Journal of Nursing Research, 9*, 9–18.

Ward, D., & Brown, M. (1994). Labor and cost in AIDS family caregiving. *Western Journal of Nursing Research, 16*(1), 10–22.

Weishut, D. (1996). Coping with AIDS in a support group: An encounter with the health system. *Harefuah, 130*(8), 521–523, 583.

Weiss, R. (1974). The provisions of social relationships. In Z. Rubin, (Ed.), *Doing unto others* (17–26). Englewood Cliffs, NJ: Prentice-Hall.

Wight, R., LeBlanc, A., & Aneshensel, C. (1995). Support service use by persons with AIDS and their caregivers. *AIDS Care, 7*(4), 509–520.

Wong, M., & Forrister, D.K. (1989). Empowerment as a group work technique with persons with acquired immune deficiency syndrome. *Free Inquiry in Creative Sociology, 17*, 193–199.

World Health Organization (1991) News about AIDS. *World Health Forum: An International Journal of Health Development, 12*(4), 296–297.

Zich, J., & Temoshok, L. (1987). Perceptions of social support in men with AIDS and ARC: Relationships with distress and hardiness. *Journal of Applied Social Psychology, 17*, 193–215.

6

Stroke and Heart Failure in Seniors: Dyadic Peer Support for Family Caregivers

Geraldine Hart, Donna Meagher-Stewart, Miriam J. Stewart, Kathleen MacPherson, Susan Doble, and Lydia Makrides

Abstract. The two studies discussed in this chapter document stresses and social support experienced by community-based seniors living with the cardiovascular conditions of stroke or heart failure and by their family caregivers. In the initial assessment study, the stroke family caregivers ranked the burden of caregiving and emotional/cognitive changes in the relative with stroke as their two main sources of stress. Although participants reported acceptable levels of social support, the least life satisfaction was experienced by the stroke survivors and stroke family caregivers. There was also evidence that stroke family caregivers perceived low reciprocity of support from their family members with stroke.

Accordingly, a support intervention was designed involving peer visitor support for new family caregivers of stroke survivors. These caregivers experienced stresses similar to those of the stroke caregivers in the assessment study. Qualitative analysis of peer visitor diaries and caregiver interviews revealed incidents of absent, insufficient, or miscarried support from family members, whereas most interactions involving peer visitors were considered supportive, appropriate, and reciprocal. Quantitative analysis demonstrated increased satisfaction with guidance support, decreased need for support, and diminished health services use.

Together, these studies indicate the need for and value of peer support for family caregivers of persons with stroke. Formal health system support will be needed for systematic implementation of similar programs.

Introduction

Cardiovascular conditions are the leading cause of death in the world and in Canada. The major cardiovascular conditions are ischaemic heart disease (including myocardial infarction (MI) and heart failure), stroke and 'other' heart and vascular conditions, representing 56 per cent, 19 per cent and 25 per cent respectively, of all deaths from cardiovascular disease (Heart and Stroke Foundation of Canada, 1997). Nevertheless, Canadian death rates from ischaemic heart disease and stroke have been reduced by almost 50 per cent over the last twenty-five years. As the large majority of strokes in Canada occur in persons over sixty-five, however, the population living with disabilities caused by stroke can be expected to increase over the next few decades, based on the age distribution of Canadians. The incidence and morbidity from all cardiovascular conditions (including stroke and heart failure, the foci of the two studies reported in this chapter) are not yet well documented in Canada or other countries. Such documentation is needed to assess the impact of health promotion efforts and new biomedical treatments (Heart and Stroke Foundation of Canada, 1997).

The expected disabilities arising from stroke and heart failure differ. The lasting effects of stroke vary widely. Depending on the part of the brain affected by the stroke, survivors may experience paralysis in one or more extremities and/or diminished ability to swallow and speak. There can be a direct impact on memory, emotions, judgment, and language comprehension and expression. These disabilities can be major or subtle, depending on the size and location of the stroke, and may partially or completely resolve. Whether or not survivors are discharged to home, a rehabilitation program, or a long-term care facility depends upon the severity of stroke deficits and the willingness and ability of family members to assist them to live in the community (MacNamara, Gummow, Goka, & Gregg, 1990).

Heart failure often follows one or more MIs and reduces a person's ability to perform activities of daily living, because of progressive fatigue and shortness of breath or coughing on exertion or even at rest (Cheitlin, Sokolow, & McIlroy, 1993). Most people with heart failure live at home, experiencing intermittent crises that may necessitate hospitalization; some with severe activity deficits may need long-term institutional care, when no family caregiver or other home support is available.

The usual family caregivers of men are their wives, while women with heart failure or stroke are more often cared for by daughters or other family members (Browning & Schwirian, 1994). This caregiving pattern relates to women's traditional role in family caregiving and to the fact that women have cardiovascular disease at a later age than men (Heart and Stroke Foundation of Canada, 1997) and thus are likely to be widowed by the time they have disabling cardiovascular disease.

Persons with stroke or heart failure and their family caregivers have been the focus of some research pertaining to stressors, support needs, and support resources (e.g., Lyons, McDonald, MacKay-Lyons, & Phillips, 1995). Studies of family caregivers of stroke survivors have focused on social support in relation to caregiver depression (Schulz, Tompkins, & Rau, 1988; Ross & Morris, 1988), caregiver strain (MacNamara et al., 1990), and caregiver burden (Silliman & Sternberg, 1988). Positive correlations between social support and functional status of community-based stroke survivors have been reported (Friedland & McColl, 1987; Glass & Maddox, 1992). If family support becomes overprotective, however, the independence of survivors may be reduced (Evans, Hendricks, Haselkorn, Bishop, & Baldwin, 1992). Conjugal support has a buffering effect on the stressors associated with stroke, but only for those who are not severely disabled (Boynton, De Sepulveda, & Chang, 1994).

According to some researchers, perceived social support can enhance coping with cardiovascular conditions by fostering beliefs in personal control, self-efficacy, and expectation of positive outcomes (Bramwell & Whall, 1986; Derenowski, 1988; Markle-Reid, 1989). In one study, perceived availability of social support, particularly affirmational support, was positively related to positive client health outcomes and spousal well-being after coronary bypass surgery (King, Reis, Porter, & Norsen, 1993). Researchers have established a positive correlation between social support and the ability of wives to cope with their husbands' cardiac illness (Bramwell & Whall, 1986; Nyamathi, 1987; Riffle, 1988). Instrumental and emotional support from family members may influence whether stroke survivors with physical and/or cognitive disabilities live at home rather than in an institutional setting (Bull, 1990).

Thus, although some persons recover from their cardiovascular conditions with no significant deficits, most receive varying degrees of family caregiving. For this reason, we view persons with these conditions and their family caregivers as a unit. Persons with cardiovascular conditions can share their perceptions of the support they need and receive from their family caregivers; and family caregivers can describe their perspectives of the support needs of their relatives with cardiovascular conditions, whether they give this support, and burdens experienced from support provision. Persons with cardiovascular conditions and their family caregivers can be assessed to uncover the presence or absence of reciprocity in their relationship and the support they receive from others in their social networks.

This approach was used in the two studies reported in this chapter. The first was a correlational study assessing stressors and the relationship of social support to the functional capacity and life satisfaction of ill persons with stroke or heart failure, and life satisfaction of family caregivers. Subsequently, a peer support intervention focused on the group with the greatest assessed support needs – family caregivers of stroke survivors – was mounted.

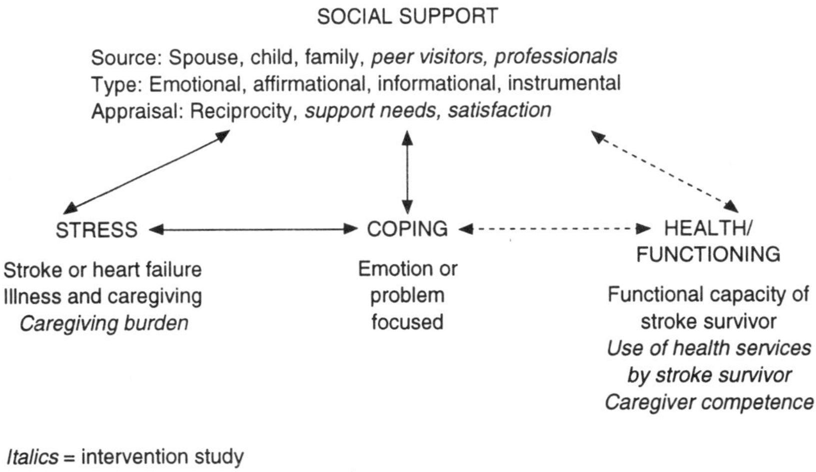

Figure 6.1 Framework for Assessment and Intervention Studies Focused on Seniors with Stroke

Fit with Framework

In the assessment study, social support was operationally defined as perceived available support. This refers to the cognitive appraisal of being connected to others, cared for, and valued (Stewart, 1993); the availability of significant others in times of stress; and satisfaction with relationships (Heller, Swindle, & Dusenbury, 1986). Social support was conceptualized in terms of Weiss's typology of social support (Weinert & Brandt, 1987), which includes the 'opportunity to nurture others' or reciprocate support, thus operationalizing social exchange theory (Tilden & Gaylen, 1987). (See figure 6.1.)

The intervention study was based on a conceptualization of social support as a coping resource or source of assistance in coping with stressful situations (Folkman, Chesney, McKusick, Ironson, Johnson, & Coates, 1991) associated with caring for a stroke survivor. This intervention was focused on provision of peer support to supplement the depleted or strained networks of the family caregivers by providing emotional, informational, and affirmational support (House, Umberson, & Landis, 1988). Peer support has a potential effect on coping by altering appraisal of caregiving stresses, sustaining caregivers' coping efforts, and influencing their choice of coping strategies (Folkman et al., 1991). Furthermore, peer support may influence the use of health services by stroke survivors.

Assessment Study: Stressors and Support Needs of Persons with Cardiovascular Conditions and Their Family Caregivers

A correlational study investigating social support as a coping resource in mediating the effect of stress on the functional capacity and life satisfaction of ill persons with stroke or heart failure, and on the life satisfaction of their family caregivers was conducted in urban and rural communities in Nova Scotia. Two research questions guided the assessment study: (1) What are the support needs, sources and types of support, and satisfaction with support perceived by persons with heart failure or stroke and their family caregivers? (2) Are there differences between ill persons with stroke or heart failure, between ill persons and their family caregivers, and between men and women in functional capacity (ill persons only), stress, social support and life satisfaction?

Assessment Design

Interviews were conducted in the homes of the individuals with stroke or heart failure and in the family caregivers' homes if they did not live with the ill persons. Participants were interviewed privately and separately on the same day; the ill person was interviewed first for consistency. The interviews took an average of ninety minutes. The data collection instruments (see appendix B for details) were administered to all participants by interview. Interviews were repeated three months later.

The *Sickness Impact Profile* (SIP), a self-report tool for assessing the effects of illness on daily activities, feelings, and attitudes, thereby giving a profile of perceived health status (Bergner, Bobbit, Carter, & Gilson, 1981), was used only with ill persons. Questions were developed to assess the specific disabilities of the ill participants. Heart failure participants were also administered the *New York Heart Association Criteria* (NYHA), used to classify cardiac functional capacity ranging from Class I (ordinary physical activity without undue fatigue, palpitations, dyspnea or anginal pain) to Class IV (inability to carry on any physical activity without discomfort, symptoms of cardiac insufficiency even at rest) (Sokolow & McIlory, 1979).

Both ill-person groups and the stroke family caregivers completed a questionnaire adapted from Gottlieb's (1978) classification scheme of informal helping behaviours, which included four categories: 'emotionally sustaining behaviours,' 'problem-solving behaviours,' 'indirect personal influence' and 'environmental action.' The twenty-three items in the first two categories were reworded in our assessment study. Participants were asked to identify all behaviours that their partner in the care receiver / caregiving dyad enacted (e.g., under emotionally sustaining behaviours, 'provides encouragement,' and 'shares respect'; under problem solving behaviours, 'provides suggestions' and 'checks that I am doing what I should be doing'). Then participants were asked to indicate if they were dissatisfied with their partner's behaviour on any of twenty-three indicators. This allowed us to identify any dissatisfaction related to enactment or absence of each indicator behaviour.

Three measures were administered to all four study groups. Stress was assessed by a self-anchoring *Cantril Ladder* (Cantril, 1965; McDowell & Newell, 1987) in which participants were asked to indicate their current position between most and least stressful time ever experienced. All participants were also asked, 'Right now, what do you find is the most difficult or stressful part of living with your (or your relative's) health problem?' Social support was assessed by the *Personal Resources Questionnaire 85* (PRQ85), a norm-referenced assessment of structural and functional components of social support (Weinert & Brandt, 1987). Life satisfaction was assessed by the *Cantril Ladder* and the *Life Satisfaction Index Z* (LSIZ) (McDowell & Newell, 1987; Wood, Wylie, & Scheafor, 1969), which evaluates general well-being, zest, self-concept, mood, congruence between desired and achieved goals, and meaning of life (see appendix B).

Descriptive analyses were completed on all questionnaire data. Multivariate analysis of variance (MANOVA) was used to test for any difference between study variables. Wilks's lambda multivariate *F*-test was then used to test for significant differences between variables. Where a significant MANOVA *F* was obtained, analyses of variance (univariate *F*) were examined for the dependent variables to determine which variables were statistically significant and contributed to the overall significant multivariate *F*. Content analysis was conducted on the qualitative data elicited by the question to the ill person, 'Right now what do you find is the most difficult or stressful part of living with your health problem?' and to the caregiver: 'Right now what do you find is the most difficult or stressful part of living with [____]'s health problem?' Responses were coded into mutually exclusive categories. The research design is summarized in table 6.1.

Profile of Participants

Participants were people with stroke or heart failure living at home and their primary caregivers, usually a family member living in the same home. The disabled participants were stratified by condition (stroke and heart failure) and sex, since women have been underrepresented in cardiovascular research. One hundred and sixty participants completed both interviews (i.e., twenty

TABLE 6.1
Research Design

	Assessment Study	Intervention Study
Sample	Purposive Stroke/family caregiver dyads ($n = 80$) Heart failure/family caregiver dyads ($n = 80$)	Purposive Family caregivers of stroke survivors ($n = 20$)
Design	Descriptive correlational	Pre-test-post-test within subjects
Measures/ instruments		
Stress	*Sickness Impact Profile* *Cantril Ladder*	*Caregiving Burden Inventory* *Job-Caregiving Conflict Scale* *Role Captivity Scale* *Global Perceived Stress Scale*
Support	*Personal Resources Questionnaire* Tool based on Gottieb's (1978) framework of informal helping behaviours	*Arizona Social Support Interview Schedule*
Health/ Functioning	*Life Satisfaction Index*	*Revised Barthel Index* *Caregiving Competence Scale* (adapted)
Data collection	3 months – 3 years post-stroke with repeat interview 3 months later	Standardized measures pre-test, post-test and delayed post-test (3 and 6 months)
Data analysis Qualitative	Content analysis of responses to 'Right now, what do you find is the most difficult or most stressful part of living with your (or your relative's) health problem?'	Content analysis of peer visitors' diaries, professionals' fieldnotes, and post-intervention interviews
Quantitative	Descriptive and MANOVA	Descriptive and paired *t*-tests

female and twenty male stroke survivors; twenty females and twenty males with heart failure; forty caregivers in each illness group).

There was a similar demographic profile for stroke and heart failure groups. The sample was predominantly Caucasian, elderly (mean age sixty-nine), and married, with equal representation from rural and urban sites.

The mean age of the family caregivers was sixty years; 68 per cent were spouses of the participants with stroke and heart failure; and the remainder were children and other relatives. Seventy-two per cent of the caregivers were female. This profile is consistent with the literature on family caregivers (Lubkin, 1992; Schafer, McCaul, & Glasgow, 1986). Most of the spousal caregivers were living with one or more chronic illnesses.

The stroke survivors had ongoing neurological deficits from a stroke that had occurred between three months to three years prior to admission to the study, as documented by chart review or confirmed by their medical practitioner. Thirty-seven per cent of the stroke participants had right hemiplegia, 54 per cent had left hemiplegia, and 9 per cent had mixed hemiplegia. Most heart failure participants (75 per cent) had had a previous MI; most of these had had at least two previous MIs. Although 70 per cent of the participants with heart failure had an ejection fraction of 30 per cent or less (i.e., high medical severity), 60 per cent reported good functional capacity on the *New York Heart Association Criteria* (NYHA), falling within Classes I and II.

Findings – Assessment Study

Illness Impact

The stroke survivors had a higher mean SIP score (meaning greater illness impact) than the heart failure group, including all physical and psychosocial scores. The only areas in which the cardiac group experienced greater impact of illness were sleep/rest and work.

Stress

The mean scores on the ill persons' and caregivers' measure of stress were mid-range. The ill persons with stroke and their caregivers, however, reported greater stress than their heart failure counterparts.

Illness-imposed change in roles was among the three most frequently noted stressors in both ill persons' groups, particularly loss of previously valued work or recreational roles. Physical dysfunction (paralysis and communication deficits for stroke survivors; energy deficits and shortness of breath for participants with heart failure) was also among the top sources of stress. Ill persons ranked dependence on other people and resources as the third stressor, in part related to perceived burden on their family caregivers.

Similarly, one of the three top stressors for caregivers was the burden of having their family member dependent on them. The continuous responsibility and confinement to home associated with care of stroke survivors was reflected in statements such as 'I feel trapped, alone.' and 'I'm on 24-hour call, cannot leave home.' Caregivers of persons with heart failure focused on the confinement that the illness imposed on both the ill person and themselves. Emotional or mental change in the ill person was the second most frequently mentioned source of stress for the stroke caregiver group, reflected in the following descriptors: 'depressed,' 'impulsive,' 'stubbornness,' 'gives up,' 'cannot carry on an intelligent conversation,' and 'not the same person he used to be.' Family caregivers and ill persons who denied experiencing stress relating to illness were primarily in the heart failure groups.

Social Support

Participants identified an average of two sources of support for each hypothetical situation and six sources over all ten situations (as measured by Part 1 of the PRQ85). Spousal pairs (ill person / caregiver) rarely noted each other as a source of available support. It seemed, however, that the participants in many spousal pairs, even though interviewed separately, responded to the ten hypothetical life situations as a member of a couple rather than as an individual. Available support from their spouse seemed to be taken for granted.

Male caregivers identified their spouses as a source of support significantly less often than did ill males. The heart failure caregivers identified their spouses as a source of support in more hypothetical situations than the stroke caregivers. Children and friends were identified most frequently by the female caregivers, while children were reported most frequently by male caregivers as a source of support. The three top needs for support were (1) 'Someone to talk to about your day-to-day personal concerns,' (2) 'felt lonely,' and (3) 'felt upset and frustrated with the conditions of your life.' The stroke caregivers also noted the need for 'help for an extended period of time in caring for a family member who is sick or disabled.'

In Part 2 of the PRQ85 (a global measure of perceived available social support), there was a striking similarity in responses of participants about the major form of perceived available support selected (i.e., 'There is someone who loves and cares about me'). In addition, many ill persons noted 'If I got sick there is someone to give me advice about caring for myself' and 'There is someone I feel close to who makes me feel secure'; whereas caregivers more often believed 'I have a sense of being needed by another person' and 'I am responsible for helping provide for another person's needs.'

All four participant groups believed that three indicators of social support were not available to them: (1) 'I spend time with others who have the same interests that I do.' (2) 'I have opportunity to encourage others to develop their interests and skills.' (3) 'There is opportunity in my life to be giving and caring for another person.' The apparent incongruity inherent in some family caregivers' observations of inadequate opportunity for giving to and caring for another person may arise from their perceived obligation to care for their family members with stroke or heart failure, which, in turn, precluded other opportunities.

Despite these common findings, there were statistically significant differences in perceived available support. Ill persons with heart failure perceived more support than stroke survivors did; family caregivers reported higher perceived support than ill persons did; and caregivers of persons with heart failure perceived higher support than their stroke caregiver counterparts did.

In response to questions adapted from Gottlieb's (1978) categories of informal helping behaviours, the stroke survivors reported significantly less satisfaction overall with support from their caregivers than persons with heart failure ($p = 0.001$). In particular, stroke survivors were more dissatisfied with (1) the absence of three emotionally sustaining behaviours: 'gives companionship', 'shows understanding,' and 'shows support'; (2) one problem-solving behaviour: 'talking about problems'; (3) the unhelpful nature of the problem-solving behaviour: 'provides suggestions' (i.e., appraisal support). Both stroke (28 per cent) and heart failure (23 per cent) participants were most dissatisfied with the problem-solving behaviour: 'tells me what to do' (appraisal support).

The informal helping behaviours questionnaire (Gottlieb, 1978) was also administered to the stroke caregiver group, allowing for assessment of reciprocal support between stroke survivors and their caregivers. Family caregivers were significantly less satisfied with the support they received from the stroke survivors than the converse ($p = 0.0003$). Caregivers indicated most dissatisfaction in relation to the problem-solving indicator: 'tells me what to do' (38 per cent) (i.e., appraisal support). Many stroke caregivers also reported being dissatisfied with miscarried or absent emotional support functions, such as 'talking about problems' (33 per cent), 'listens to me' (30 per cent), 'shows understanding' (27 per cent) and 'talking about general feelings' (25 per cent).

Life Satisfaction

All participants appeared to be moderately satisfied with their lives, although persons with heart failure and their caregivers reported higher satisfaction than the participants living with stroke did. There was agreement among participants on the item that received the most positive rating: 'As I look back on my life I am fairly well satisfied'; and the most negative rating: 'I have [not] made plans for things I'll be doing a month or a year from now.'

Key Findings from the Assessment Study

Family caregivers of stroke survivors:

- identified continuous responsibility of caregiving and emotional and cognitive changes in stroke survivors as major sources of stress
- perceived more stress than cardiac caregivers or stroke survivors
- reported lack of reciprocity in their relationship with the stroke survivor
- expressed least satisfaction with support.

Implications for Intervention Study

The participants who reported the most stress and the least satisfaction with support from their partner in the caregiver / care receiver relationship were the family caregivers of stroke survivors. These findings are consistent with some recent research with family caregivers of persons with stroke. When a close relative has a stroke and becomes physically and emotionally dependent on a family caregiver, the loss of previous social support from the ill person is added to the direct burden of caregiving (Enterlante & Kern, 1995). The stress associated with emotional and behavioural changes in the relative with stroke (Anderson, Linto, & Stewart-Wynne, 1995; Draper, Poulos, Cole, Poulos, & Ehrlich, 1992) may lead to negative role changes (Periard & Ames, 1993), unhappiness (Enterlante & Kern, 1995), and diminished health (Vanetgian & Corrigan, 1995) for family caregivers. Social support can help to decrease negative reactions to caregiving (Pohl, Given, Collins, & Given, 1994).

Studies suggest that family caregivers of frail elderly persons are in need of support and guidance as they cope with caregiving demands (Williams, 1994). Yet support interventions for caregivers of the elderly have not been matched to demands, and such interventions are virtually non-existent for caregivers of stroke survivors. Furthermore, interventions have emphasized professional rather than lay supporters who have first-hand experience with caregiving and who can provide less costly and most effective support (Forster & Young, 1996).

Intervention Study: Peer Visitor Support for Family Caregivers

The three objectives of the intervention study were to (1) implement a home visiting support program, involving experienced peers, for family caregivers of seniors with a recent stroke; (2) monitor, describe, and evaluate the support intervention processes; and (3) measure the impact of the peer support intervention on caregivers' perceptions of their social support, burden, stress, and competence and on the use of health care services by stroke survivors.

Intervention Design

Participants received two home visits per week, for a period of twelve weeks. The support intervention was planned to be implemented soon after an elderly person who had had an initial stroke was discharged from the hospital. This is a time when new family caregivers are fearful, lack confidence, need someone to listen to their apprehensions about caregiving burden, and need ongoing reinforcement of tasks and other aspects of care. This intervention introduced guidance and information on caregiving within the context of a supportive relationship with a peer who had cared for a person recovering from stroke. Most peer visitors had cared for mothers and a few had cared for their husbands following a stroke. Although this was not a criterion, all of the peers were women. The selection of peers was based, in part, on geographical proximity to the family caregivers.

A guide for peer visitors encompassed specific issues and strategies pertaining to each of four caregiver burden domains – physical care, changes in family life, changes in caregiver roles, and emotional needs of caregivers – which might be raised in peer-caregiver interactions. These demands were consistent with the stressors identified in the assessment study. The peer helper was expected to listen empathetically to the caregiver, offer suggestions concerning coping with different burden domains, encourage problem solving, and deal with any interpersonal tensions that existed between the caregiver and care recipient that might increase the stress felt by the caregiver. It is noteworthy that caregivers in the initial assessment study rarely identified the ill spouse as a source of support.

Health professionals – nurses and occupational therapists – conducted the initial assessment of the home environments and the stroke survivors' functional status, using the *Revised Barthel Index* (Shah, Vanclay, & Cooper, 1989), and introduced peers to caregivers and provided ongoing support and guidance to the peer visitors. The professionals were also on call (as consultants) for problems or concerns raised by either peers or family caregivers. Professionals used their assessment, communication, teaching, and coaching skills to help peer visitors to (1) maintain the major focus on the family caregivers' needs, (2) encourage caregivers to share their experiences, and (3) provide emotional support by listening to caregivers' stories. By providing situation-specific feedback, the professionals enabled the peers to further hone their interaction skills and boost their confidence in their ability to provide effective support.

The peer visitors provided ongoing emotional, affirmational, and informational support to family caregivers. Furthermore, the peer visitors monitored the caregiver's needs and any unanticipated effects of the intervention on both family caregivers and stroke survivors.

Several steps were taken to control sources of bias and other potential problems: (1) The professionals received specific project-related training in observation techniques and assessment criteria. (2) The professionals and peers had a joint day of empathy training. (3) Peer visitors were taught how to document support processes. (4) Objective research assistants conducted pre- and post-intervention interviews, and other research assistants helped with data analysis.

Key Features of the Intervention

- Two weekly home visits to new family caregivers of stroke survivors were made by experienced peers over a period of twelve weeks.
- Peers provided emotional, affirmational and informational support.
- Health professionals did initial assessments of stroke survivors at home and were available for consultation to peer visitors.
- Peers and professionals trained jointly.
- Peers recorded diary accounts of conversation topics and types of support provided.
- Professionals documented contacts with peers and family caregivers.
- Standardized measures were administered pre-test, post-test, and delayed post-test (social support, confidence, burden, stress).
- The post-test interview concerned perceived impact of the intervention.

Documentation of Processes and Outcomes

After each visit, peer visitors recorded a diary account of the visit, describing subjects of conversation and documenting types of support provided. The professionals kept records of contacts with peers and family caregivers. The family caregivers also commented on types of support received and satisfaction with the intervention during the post-intervention interviews and at three- and six-month follow-ups. Both the transcripts from the taped post-intervention interviews and the peer and professional diaries/logs were content analysed using a category system that was developed inductively from the data (Waltz,

Strickland, & Lenz, 1991). The data were analysed for both manifest and latent content. The units of analysis were full references to any content related to (1) nature of the demands involved in caring for an elderly relative with a chronic condition; (2) caregivers' reactions to those demands; (3) types, sources, and appraisal of support; (4) coping strategies; and (5) perceived impact of the intervention. All of these mutually exclusive categories and subcategories were fully and clearly defined.

Six standardized measures were administered pre-test, post-test, and delayed post-test (three and six months later). The *Arizona Social Support Interview Schedule* (ASSIS) (Barrera, 1981) was used to assess the family caregivers' social support with emphasis on support related to their caregiving demands. A measure of caregiving competence and confidence was developed for the intervention study. This was adapted from the *Caregiving Competence Scale* (Pearlin, Mullen, Semple, & Skaff, 1990) and supplemented by a question about caregivers' perceived competence in major roles other than caregiving. The *Caregiver Burden Inventory* (Novak & Guest, 1989), a multidimensional measure of caregiver burden, was used to assess three of the four burden domains in this study: (1) physical care, (2) family disruption and caregiver relationship with relative with stroke, and (3) socio-emotional burden. The remaining burden domain was assessed using the *Job-Caregiving Conflict Scale* and *Role Captivity Scale*, two subscales of a caregiving stress measure (Pearlin et al., 1990). The *Global Perceived Stress Scale* (Cohen, Kamarck, & Mermelstein, 1983) was administered to assess the degree to which situations in caregivers' lives were appraised as stressful. The *Revised Barthel Index* (Shah et al., 1989) was used to measure functional status of stroke survivors (see appendix B for a description of these measures). Use of health services by the stroke survivor was measured through questions posed during pre-test, post-test, and delayed post-test interviews. In addition to simple descriptive statistics for all variables (comprising the six standardized measures) showing mean values over time, quantitative analysis consisted of paired *t*-tests comparing pre-test versus post-test and pre-test versus six-month delayed post-test measure (table 6.1 summarizes the research design).

Profile of Participants

Of the twenty female caregivers who participated in the study, eighteen were married. Education levels varied, with twelve caregivers having less than high school. The mean age of the caregivers was fifty-nine years. Thirteen were spouses of the stroke survivor, four were daughters, and one was a daughter-in-law. Seventeen caregivers resided with the stroke survivor. The mean length of residence with the stroke survivor was thirty-two years. Four caregivers noted a change in their work status following the stroke: three had changed from full- to part-time work and one had left work completely. Like the caregivers in the assessment study, the majority reported having their own health problems. The stroke survivors were sixteen males and four females who had a mean age of seventy-one years. The average amount of time between the date of the stroke and the date of the first visit by a peer was nine months.

Findings – Intervention Study

Caregivers experienced numerous primary demands. All caregivers expressed considerable concern to the peer visitors about managing the symptoms and deficits experienced by their family member with stroke. Many spoke of the constancy of worrying about the stroke survivor, and their need for vigilance. The constancy of caregiving was reflected in fears of leaving the stroke survivor alone, and feeling 'tied down.' Caregivers performed a variety of physical tasks (e.g., assisting the stroke survivor with personal activities of daily living). Caregivers often reported that they wished stroke survivors would 'do more for themselves,' and they attempted to facilitate the survivor's participation in self-care, meaningful activities, and social activities.

Caregivers indicated that sometimes stroke survivors behaved towards them in ways that were unappreciative, unkind, and even abusive. Caregivers found it difficult to deal with the stroke survivors' frustrations and fears. Caregivers also reported some negative experiences in their interactions with health professionals and the health care system.

Secondary caregiving demands described by these caregivers included the devastating impact of the stroke on their own personal needs, other ongoing role involvements, and the family unit. Family caregivers contended that the additional role of caregiving interfered with their rest and freedom to engage in personal activities and social occupations. They also had to deal with the emotional impact of the stroke on their own and their family member's life, relationship changes with the stroke survivor, and their own emotional reactions to their caregiving responsibilities. Caregivers also expressed concerns related to family relationships and sought strategies for reducing and managing conflict.

The expressed concerns of these family caregivers, recorded in peer visitor diaries, were strikingly similar to the three major stressors identified by the (different) group of family caregivers of stroke survivors in the assessment study: (1) burden of caring for a dependent family member, (2) coping with negative changes in their emotions and behaviour, and (3) the resulting role changes imposed on the family caregivers.

Caregivers in the intervention study spontaneously discussed support from members of their social network with the peer visitors. To meet their needs for instrumental support, a few had hired help, while others relied on persons in their natural network, primarily family members. Forty per cent of the caregivers, however, contended that they did not have persons available within their networks who could meet their needs for emotional, affirmational, and informational support. Even when potential support providers were available, 35 per cent reported that these persons were either not able to provide any help or provided insufficient help. Another 15 per cent did not believe that the support they received was helpful (i.e., miscarried helping). These findings are consistent with the assessment study, in which the group of family caregivers of stroke survivors was least satisfied with social support.

Clearly, the caregivers in the intervention study had unmet emotional, affirmational, and informational support needs. There was a strong need for supplementary support from the project peers and professionals.

Types of Social Support Provided by Intervention

Peer visitors provided emotional, affirmational, informational, and occasional instrumental support. Project professionals primarily offered informational support.

Active listening was a central component of *emotional support* in every caregiver/peer relationship. The presence of the peer provided caregivers with an opportunity to tell their 'stories' and to vent anger and frustration. Caregivers confirmed that understanding based on peers' common experience as caregivers was a very important element in the support provided. Interactions with peer visitors served both as a point of social comparison regarding the behaviour and functioning of their relative and as a foundation for rapport. The peer visitors attempted to create an atmosphere in which caregivers would feel comfortable in expressing themselves. Peer visitors provided comfort in conjunction with listening, understanding, sharing similar experiences, and 'just being there': '*Before she started coming I ... didn't have anybody to really talk to that would understand*' (caregiver).

Affirmational support such as positive feedback or encouragement was sometimes general, and sometimes focused on particular aspects of caregiving or specific caregiving activities. In addition, peer visitors offered affirmation that caregivers' decisions or strategies were appropriate and that they were not alone in their caregiving experiences and feelings. Peer visitors also related difficulties that they themselves had experienced, so that family caregivers could see that they were handling similar situations effectively.

Seventy-five per cent of the caregivers reported receiving *informational support* from peers and/or professionals. Peers provided informational support based on their own experiential knowledge, whereas project professionals provided information from a professional perspective either directly to the caregiver or indirectly through the peer. The peers offered information about local formal and informal resources, which many caregivers had not been aware of. Oral information focused on stroke symptoms, the effects of stroke therapy, modifications to living spaces, and strategies for promoting self-care. Peer visitors suggested strategies for managing reactions of stroke survivors, respite needs, caregiver stress, and family conflict/demands. Peer visitors also offered problem-specific suggestions for meaningful activities for stroke survivors and suitable solutions to caregiving problems. Moreover, peers recommended equipment and strategies to enhance the safety and comfort of the stroke survivor.

Consistent with the purpose of the support intervention, project personnel provided *instrumental support* infrequently. On a few occasions, peer visitors assisted with transportation or obtaining equipment for stroke survivors or family caregivers.

Caregivers' Perceptions of Intervention Processes

Most support from peer visitors was viewed as supportive, reciprocal/bidirectional, appropriate, and timely. Caregivers noted that peer support helped them to feel more confident in their role. Elements that contributed to the success of a caregiver/peer match included similarities in caregiving experience, personality factors, age, and interests. A feeling of mutuality (reciprocity) in the relationship was also important: '*You just feel connected to other people who are going through the same thing. I felt connected to peer*' (caregiver).

The caregivers' comfort in talking freely and openly with peer visitors as well as the process of establishing comfort in the caregiver/peer relationship were significant. Trust developed over time. Caregivers looked forward to the peer visits as an opportunity to talk openly about their experiences with someone who understood their reactions: '*I was talking to peer and she realized that I was doing more than ... I expected a lot from myself ... talking to her, I knew that I had to start taking more time for me. It was good to have somebody that wasn't in the family that you could vent your frustrations and you knew that they weren't going back and telling'* (caregiver).

Many family caregivers saw the professional as a source of information and as a liaison with the peer visitor, although others noted that the professional's role seemed to be restricted to initial assessment. Family caregivers were asked during the post-intervention interviews whether they would choose a peer or a professional visitor in a future intervention. Of those who responded, 67 per cent indicated a preference for a peer visitor, while 33 per cent preferred to have both a peer and professional; none selected the option of professional alone: *'I just think that somebody who is living with it, day in and day out, sees it on a different level because they have to experience the emotional side of it, not just the clinical side of it'* (caregiver).

Some peers and family caregivers found it difficult to terminate the visits. In an effort to fill the void, however, several reported joining peer support groups or exploring respite care options. During the follow-up interviews, most caregivers indicated that they still kept in touch with their peer visitors: *'She keeps in contact with me though, like through the phone just to say 'Hi'... It's good that you can feel that you can talk to her from time to time'* (caregiver).

The intervention was not without perceived costs. Some caregivers reported that their relatives with stroke seemed suspicious about the purpose of the intervention and jealous of the attention they received. Although the intervention was valued, some caregivers noted that it added to their time constraints.

Caregivers' Perceptions of the Impact of Intervention on Burden and Coping

Some reductions in burden were reported by family caregivers following the intervention, due, in part, to positive changes in the stroke survivor (e.g., acceptance of functional deficits, more self-care, engagement in physiotherapy or speech therapy). Some family caregivers indicated that the peer visitor helped to decrease their burden.

During their discussions with peer visitors, family caregivers reported using a wide array of coping strategies – support seeking, protective buffering, acceptance – to manage the demands of caregiving. Caregivers sought practical and emotional support from others in their network, such as family and friends. Caregivers hid concerns, denied worries, and yielded to the stroke survivor to avoid disagreements (i.e., protective buffering). Generally, family caregivers accepted their relatives' illness and their need for care: '*There are days I'm really, really nervous with him. Not that I can't care for him ... But my nights are worse. I go to bed and I wake up, and I hear him also coughing ... I'll get up and see if he's alright. That is just what goes on with me. That's the way it's going to be*' (caregiver).

There were changes in coping following the intervention. Nearly all caregivers reported that coping with caregiving was easier because of the support intervention, and almost half indicated that the visits by peers offered a distraction from their caregiving roles: '*It was a very ... Well, I wouldn't call it informal. I mean she made you feel, "Well here is somebody coming in to give support," and while we talked about the stroke part, there were other things that she talked about which was good too. It's kind of depressing just to talk about one thing*' (caregiver).

Peer visitors may have helped family caregivers to select more effective coping strategies, leading to a more positive appraisal of caregiving stress: '*It made it easier because I had somebody to talk to. I didn't know where I was going from one day to another, so it was nice. It would relieve some of the pressures. I guess it helped me in different ways. It helped me to understand stroke survivor's problems*' (caregiver).

Impact of the Intervention

From pre-test to six-month delayed post-test, there were significant decreases in overall support need, need for material aid, and need for guidance and a significant increase in satisfaction with guidance. The decreased need for feedback and for discussion of personal feelings, while short of statistical significance, were of note given the small sample size. There were no significant changes over the study period in confidence, stress, and burden measures, although one-third of the family caregivers reported that the support intervention had increased their confidence and self-esteem and reduced their uncertainty.

A paired *t*-test of pre-intervention versus six-month follow-up identified a significant decrease in perceived network size, and some decrease in the actual network size. Analysis of the network composition revealed that, prior to the intervention, these caregivers' social networks were composed primarily of family members; the second-largest category was friends. Over half identified physicians and only a few named neighbours, other health professionals, or clergy as network members. Over time, from pre-test to post-test to delayed post-test, there was a notable decline in the number of most of these social network members; only the number of persons classified as friends (including peer visitors) increased.

It was anticipated that caregivers who received peer support would be less likely to seek professional intervention for stroke survivors. From pre-intervention to six-month delayed post-test interviews, there was a significant decline in the number of visits to hospital outpatient departments and in admissions to hospital for the stroke survivor.

Key Findings from the Intervention Study

- Caregivers identified family (including ill members) as the major source of conflictual or absent support.
- All caregivers expressed satisfaction with the intervention.
- Key benefits of the intervention were identified by caregivers:
  - receiving emotional and affirmational support
  - access to knowledge of experienced peers with similar caregiving experiences.
- Perceived disadvantages were reported by caregivers:
  - stroke survivors were uncomfortable or jealous
  - time demands.
- There were increased support satisfaction, decreased support need, and decreased perceived network size but increased friend support (including peers) following intervention.
- There were reduced contacts with hospitals regarding stroke survivors' health following intervention.

Similarities between the Assessment and Intervention Studies

There were significant similarities in the findings of both the assessment and the intervention studies. The centrality of the burden of daily care and caregiver stress caused by emotional changes in the stroke survivor were evident in both studies. In this context, it is interesting that life satisfaction was mid-range in the assessment study. This finding is consistent with the fact that acceptance was the dominant coping style used by caregivers in the intervention study. Both studies also showed that family members, friends, and care partners were sources of both support and conflict. Furthermore, stroke caregivers indicated that support from their natural network was often absent, non-reciprocal, or conflictual. Peer visitors, as sources of supplementary support, were viewed as supportive in the intervention study.

Implications for Programs and Policies

Although potential peer visitors and professionals for the intervention study were identified easily through stroke clubs and newspaper ads, it was impossible to recruit sufficient stroke caregivers to mount the originally planned randomized controlled study within the Maritime region. Despite multiple recruitment avenues (print and electronic media, church bulletins, neurologists and family physicians, stroke clubs, hospitals, VON, Heart and Stroke Foundation, etc.) and interest expressed from all groups, few referrals resulted. The lack of initiative by health professionals approached for referrals may have been due to their busy schedules and other priorities. The current era of health funding cutbacks may limit the capacity of health professionals to be involved in voluntary activities not covered directly by their job descriptions.

Some peer visitors were not as well matched with the family caregiver as others were. Caregivers expressed a clear preference for peer visitors whose situations were most similar to their own experience. Caregivers and peer visitors recommended that, in future programs, the peer should be matched as closely as possible to the family caregiver, particularly in terms of experience with specific stroke disability and relationship between the caregiver and the stroke survivor (i.e., spouse, daughter, daughter-in-law). Peer visitors who did not meet these criteria were uniformly viewed as less effective than those who had had similar personal experiences.

Some seniors with stroke were uncomfortable or jealous about the home visits by the peers and professionals and the attention paid to the family caregiver. Although the intervention was focused on the needs of family caregivers, it was clear that the peer visitor also needed to interact with the stroke survivor, reflecting the importance of the familial dyad.

It is not surprising, given the mean age of caregivers in both studies, that many family caregivers themselves had chronic illnesses. The stressors of caregiving increase the potential for deterioration in their health, which can have a detrimental impact on their ability to keep stroke survivors at home. Community-based support programs, such as the peer visitor program evaluated in this intervention study, offer needed support at a modest cost. A peer intervention based on a combination of visits and telephone or on telephone alone might have a similar impact with less cost.

Participants in the two studies reported in this chapter represent the growing number of caregivers who are given responsibility for home care of family members with complex psychological and physical deficits. Family caregivers in the intervention study suggested that the peer visitor program should start within a month after the stroke survivor is discharged from hospital, since this was a time when they experienced the greatest uncertainty. More proactive programs prior to discharge from hospital settings are needed to help to reduce the uncertainty and stress of new family caregivers. These programs might include family conferences, regular educational sessions for family members using experienced family caregivers as resources, and pre-discharge passes to the home so that family caregivers can identify unmet learning or support needs before discharge.

Given the current practice of early discharge from hospitals and the expectation that families will provide home-based care, health professionals need to assume a more proactive role in educating and supporting family and other lay caregivers in their home-based care of persons with chronic illnesses and disabilities. In order to achieve these goals, professional educational programs must assume responsibility for enabling students to undertake these expanding roles in their communities.

Lessons Learned

- The study supports the value of peer visitor interventions for family caregivers of stroke survivors.
- There is potential for peer support of similar value and less cost via telephone contacts instead of home visits.
- Programs should be launched soon after the stroke.
- A close caregiver/peer match increases the effectiveness of intervention.
- Parallel intervention for stroke survivors may be desirable.
- Formal health system support is needed for widespread implementation.

Acknowledgments

Both studies were funded by the Heart and Stroke Foundation of Nova Scotia. The intervention study was funded, following review, by the Canadian Heart and Stroke Foundation.

Note

A report of the assessment study has been submitted to *Canadian Journal of Cardiovascular Nursing*, and a partial report of the intervention study has been published (Stewart, Doble, Hart, Langille, and MacPherson (1998).

References

Anderson, C., Linto, J., & Stewart-Wynne, E. (1995). A population-based assessment of the impact and burden of caring for long-term stroke survivors. *Stroke, 26*, 843–849.

Barrera, M. (1981). Social support in the adjustment of pregnant adolescents. In B. Gottlieb (Ed.), *Social networks and social support* (69–96). Beverly Hills, CA: Sage.

Bergner, M., Bobbit, R., Carter, B., & Gilson, B. (1981). The sickness impact profile: Development and final revision of a health status measure. *Medical Care, 19*, 787–805.

Boynton De Sepulveda, L., & Chang, B. (1994). Effective coping with stroke disability in a community setting: The development of a causal model. *Journal of Neuroscience Nursing, 26*, 193–203.

Bramwell, L., & Whall, A. (1986). Effect of role clarity and empathy on support role performance and anxiety. *Nursing Research, 35*, 282–287.

Browning, J.S., & Schwirian, P.M. (1994). Spousal caregivers burden: Impact of care recipient health problems and mental status. *Journal of Gerontological Nursing, 20*(3), 17–22.

Bull, M. (1990). Factors influencing family caregiver burden and health. *Western Journal of Nursing Research, 12*, 758–776.

Cantril, H. (1965). *The pattern of human concerns.* New York: Rutgers University Press.

Cheitlin,, M., Sokolow, M., & McIlory, B. (1993). *Clinical cardiology* (6th ed.). Norwalk, CT: Appleton Lange.

Cohen, S. Kamarck, T., & Mermelstein, R. (1983). A global measure of perceived stress. *Journal of Health and Social Behaviour, 24*, 385–396.

Derenowski, J.M. (1988). The relationship of social support systems, health locus of control, health value orientation and wellness motivation in the post myocardial infarction patient during three phases of rehabilitation. *Progress in Cardiovascular Nursing, 3*, 143–152.

Draper, B., Poulos, C., Cole, A. Poulos, R., & Ehrlich, F. (1992). A comparison of caregivers of elderly stroke and dementia victims. *Journal of the American Geriatrics Society, 40*, 896–901.

Enterlante, T., & Kern, J. (1995). Wives reported role changes following a husband's stroke: A pilot study. *Rehabilitation Nursing, 20*, 156–160.

Evans, R., Hendricks, R., Haselkorn, J., Bishop, D., & Baldwin, D. (1992). The family's role in stroke rehabilitation: A review of the literature. *American Journal of Physical Medicine and Rehabilitation, 71*, 135–139.

Folkman, S., Chesney, M., McKusick, L., Ironson, G., Johnson, D., & Coates, T. (1991). Translating coping theory into an intervention. In J. Eckenrode (Ed.), *The social context of coping* (240–260). New York: Plenum Press.

Forster, A., & Young, J. (1996). Specialist nurse support for patients with stroke in the community: A randomized controlled trial. *British Medical Journal, 312,* 1642–1646.

Friedland, J., & McColl, M. (1987). Social support and psycho-social dysfunction after stroke: Buffering effects in a community sample. *Archives of Physical Medicine and Rehabilitation, 68,* 475–480.

Glass, T., & Maddox, G. (1992). The quality and quantity of social support: Stroke recovery as a psycho-social transition. *Social Science & Medicine, 34,* 1249–1261.

Gottlieb, B. (1978). The development and application of a classification scheme of informal helping behaviours. *Canadian Journal of Behavioural Science, 10,* 105–115.

Heart and Stroke Foundations of Canada (1997). *Heart disease and stroke in Canada.* Ottawa: HSFC.

Heller, K., Swindle, R., & Dusenbury, L. (1986). Component social support processes: Comments and integration. *Journal of Consulting & Clinical Psychology, 54,* 446–470.

House, J., Umberson, D., & Landis, K. (1988). Structures and processes of social support. *Annual Review of Sociology, 14,* 293–318.

King, K., Reis, H., Porter, L., & Norsen, L. (1993). Social support and long term recovery from coronary artery surgery: Effects on patients and spouses. *Health Psychology, 12,* 54–62.

Lubkin, I.M. (1992). *Chronic illness: Impact and interventions* (2nd ed.). Boston: Jones & Bartlett.

Lyons, R., McDonald, A., MacKay-Lyons, M., & Phillips, S. (1995). *Stroke: A needs analysis in Nova Scotia.* Halifax, NS: Heart and Stroke Foundation of Nova Scotia.

MacNamara, S., Gummow, L., Goka, R., & Gregg, C. (1990). Caregiver strain: Need for late post-stroke intervention. *Rehabilitation Psychology, 35,* 71–78.

Mahoney, F., & Barthel, D. (1965). Functional evaluation: The Barthel Index. *Maryland State Medical Journal, 12*(1), 61–65.

Markle-Reid, M. (1989). Social Support and perception of illness in the early discharge phase for the MI patient. *Canadian Journal of Cardiovascular Nursing, 1*(2), 9–18.

McDowell, I., & Newell, C. (1987). *Measuring health: A guide to rating scales and questionnaires.* New York: Oxford University Press.

Novak, M., & Guest, C. (1989). Application of a multidimensional caregiver burden inventory. *Gerontologist, 29,* 798–803.

Nyamathi, A. (1987). The coping responses of female spouses of patients with myocardial infarction. *Heart and Lung, 16*, 86–91.

Pearlin, L., Mullen, J., Semple, S., & Skaff, M. (1990). Caregiving and the stress process: An overview of concepts and their measures. *Gerontologist, 30*, 583–594.

Periard, M., & Ames, B. (1993). Lifestyle changes and coping patterns among caregivers of stroke survivors. *Public Health Nursing, 10*, 252–256.

Pohl, J., Given, C., Collins, C., & Given, B. (1994). Social vulnerability and reactions to caregiving in daughters and daughters-in-law caring for disabled parents. *Health Care for Women International, 15*, 385–395.

Riffle, K. (1988). The relationship between perception of supportive behaviours of others and wives' ability to cope with initial myocardial infarctions in their husbands. *Rehabilitation Nursing, 13*, 310–315.

Ross, S., & Morris, R. (1988). Psychological adjustment of the spouses of aphasic stroke patients. *International Journal of Rehabilitation Research, 11*, 383–386.

Sandin, K., Cifu, D., & Noll, S. (1994). Stroke rehabilitation: Psychologic and social implications. *Archives of Physical Medicine and Rehabilitation, 75*, S52–S55.

Schafer, L., McCaul, K., & Glasgow, R. (1986). Supportive and nonsupportive family behaviours: Relationship to adherence and metabolic control in persons with type I diabetes. *Diabetes Care, 9*, 179–185.

Schulz, R., Tompkins, C., & Rau, M. (1988). A longitudinal study of the psychosocial impact of stroke on primary support persons. *Psychology and Aging, 3*, 131–141.

Shah, S., Vanclay, F., & Cooper, B. (1989). Improving the sensitivity of the Barthel Index for stroke rehabilitation. *Journal of Clinical Epidemiology, 42*, 703–709.

Silliman, R., & Sternberg, J. (1988). Family caregiving: Impact of patient functioning and underlying causes of disability. *Gerontologist, 28*, 377–382.

Sokolow, M., & McIlroy, M. (1979). *Clinical cardiology*. Los Altos, CA: Lange Medical.

Stewart, M., Doble, S., Hart, G., Hirth, A., Langille, L., & MacPherson, K. (1998). Peer support for family caregivers of seniors with stroke. *Canadian Journal of Nursing Research, 30*(2), 87–117.

Stewart, M. (1993). *Integrating social support in nursing*. Newbury Park, CA: Sage.

Tilden, V., & Gaylen, R. (1987). Cost and conflict: The darker side of social support. *Western Journal of Nursing Research, 9*, 9–18.

Vanetzian, E., & Corrigan, B.A. (1995). A comparison of the educational wants of family caregivers to patients with stroke. *Rehabilitation Nursing, 20*(3), 149–54.

Waltz, C., Strickland, O., & Lenz, E. (1991). *Measurements in nursing research* (2nd ed.). Philadelphia: F.A. Davis.

Weinert, C., & Brandt, P. (1987). Measuring social support with the personal resource questionnaire. *Western Journal of Nursing Research, 9*, 589–602.

Williams, A. (1994). What bothers caregivers of stroke victims? *Journal of Neuroscience Nursing, 26*, 155–161.

Wood, V., Wylie, M., & Scheafor, B. (1969). An analysis of a short self-report measure of life satisfaction: Correlation with rater judgement. *Journal of Gerontology, 24*, 465–469.

7

Support Needs of Nurses: Telephone Support for Professional Supporters

Gail G. Tomblin Murphy, Miriam J. Stewart, Judith A. Ritchie, Andrew Johnson, and Patty J. Weld Viscount

Abstract. We conducted assessment and intervention research with Canadian nurses in HIV/AIDS (n = 177) and community health (n = 100) care to determine how social support influences the relationship between perceived job stress and mental and physical health. We found that both social support and coping moderate the effects of these stressors on nurses' health and functioning outcomes (i.e., job satisfaction and burnout). Given the potential harmful effects of stress and burnout, we recognized the importance of developing strategies that reduced the cost to nurses, clients, and the health system. We examined how social support can buffer the debilitating effects of stress and burnout. Accordingly, our follow-up intervention study tested the effectiveness of an intervention designed to enhance social support, promote the use of certain coping strategies for managing occupational stress and prevent burnout in nurses. Telephone support groups, co-led by an expert facilitator and an expert 'AIDS nurse,' were tested in a demonstration project for nurses in HIV/AIDS care (n = 30). Lessons learned include the merits of a multifaceted recruitment strategy, specifically designed training sessions that reflect changing challenges in AIDS care and the necessity to maintain confidentiality and full participation in the sessions.

Introduction

Acquired Immune Deficiency Syndrome (AIDS) is a chronic illness that is escalating globally at an alarming rate. In Canada, nurses are the largest group of professionals who provide support to persons living with HIV/AIDS (PWA). It is evident that nurses are increasingly likely to encounter stressors associated with AIDS care, regardless of their work setting. Accordingly, nurses, as 'professional supporters,' themselves require support.

The treatment of AIDS and the prevention of Human Immunodeficiency Virus (HIV) infection will continue to challenge the health system (Grady,

1989). In 1995 Health and Welfare Canada received reports of 11,664 cases of AIDS (Laboratory Centre for Disease Control, 1995). The World Health Organization (WHO) predicts that the number of people with AIDS in the world will increase tenfold, from an estimated 1.5 million to 12-18 million by the year 2000. Consequently, the potential for occupational stress in HIV-care workers can be expected to increase in the near future (Bennett, Miller, & Ross, 1995).

Despite the alarming worldwide increases in HIV/AIDS and the fact that nurses are the largest group of professional caregivers who have contact with HIV/AIDS, there has been very little research on the impact of working with PWA on nurses or nursing care. To date, only two pertinent studies of nurses working in HIV/AIDS care have been conducted in Canada. Pickhall (1984) identified many work-related stressors in a qualitative study of eight nurses in HIV/AIDS care. Tomblin-Murphy, Stewart, Ritchie, and Johnson (1995) conducted a nationwide survey of 177 nurses working in HIV/AIDS care, in a variety of hospital and community-based settings, in order to examine work-related stress, social support, coping, job satisfaction, and burnout. This assessment study, reported in this chapter, demonstrated a clear need for a support intervention to help nurses to cope with the stresses of AIDS care.

Present State of Knowledge

Nurses working with persons living with PWA are exposed to diverse stressors related to counselling, social support, sexuality and homophobia, ethics, death, dying, and grieving (Ferris, Flannery, McNeal, & Morrisette, 1995; Hearn, Nihill, & Ong, 1991; Macks & Abrams, 1992; Martin, 1990; Meisenhelder, 1993). According to numerous authors, however, prior to our assessment study there had been limited research regarding the impact of occupational stress on nurses working in HIV/AIDS care (Barbour, 1994; Crawford, 1991; Kleiber, Enzmann, & Burkhard, 1992; Hearn et al., 1991; Miller, 1991; Morrison, 1991; Silverman, 1993). Many authors have examined the relationships among job stress, job satisfaction, and turnover in nursing. Two meta-analyses found a strong inverse relationship between stress and job satisfaction (Blegen, 1993; Irvine & Evans, 1992). In another study job stress is identified as a precursor to nursing burnout (Martin, 1990).

The consequences of burnout are detrimental to clients, health professionals, and health organizations. Previous research suggests that professional burnout can lead to deterioration in the quality of health care. Burnout is correlated with job turnover, absenteeism, low morale, reduced productivity, poor organization, increased accidents, physical exhaustion, insomnia, use of drugs and alcohol, marital and family problems, and illness among professionals (Bennett et al., 1995; Maslach, 1982; Maslach & Jackson, 1986; Pines & Maslach, 1977). Macks and Abrams (1992) report that the emotional and psychological demands of HIV/AIDS work have taken a toll on health care providers and their organizations. Martin (1990) concluded that many nurses in HIV/AIDS care are using ineffective, negative coping strategies, including behavioural and mental disengagement and alcohol to cope with work-related stress.

The high cost of professional burnout, in human, economic, and administration domains, points to the need to reduce burnout in order to enhance the quality of care provided to PWA. Reports of social support interventions (AIDS Alert, 1994a, b; Garside, 1993; Grossman & Silverstein, 1993; Jamieson, 1994; Lego, 1994; Pasacreta & Jacobsen, 1989; Read, 1991; Simpson, 1994) and educational/informational interventions (Knox & Gages, 1990; Nodes, 1994) established for workers in HIV/AIDS care are largely anecdotal or descriptive. Empirical evidence regarding the effectiveness of these interventions is absent.

Several authors have begun to develop models of interventions for professionals in HIV/AIDS care to prevent and manage burnout such as education programs, group discussions, staff support, and social-psychological support groups (Bolle, 1988; Brewington, 1994; McAbee, 1991; Miller, 1993, 1994; Ross, 1993; Silverman, 1993). These authors agree that burnout affects the whole person and is experienced as a continuum of symptoms resulting from chronic, unmanaged exposure to stress (Miller, 1993; Ross, 1993). Investigation of the effect of interventions intended to reduce burnout is preliminary (Miller, 1995). In one study, diminished burnout in hospital workers who work with PWA was correlated with membership in a support group (Oktay, 1992).

It is timely to investigate one element consistently linked in the literature to diminished burnout. Social support is central to any work on decreasing burnout, through either a buffer or direct effect. An earlier study in our research program revealed that an increase in support was significantly related to increased job satisfaction and to decreased nursing stress and burnout among community health nurses ($n = 100$). As work-related support increased, their burnout decreased (Stewart & Arklie, 1994). Perceived lack of support from supervisors, however, was frequently identified as a source of stress for these community health nurses. Furthermore, although work associates were among their key sources of support, these community-based nurses reported little socializing with their associates (Stewart & Arklie, 1994). Consequently, support interventions were needed.

Support interventions can create new sources of support, decrease conflict, enhance the quality of support (Barrera, 1991), or moderate the costs of providing and seeking support (Fisher, Goff, Nadler, & Chinsky, 1988). Support interventions are most useful when they restore or enhance role functioning, develop new skills, and enable coping with stressful transitions (Heller, 1990).

In summary, support interventions for health professionals working in HIV/AIDS care have typically not been tested. The support needs and stressors experienced by nurses in HIV/AIDS care are unique. Canadians need to understand more clearly the complex interactions among societal, organizational, and individual forces that influence professional caregivers' burnout and the role of social support and support interventions.

Fit with Framework

The assessment study explored the relationships among social support, stressful situations, coping strategies, work satisfaction, and burnout as experienced by Canadian nurses in HIV/AIDS care. *Social support* was conceptualized in both assessment and intervention studies as nurses' interactions with family members, friends, health professionals, co-workers, and peers that communicate information, reliable alliance, aid and affirmation (House, 1981; Cutrona, 1990). These communications improve coping and moderate the impact of stressors associated with HIV/AIDS care.

The assessment and intervention studies were based on a conceptualization of social support as a *coping* resource (see figure 7.1). Social support is one of the most important resources for coping with stress in HIV/AIDS care (Ferris et al., 1995). Social support influences adaptation to stressful situations in that supportive persons can alter appraisal of stressors, sustain coping efforts, influence choice of coping strategies (Stewart & Arklie, 1994), and bolster confidence in such a way that coping is facilitated (Cormier-Daigle & Stewart, 1997). Conversely, the ways that individuals cope influence the support they seek and receive (Silver, Wortman, & Crofton, 1990). This implies a bidirectional relationship between social support and coping of nurses in HIV/AIDS care.

Nurses working with PWA experience at least two types of *stressful situations*; (1) AIDS impact (gay affiliation, stigma, discrimination, identification with PWA, grief, loss, social reward and recognition), and (2) cumulative loss (exposure to numerous deaths of young people). Multiple losses and cumulative grief resulting from AIDS appear to be unique (Carmack, 1992; Ferris et al., 1995).

According to the framework guiding our two studies, social support indirectly modifies the relationship between perceived job stress and mental and physical health. Both social support and coping moderate the effects of job stressors on nurses' health and functioning outcomes (i.e., job satisfaction and burnout).

Job satisfaction includes workers' attitudes towards job stress, task requirements, time, and interest in the job (Stamps, Piedmont, Slavitt, & Hause, 1978) and for health professionals the provision of high quality care (Hinshaw & Atwood, 1983).

Emotional exhaustion is common to most definitions of *burnout* (Bennett, Milchie & Kippox, 1991). According to Maslach and Ozer, 'Burnout ... [is] an individual stress experience that is embedded in a context of social relationships, and thus involves the person's conception of both self and others' (1995, 1). Burnout was operationalized in both studies as a syndrome of emotional exhaustion, depersonalization, and diminished personal accomplishment, which develops in response to the demands of working closely and intensely with people (Maslach, 1982; Maslach & Jackson, 1986). Burnout has been linked to emotional and physical illness in health care providers (Maslach & Jackson, 1986).

Assessment Study: Support Needs of Nurses in HIV/AIDS Care

Aims of the Study

This exploratory descriptive study was designed to: (1) describe types of social support, stressors, coping strategies, work satisfaction, and burnout experienced by Canadian nurses who work in HIV/AIDS care; (2) explore the relationships among social support, stressors, coping strategies, work satisfaction, and burnout experienced by these nurses; (3) examine how personal factors (age, years of HIV/AIDS experience, urban/rural location, employment site), social support, stressors, coping strategies, and work satisfaction influence burnout.

Using the theoretical framework and review of related literature, four hypotheses were tested: (1) Social support would be positively related to total coping and work satisfaction. (2) Social support would be negatively related to AIDS impact, burnout, and stress. (3) Controlling for other personal factors – as total social support increased, coping increased, AIDS impact and cumulative losses decreased, and age increased, then work satisfaction would increase. (4) Controlling for other personal factors – as total social support

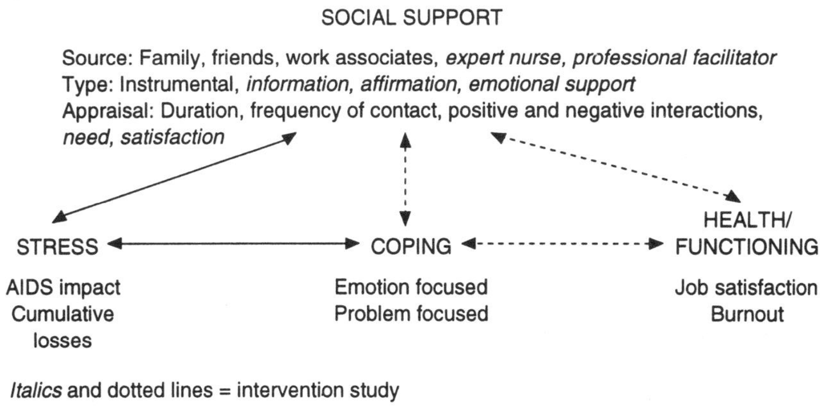

Figure 7.1 Framework for Assessment and Intervention Studies Involving Nurses in AIDS Care

increased, coping increased, AIDS impact and cumulative losses decreased, age increased, and work satisfaction increased, then burnout would decrease. As suggested by other studies, increasing age is related to lower levels of burnout (Bennett et al., 1991; Bennett, Kelaher, & Ross, 1994; Maslach & Jackson, 1981; Maslach, 1982). Our pilot study indicated that there were correlations between age and burnout and between age and work satisfaction.

In addition to testing these hypotheses based on the relationships depicted in the theoretical model, we explored two relevant but secondary research questions: (1) Which coping strategies do nurses caring for persons living with HIV/AIDS use to respond to specific stressors? (2) What are the sources and types of social support for these nurses?

Participant Profile and Recruitment

Two sampling techniques were used. The first was a convenience sample that included members of the Canadian Association of Nurses in AIDS Care (CANAC). Questionnaire packages were mailed to each member on the Association's mailing list (n = 135). The second technique involved the identification of potential participants by key informants, who were recognized leaders in the field of HIV/AIDS nursing care. These key informants were selected through consultation with CANAC. The role of key informants was considered vital to the sampling process in that many nurses who practice HIV/AIDS care are often hidden within the larger population of nurses.

The 177 participants (153 English, 24 French) were registered nurses employed as full-time or part-time staff in community settings (community health, public health, VON, home care, visiting nursing, independent practice, community-based organizations, private agencies, walk-in clinics, hospice in the home) and institutional settings (acute care, critical care, ambulatory care, outpatient clinics, clinical trials, palliative care units, psychiatric settings, hospice, hospital occupational health departments) in all provinces and territories of Canada. Nineteen per cent were living in British Columbia / Yukon, 11 per cent in Prairies / Northwest Territories, 34 per cent in Ontario, 12 per cent in Quebec, and 24 per cent in Atlantic Canada. Nearly all (91.4 per cent) lived in urban areas.

The mean age of the nurses was 39.9 years and the majority were female (86.9 per cent). Most (87.4 per cent) were heterosexual and married. The mean number of dependent children per household was two. Most nurses (73.7 per cent) had a diploma in nursing; 26.3 per cent had a degree. The average length of experience in nursing was sixteen years, with a mean of 5.1 years in HIV/AIDS experience. Average cumulative losses due to HIV/AIDS were 19.3 in the previous twelve months. Most nurses (79.4 per cent) were full-time employees, and most (73 per cent) worked in hospitals.

Methodology

Given that there has been very little research focused on nurses in HIV/AIDS care and no research to determine the relationships among coping, social support, job satisfaction, and burnout in HIV/AIDS nurses, we conducted a cross-sectional, exploratory, nation-wide survey. As HIV nursing may be unique and as research in this area is in the early stage of development, we believed it was premature to select a comparison group that could provide matched controls.

The key informants distributed sealed questionnaire packets to all eligible nurses. We also mailed questionnaire packages to each member of the CANAC group. Each package incorporated a brief letter of introduction that explained the purpose and nature of the study and a demographic data sheet. We assessed personal factors – age, HIV/AIDS experience, urban/rural location, employment site, and sex – using a demographic data form developed for this study. We presented the questionnaires to measure stressors (*AIDS Impact Scale*), coping strategies (*Ways of Coping*), sources and types of social support (*Norbeck Social Support Questionnaire*), job satisfaction (*Nursing Job Satisfaction Scale*), and burnout *(Maslach Burnout Inventory*) in random order to control for bias that might be introduced through responding to previ-

TABLE 7.1
Research Design

	Assessment Study	Intervention Study
Sample	Canadian nurses in HIV/AIDS care ($n = 177$)	Canadian nurses in HIV/AIDS care ($n = 30$)
Design	Descriptive, correlational	Demonstration intervention, within subjects
Measures/ Instruments		
Stress	*AIDS Impact*	*AIDS Impact*
Coping	*Ways of Coping*	*Ways of Coping*
Support	*Norbeck Social Support Questionnaire*	*Arizona Social Support Interview Schedule*
Health/Functioning	*Maslach Burnout Inventory* *Nursing Job Satisfaction*	*Maslach Burnout Inventory* *Nursing Job Satisfaction*
Data collection	T_1 (cross-sectional)	T_1 pre-test T_2 post-test T_3 delayed post-test (3 mos) T_4 delayed post-test (6 mos)
Data analysis		
Quantitative	Descriptive statistics, *t*-tests, multiple regressions (forward and backward step regressions)	Descriptive statistics, means, *t*-tests
Qualitative		Thematic content analysis of facilitators' field notes, participants' diaries, and post-intervention interviews with participants and facilitators

ous questionnaire(s) (A description of these measures appears in appendix B). The nurses were instructed to return the completed questionnaires in the self-addressed envelope one week following receipt of the package. We sent follow-up reminders to nurses who had not returned packages three weeks after the initial mail-out (see table 7.1 for a description of the design).

Key Findings from the Assessment Study

Similar to findings from our early study of community health nurses, those from our assessment study of Canadian nurses working in HIV/AIDS care revealed that social support is positively related to job satisfaction and that nurses with less informational and affirmational support report higher burnout scores. Thus, inadequate support seemed to be a key determinant of burnout.

Another major determinant of burnout in this population of nurses appeared to be coping skills (Bennett et al., 1994). In our assessment study, we found that emotional exhaustion and depersonalization increased when these nurses used 'escape-avoidance' coping strategies. In addition, sense of personal accomplishment increased when these nurses used planful problem solving and positive reappraisal. When nurses accepted responsibility as a coping strategy, their emotional exhaustion and depersonalization increased, but so did their sense of personal accomplishment. The fact that experienced Canadian nurses in HIV/AIDS care used accepting responsibility and escape-avoidance coping to deal with stressors in AIDS care raises concerns. Martin (1990) described ineffective coping strategies employed by American nurses in HIV/AIDS care to manage stress and burnout. It seemed that these coping behaviours became a survival tactic for nurses who want to continue to practise in HIV/AIDS care. The difference in level of burnout between new and experienced nurses in our assessment study supports this notion.

Our findings suggested that informational and affirmational support should form the basis of an intervention to reduce burnout. It is expected that if such support is enhanced, nurses will have an increased capacity to mobilize support and use planful problem solving and positive reappraisal coping strategies.

Key Findings from the Assessment Study

- Nurses who received work-related social support were more likely to seek out social support from varied sources and to reappraise stressful situations.
- Higher levels of job satisfaction were related to higher levels of social support.
- Most common coping strategies were planful problem solving, seeking support, and self-controlling.
- Nurses with higher levels of social support were less likely to use distancing coping.
- Nurses with more nursing experience and nurses with less experience in HIV/AIDS care but more affirmational support (e.g., feedback) reported higher levels of burnout.
- Social support had an indirect influence on stress and burnout.

Given the potential harmful effects of stress and burnout, it is important to develop strategies that reduce the cost to nurses, clients, and the health system. It is timely to explore factors, such as social support, that buffer the potentially debilitating effects of stress and burnout. Accordingly, in our follow-up study we tested the effectiveness of an intervention designed to enhance social support and promote the use of certain coping strategies for managing occupational stress and preventing burnout in nurses working in AIDS care.

Intervention Study: Telephone Support Group

Aims

The findings from the assessment study and data from subsequent focus groups that we conducted with nurses in HIV/AIDS care revealed the clear need for a support intervention to help nurses to cope with the stressors of AIDS care. Therefore, the purpose of the intervention study was to develop and test a social support intervention for nurses working in HIV/AIDS. One of the investigators recently conducted a pilot test of a telephone support group intervention that met the assessed support needs of persons with hemophilia and HIV/AIDS and their family caregivers (Stewart, Hart, & Mann, 1995; reported in chap. 5 of this text). This intervention study for professional (formal) caregivers of PWA was modelled after the intervention for PWA and informal caregivers.

The two objectives of this study were (1) to design and implement an accessible peer support group intervention directed at the assessed support needs of Canadian nurses in HIV/AIDS care; and (2) to determine the impact of telephone support groups on the nurses' experiences of stress, job satisfaction, burnout, coping, and social support. It was hypothesized that, following the intervention, nurses who participated in the telephone support groups would have decreased perceived stress, increased job satisfaction, and lower burnout than at pre-test. Furthermore, we predicted that nurses would be more satisfied with support and be better able to cope with the stressful demands of HIV/AIDS care following the twelve-week intervention.

Intervention Design

The advantages of telephone support include the ability to bring people together who are unable to connect geographically or logistically or who would not choose to participate in a face-to-face group. As a result of our earlier work, we knew that nurses working with PWA would prefer to meet over the telephone, in the comfort of their own homes, rather than go to a meeting place. Telephone support is appealing because it protects anonymity and confidentiality and promotes accessibility. Findings from three focus groups that included Canadian nurses in HIV/AIDS care (n = 30) reinforced the need for a telephone intervention to enhance both knowledge and support. Using recommendations from our focus groups and the results of our assessment study, we designed a telephone support intervention for thirty nurses from Toronto, Calgary, and Vancouver. These three locations were chosen as the highest number of anglophone nurses in HIV/AIDS care are employed in these cities.

Separate telephone support groups were formed in each of the three cities. Each support group included a maximum of six members linked by telephone once every two weeks, over a six-month period, for a total of twelve sessions. The support groups met for approximately one hour and were co-led by an experienced nurse in HIV/AIDS care (peer/mentor) and a professional with expertise in facilitating groups (e.g., psychologist, pastor, social worker, nurse). In these groups, nurses were given the opportunity to discuss issues such as changes in HIV/AIDS care, living with HIV/AIDS, caring for the caregiver, coping strategies, and support needs and resources.

The study employed a modified participatory experimental design.The project was participatory in several ways: (1) Key stressors and sources and types of support were identified in the preliminary assessment study of 177 nurses in HIV/AIDS care. (2) We conducted focus groups with 30 nurses in HIV/AIDS care to determine the preferred strategy for the intervention study. (3) During the initial telephone group session, participants provided input to and approved issues and topics to be discussed by the group; in the subsequent sessions, the topics of discussion were altered by group members. (4) Leadership was shared by facilitators and participants. (5) One of the investigators has an active practice in HIV/AIDS care and helped to keep the research team focused on current and emerging issues and important factors in the workplace.

Participants were recruited from the available population of Canadian nurses in HIV/AIDS care working in the identified urban centres. Once participants completed demographic data forms and pre-tests (baseline), they received the intervention. Post-tests were conducted at zero, three, and six months after completion of the intervention.

Participant Selection and Recruitment

The sample consisted of thirty registered nurses employed as full-time or part-time staff in a variety of work sites where care is provided for PWA, in

Vancouver, Calgary, and Toronto. The inclusion criteria were ability to speak, read and write in English and having worked either full time or part time in HIV/AIDS care for one year. (The design is summarized in table 7.1.)

We approached nurses whose practice involved some aspect of HIV/AIDS care and considered several practice settings. These included acute and chronic care institutions, public health agencies and their satellites, provincial home care programs, other community-based settings, and independent practice settings.

The thirty participants were registered nurses employed as full-time or part-time staff in community settings (community health, public health, VON, home care, visiting nursing, community-based organizations, private agencies, walk-in clinics, hospice in the home) and institutional settings (acute care, ambulatory care, outpatient clinics, clinical trials, palliative care units, psychiatric settings, hospice, hospital occupational health departments) in the three provinces. Fifty-three per cent of participants were living in Ontario, 27 per cent in British Columbia, and 20 per cent in Alberta. Nearly all (93 per cent) lived in urban areas.

The mean age was 40.5 years and the majority were female (93 per cent). Most (80 per cent) were heterosexual and 56 per cent were partnered. The average length of nursing experience was eighteen years, with a mean of six years in HIV/AIDS experience. Most nurses (72.4 per cent) were full-time employees, and most (70 per cent) worked in community-based organizations.

We experienced two key challenges to recruitment during the initial stages of the intervention study. First, because nurses in HIV/AIDS care are often difficult to identify, promoting the study to potential participants relied on re-establishing close links with the Canadian Association of Nurses in HIV/AIDS Care (CANAC). As CANAC's assistance with recruitment during the initial assessment study proved to be very successful, the intervention study was introduced to CANAC members during their 1997 annual conference, at a booth displayed throughout the conference and through a presentation. The presentation was designed as an informal 'focus group.' More than thirty nurses in HIV/AIDS care attended. Following a brief description of the project, participants identified potential discussion topics for the telephone groups and recruitment strategies and confirmed the desirability of a heterogeneous composition of groups (comprising HIV/AIDS nurses from diverse practice settings). Attendees also reviewed the recruitment brochure and were given draft copies to distribute to their workplaces. Further, participants developed a list of 'key informants' in HIV/AIDS nursing (e.g., persons in managerial or coordinator roles).

Following the conference, the brochure was modified to incorporate clearer language and was reformatted by a graphic designer to add visual appeal. A professionally designed logo was included in the brochure, letterhead, and business cards for the project. Several copies of the brochures were then mailed to key informants for distribution. Short articles describing the study were accepted by *Canadian AIDS News* and *Canadian Nurse*. Press releases and brochures were forwarded to the communications departments of major hospitals with HIV/AIDS units or clinics in each of the three study sites.

CANAC members also were sent personalized letters inviting them to participate. Each member received a package that included a detailed covering letter, study brochure, and stamped postcard. CANAC members who were *not* interested in being involved in the project were asked to explain why and to return the postcard. Approximately 60 per cent of the postcards were returned. The project coordinator then contacted members who did not return the postcard within three weeks, discussed the project in more detail, answered questions, and invited them to participate.

The second challenge to recruitment involved the difficulty of coordination from only one centre (i.e., Halifax). It became apparent that effective recruitment in each site required someone from the local area. Accordingly, site coordinators were hired in Toronto and Calgary to develop extensive contact lists of key informants, manage mail-outs, and, most important, to discuss the project with groups of HIV/AIDS nurses. This intensive recruitment strategy took place over a time-frame of six to eight weeks. The research team member in Vancouver coordinated key players in HIV/AIDS care, many of whom had been trained as group leaders for the telephone sessions. This group distributed brochures, made important linkages, and recruited nurses during the annual HIV/AIDS conference in British Columbia. The project coordinator then followed up with every interested nurse to confirm her/his involvement and discuss participant responsibilities.

Clearly, this study required a multidimensional approach to reach the target population of nurses in HIV/AIDS care in three sites across Canada. Indeed, development of a succinct and attractive brochure, contact of key informants in all regions, and day-to-day recruitment by the site coordinators resulted in a comprehensive recruitment strategy on a national level.

Telephone Support Group Composition, Format, and Content

Each support group included a maximum of eight participants (including co-facilitators). There were four groups in Toronto, one group in Calgary, and two groups in Vancouver. The support groups, each sixty to ninety minutes long, were designed to convey emotional, informational, and affirmational support specific to stressful situations encountered by nurses working in HIV/AIDS care. In our earlier study, nurses' burnout was linked to low informational and affirmational support.

An outline for twelve sessions was developed, using input from the focus groups, the needs expressed in the assessment study, the literature, and Canadian documents published for nurses in HIV/AIDS care (CNA, 1992; CHA, 1992; *Module 3: Nursing Care* (CANAC)).

During the first group meeting, members were invited to discuss key issues and support needs in HIV/AIDS nursing and recommend modifications and additions to the tentative content and potential topics. Each of the support groups assessed its own needs and determined the content and the order and extent of discussion of specific topics. The following topics were suggested initially in the facilitators' guide:

- *Changes in HIV/AIDS:* epidemiology; immunology; natural history of HIV; advances in HIV/AIDS treatment; complementary therapies
- *Living with HIV/AIDS:* physiological aspects; social-psychological aspects; cultural diversity (e.g., women, children, IV drug users, gay men, First Nations)
- *HIV/AIDS Nursing Care:* role of nursing in multidisciplinary team; mental health care (substance use and HIV); pain management
- *Decision-Making Process:* ethical and other dilemmas
- *Challenges in AIDS Care:* unique challenges in HIV/AIDS nursing care; challenges related to the disease; challenges related to the context of the disease; death and dying; assisted suicide; challenges related to the professional context
- *Caring for Caregiver:* stressors unique to AIDS care; job satisfaction; burnout; occupational exposure to HIV
- *Closure of Group.*

Group members were invited to discuss these and other stressful situations, associated coping/managing strategies, and support that was available, helpful, or needed. The sessions could move from a phase of experience swapping and social comparison regarding feelings and emotion-focused coping to a phase of problem solving and exchange of ideas for enhanced coping with AIDS-related stressors. Following from our assessment study findings, which demonstrated the relationship between coping strategies and level of burnout, we asked facilitators to explore ways to increase 'planful problem solving,' and to reduce 'accepting responsibility' and 'escape-avoidance' strategies.

Group Facilitation

Each of the telephone support groups was co-facilitated by an expert facilitator and an HIV/AIDS nurse expert. As we did in the other intervention studies in the Social Support Research Program, we promoted co-leadership and co-facilitation by (1) joint training of leaders in face-to-face or videoconference sessions, (2) monitoring of leadership 'balance' through review of transcripts of group discussions, (3) field notes prepared by both group leaders, and (4) one-to-one interviews with all leaders following the sessions.

Experientially based coping strategies and sources of support were expected to be primarily the domain of the experienced HIV/AIDS nurse (peer/mentor). The other professional facilitator typically supplemented participants' experiential knowledge with expertise about the group process and some coping strategies (Gottlieb, 1988). Some facilitators augmented group discussions with varied techniques and resources, depending on the topic (e.g., role playing, invited speaker). To monitor co-leadership, facilitators participated in two group 'check in' teleconferences with the trainer and research team after about their fourth and eighth biweekly sessions.

Documentation and Evaluation

The co-facilitators documented the support processes in the telephone group sessions by completing field notes that identified topics/issues discussed and the extent to which members compared their situation with that of others (social comparison), shared personal experiences with others (social exchange/reciprocity), and learned from each other (social learning). Second, participants completed diaries after each biweekly group discussion. Third, group members participated in follow-up telephone interviews in which open-ended queries focused on mediating support processes (e.g., social comparison, social learning, reciprocity), on satisfaction with and perceived impact of the intervention, and on continuing contacts with support group members. These interviews were conducted by a trained research assistant immediately following the intervention and again six months later.

We measured the hypothesized impact on social support, stress, and coping and on health/functioning outcomes with standardized measures administered at four points (baseline, completion of the intervention, three and six months following termination of group meetings). The instruments included the *AIDS Impact Scale* (stress), *Ways of Coping Questionnaire* (we asked the nurses to respond in relation to a specific AIDS work-related stressor), *Arizona Social*

Support Interview Schedule (ASSIS), Nursing Job Satisfaction Scale (job satisfaction), and the second edition of the *Maslach Burnout Inventory (MBI)* (burnout). We substituted the support measure used in the earlier assessment study because it was difficult to identify the amount of support received from reported sources, negative interactions (i.e., appraisal of support), support needs and support satisfaction with the earlier measure *(NSSQ).* Measures were mailed out to all participants, along with stamped, self-addressed envelopes. Participants who had not returned the completed measures were contacted by telephone three weeks after initial mail-outs.

Key Features of the Intervention

- Telephone support groups were created.
- There were seven groups of nurses at three sites: Vancouver, Calgary, and Toronto.
- Professional facilitators were nurses, clergy, social workers.
- Expert HIV/AIDS nurses worked in acute, tertiary care, long-term care, palliative care, public health, VON, needle-exchange programs.
- Varied themes were identified in the facilitator guide for twelve sessions.
- Co-facilitators trained together.
- Support processes were documented through diaries, field notes, and transcripts of taped sessions.
- Health-related outcomes were measured pre- and post-intervention.
- Post-test interviews focused on satisfaction and suggested changes.

Key Findings of the Intervention Study

Topics Discussed in Support Groups

Stressful Situations: The leaders reported addressing a wide range of issues with their groups. Some of the preplanned topics covered included stress, coping strategies, burnout, social support, the changing face of HIV/AIDS (including advances in treatment of HIV, complementary therapies, mental health care, and substance use), death and dying, pain management, occupational exposure to HIV, cultural diversity, euthanasia and assisted suicide, resources in HIV/AIDS, and problem solving. Other issues raised spontaneously by members included health care restructuring, management/staff relations, confidentiality, and group process and dynamics. Indeed, in many groups, preplanned and scheduled topics were replaced gradually with flexible topics and agendas set by members at the beginning of each session. Except for the emphasis on the changing health system, topics in the facilitator guide matched the discussion topics.

Topics most frequently discussed by group members included changing health care system, changing face of AIDS (particularly HIV arising from substance use), resources in HIV/AIDS care, moral/ethical issues associated with HIV/AIDS, death and dying, assisted suicide, and coping strategies. In addition to HIV/AIDS care experiences, one leader commented that participants '*shared experiences of ... their nursing practice ideals being eroded by health care restructuring*.' The impact of health care restructuring, a source of stress for many participants, seemed to dominate some sessions. As one leader described, '*We spent more time than I anticipated on talking about stresses that are arising out of changes that people are experiencing in the workplace ... and how that impacted on people's practices, and how it impacted on how people were feeling*.'

Coping Strategies Discussed: The leaders reported that participants shared coping strategies during the sessions. For example, one group discussed a team-based approach as a coping strategy. Other strategies discussed included peer support, advocacy, education, exercise, humour, denial, introspection, and personal growth. While most of the coping strategies dealt with the stress of HIV/AIDS care, others allowed them, in the words of one leader, 'to renew their sense of professionalism and passion for nursing.'

Support Processes

Social Comparison: A key strength of the intervention process was social comparison among the members in the telephone support groups. One leader explained, '*It provided a ... forum where people would come to expect, after a few sessions, that they would get some support from other people who were in similar circumstances*.' Participants reported comparing their experiences with those of the other participants. The words used by participants to describe the perceived impact of comparing situations with those of others included acknowledged, encouraged, connected, validated, normality, safe, felt a boost, less alone, hopeful, optimism, autonomy, reassured, rejuvenated, relieved, respectful (of knowledge and commitment of other nurses), supported.

Social Exchange: In their diaries, the leaders reported that participants shared their experiences with each other. One leader wrote, '*By sharing experiences, members got beneath the surface methods of coping ... to the 'meatier' dy-*

namic of reflecting upon personhood.' By sharing their experiences, the participants were able to discuss '*commonalities, thus reinforcing strengths identified by members.*' The leaders facilitated these discussions in a sensitive manner and encouraged disclosure by sharing personal experiences from time to time. For example, one group '*struggled together*' to deal with '*requests for end of life help from patients.*' More participants described what they gave to the group than what they received. One nurse commented, '*I was able to clarify a lot of things ... and I know [I gave] a lot of humour to the group ... I also shared a lot of my experience.*'

Social Learning: In many groups, members frequently exchanged experiential knowledge. One leader said, '*I think the most significant learning that happened in the group was just people hearing of other people's work experience and the challenges and barriers that exist in all of that. You know, the good solid learning that happens in a peer support group where people find out that other people have similar experiences.*' Experiential knowledge was often exchanged about (1) stress identification and management, (2) client care, (3) problem solving strategies, and (4) the changing face of AIDS.

Group Process: According to the participants' feedback, they valued the flexibility and the member-driven approach of the group process. One participant explained it best by saying, '*We chose [the topic] the week before, and then when the sessions started, we revisited whether or not that was an appropriate one ... but we'd just say "Is this what we want to talk about today? Is there anything else that's come up in the week?" and then we'd go on with a new topic, rather than the one that was originally planned.*' Establishing ground rules at the first session seemed to facilitate positive group interactions. Overall, the leaders reported mutual support, sharing, and listening among the participants.

Most leaders and participants commented on the evolution of the group process and dynamics over the six-month time-frame. In the early sessions, most members sought and shared informational support, whereas emotional and affirmational support emerged in later sessions. As one leader recalled, '*It started out very specifically around HIV and AIDS issues and then as we got to know each other ... by the end of it, we were almost an informal support group where we just kind of talked about everything and nothing.*' Most groups reported that group cohesion developed gradually. For example, one leader noted, '*over time they developed more trust and intimacy, so that they were able to talk about matters that were work related but more per-*

sonal, in terms of my heart hardening at work and my burning out, and that type of thing. The tone and flavour changed. But in terms of how they supported each other, they were fairly consistent in that.'

Facilitator Roles and Co-leadership: All leaders believed that shared leadership was an a positive feature of the intervention. A few HIV/AIDS' nurse experts, however, described their role as confining; this perception may have influenced the dynamics in the groups. One leader benefited personally from involvement with the group, which created some role confusion: '*At times I was unclear about my role ... I felt like a participant benefiting from the support process.*' In addition, a few nurse facilitators reported that maintaining their expert role may have added to their personal stress, because worklife issues, such as health system reform and nursing shortages, were affecting their own worklives. The responsibility to the facilitative role prevented leaders from seeking social support from the group members. The leaders used their diaries to keep track of participation levels in the group and made concerted efforts to encourage all members to participate in the discussion.

Perceived Impact of the Intervention (Qualitative Results)

Participants: Overall, the participants reported that their participation in the telephone support groups both enhanced their coping strategies and met their support needs. During her six-month post-test interview, one nurse reflected, '*I'm coping better because I'm taking a little bit better care of myself ... and also just sharing with my co-workers is helping me to cope. Those are two things I'm employing to cope on a day-to-day basis, versus letting things build up.*' Another participant stated that, '*It really made a difference in my overall feeling as a person, not just professionally. Just in general. I got a sense of more energy, actually ... it really gave me a sense of support and strength.*'

In their interviews and diaries, many participants referred to the benefits of the discussions in the sessions. For instance, one nurse said that the sessions gave her, '*just a bit of go get em, or support, or validation, and then you can shake off whatever you've been carrying, and you can start off again with the week almost brand new.*' When asked to compare his feelings before and after the session, one participant wrote, '*Before: frustrated – more questions than answers. After: supported, respected, affirmed, pumped.*' Another explained that she was, '*grateful for a forum to discuss my feelings.*'

The participants reported that they were very satisfied with the intervention, which met their expectations. When asked to describe satisfaction with the group, one participant said, '*There was a sense of support. I felt like the talking on the phone with other people spilled over to a more productive day-to-day life for myself. I really felt good about it.*' The most common benefits mentioned by nurses were an enhanced appreciation for nursing in different sectors and the sense of being better connected to the HIV/AIDS nursing community. For example, one nurse said that the most important benefit of participating was '*Probably the relationships that are maintained now six months later. People, like the acquaintances that I didn't know, and now I am able to call on them, and they on me - we have a relationship professionally that we didn't have before.*' For some nurses, the groups enhanced previous relationships. When asked whether existing relationships had changed, one member replied, '*I think there is a better bond – we can talk and be much more at ease. I am not afraid to ask them for support.*'

Not all participants' experiences, however, were positive. Some participants reported that some of the topics discussed added to their feeling of frustration and stress. One nurse wrote that the sessions made her feel '*a bit weary – obviously the problems I face are everywhere, and that's depressing.*' Negative feelings were also reported by participants who felt that their specific group had poor dynamics. Lack of participation and confidentiality issues were problematic for some other groups.

Leaders: The leaders reported that the intervention was meaningful and that it enhanced participants' coping strategies. They contended that participation in the intervention was very positive. For example, one leader said, '*I think they felt more comfortable in challenging their co-workers, especially those who came in from hospitals who were frustrated to exhaustion because of patients and physicians who were not part of the team ... And so, I think through our encouragement, they either felt more empowered to confront and challenge or learned how to disengage or let that kind of stressor go.*'

Factors Influencing the Impact of the Intervention

Overall, concerns about confidentiality and trust hindered participation in the support groups, especially during the first few sessions. One nurse who said she felt disconnected from her group elaborated, '*I probably had met half of them and one I work with. She had some very difficult issues that I had to keep sacred and not even acknowledge them to her. She and I know that we were both in the same group but it was not appropriate to acknowledge our work that we were doing in the group ... Or for me to acknowledge her issues and so on. And I find that really difficult. It interfered in my interactions in the group as well.*' Indeed, anonymity and confidentiality were not always possible. Other barriers to positive group interactions included the following: participants' absence, insufficient commitment to the group, frequency and length of intervention, and disloyalty to their employers and colleagues.

Most nurses liked the telephone mode of support groups and commented on unanticipated benefits, '*I always feel like when you're in a group ... there has to be eye contact. But in this way, I was free.*' In contrast, one leader suggested that the telephone made it 'hard to know whose voice belonged to whom. Difficult for continuity of issues.'

Absenteeism seemed to affect the dose of the intervention. The leaders reported that everyone could not attend every session. In contrast, one leader noted, '*there was so much significant movement in people's lives, and so they stayed because they made the commitment.*'

The leaders stressed the importance of having a trained facilitator or group leader who was sensitive to the needs of the group, an expert in facilitation, and an active listener. A focus on group process and familiarity with HIV/AIDS nursing care issues were considered important. Future telephone support groups should be member driven, co-led by expert facilitators, and confidential.

Even though the leaders worked diligently to bring meaningful closure to the groups, four participants reported feeling abandoned at the end of the twelve sessions: '*I felt grateful for the support and the respect and the care we were able to experience with each other. But also felt the frustration of the fact that it is over. I personally came out with the sense that phone support absolutely works, and it is too bad that it is discontinued because it is a research project ... I came out feeling really warm towards the members and great respect.*' Another nurse commented, '*I felt almost abandoned. Like a huge part of my support network was gone. Not that I don't feel very supported at work, but the sessions for this particular group were very important to me.*'

Impact of the Intervention (Quantitative Results)

The quantitative analysis of data collected pre- and post-intervention using five measures suggests that the intervention had some limited effects. Although there was no statistical significance, analysis of the *AIDS Impact Scale* demonstrated four trends following the intervention: less stigma, less discrimination, less grief, and more reward. The intervention appears to have strengthened the nurses' ability to use effective coping strategies, such as seeking social support, positive appraisal, and planful problem solving. There was an increase in total support satisfaction post-intervention. Our findings also suggest increase in personal accomplishment (reflecting diminished burn-out) post intervention. The burnout scores were within the normal range, however, consistent with the findings from Topf (1989) and Servellen & Leake (1994) studies. Our findings indicate an increase in job enjoyment post-intervention.

Key Findings from the Intervention Study

- Interesting trends in impact on stress include decreased stigma, decreased discrimination, decreased grief, and increased reward.
- Key coping strategies include seeking social support, positive appraisal, and planful problem solving.
- Total support satisfaction increased.
- Personal accomplishment increased.
- Participants perceived the following impact: enhanced coping, feelings of validation, sense of belonging, decreased isolation, learning about stress identification and management skills.

Lessons Learned

The challenge of conducting intervention research immediately following an assessment study is difficult. During the twenty-four months over which we developed the proposal and awaited funding, the 'face' of HIV/AIDS changed dramatically. These profound changes have had an impact on PWA, and on family and professional caregivers. 'Willingness to care for people with AIDS combined with burnout are probably going to be compounded among health care providers, particularly nurses, as the demographics of the epidemic have moved more to the urban poor, who have access to fewer resources and a more complicated insurance structure' (Holzemer, 1997, 64).

Time Warp from Assessment to Intervention: The Changing Face of AIDS

Changes in the Health System

In addition to the ongoing challenges of providing quality care, nurses involved in AIDS care now have to cope with health system reform, reduced government health care funding, research developments, and new technology. Within the context of budget cutbacks, nurses report that they are caring for more clients, families, and communities with complex needs, working longer hours, and receiving less informational support. The impact of the burden of dwindling resources on nurses and their ability to provide quality care and strategies to reverse burden and burnout should be investigated.

Advances in the Treatment of HIV

Advances in treatment have been dramatic over the past few years. With the advent of new antiretroviral agents, along with suppressive and preventive therapies for opportunistic infections, people are 'living with' HIV disease, instead of 'dying from' AIDS (Ungvarski, 1997). Knowledge of the pathogenesis of the disease has evolved, and the availability of HIV-RNA viral loading has dramatically changed diagnoses and treatment. New behavioural patterns seem to be emerging with use of protease inhibitors. For instance, reduction in condom use among gay men and the use of protease inhibitors as a 'morning-after pill' have been reported (Ungvarski, 1997). There is a concomitant risk that new infections will occur and that reduction in AIDS cases and AIDS mortality rates may be short lived. As nurses are a primary source for providing information and support to PWA for decisions about treatment, they are accepting responsibility to stay abreast of developments.

Complementary Therapies

Concurrently, the use of complementary therapies is proliferating. According to a recent review by Health Canada, complementary therapies among PWA range from 40 per cent to 78 per cent, compared with 20 per cent and 50 per cent among the general population (Garmaise, 1997). Lack of empirical evidence and available literature on their use, benefits, efficacy, and safety, as well as insufficient funding for research, have a negative impact on the access of quality information for PWA and nurses.

Mental Health

As PWA live longer and more 'functional' lives, nurses will be more involved in the provision of mental health care. Anxiety and depression are often experienced by PWA (Cabaj, 1996). HIV disease may also reflect comorbidity in people who have mental illness or chemical dependence and may exacerbate pre-existing mental illnesses. Conversely, pre-existence of mental disorders complicates interventions (McEhany, Hughes, & Lee, 1996). Neuropsychological complications of HIV disease lead to mental health symptoms (e.g., apathy, withdrawal, loss of memory and concentration, impaired cognition). Moreover, side-effects of many antiretroviral, antibiotic, and chemotherapeutic agents may mimic mental health problems (McEhany et al., 1996).

Little is known about the impact of physical and social-psychological adjustments on quality of life of PWA. A higher incidence of suicidal ideation, suicide attempts, and suicide has been reported among PWA than among the general population. Meeting the psychiatric and neuropsychological needs of PWA calls for varied interventions, depending on population groups, psychiatric diagnosis, and stage of HIV disease. There is current public debate regarding euthanasia and assisted suicide for those suffering from HIV/AIDS. As people live longer and healthier lives and as self-control is restored with protease inhibitors, more PWA are taking charge of decisions about their living and dying.

Substance Use and HIV

There is mounting evidence that HIV/AIDS is a concern for people living with addiction. Professionals who provide care for drug users and ex-users affected by HIV/AIDS must face fears, anxieties, and attitudes related to drug consumption and must cope with unique management problems in in-patient settings (e.g., use of illicit drugs on the ward, aggressive or violent behaviour). Furthermore, nurses are confronted with ethical or legal dilemmas when they are aware of clients' involvement in illicit activities. Providing care necessitates learning about substance use and its effects on traditional therapeutic approaches (i.e., pain management). Dealing with the complexities and frustrations related to compliance is one of the most profound issues facing nurses in the community setting.

Although the next wave of the AIDS epidemic will involve the intravenous-drug user population, there is virtually no in-depth attention to substance use issues in the formal education of nurses and few continuing education opportunities. This is yet another source of profound stress in the workplace.

According to our findings, these issues associated with the changing context are real. Therefore, the training of facilitators had to be designed to reflect the challenges in HIV/AIDS nursing unique to each region. In addition, the training sessions for each site had to be re-evaluated to fit the changing needs of HIV/AIDS nurses.

Lessons Learned

- Training should be redesigned to reflect the challenges in the changing 'face' of HIV/AIDS.
- Nurses in HIV/AIDS care are difficult to identify: links with CANAC, poster board displays, focus groups, a visually appealing brochure, and short articles in Canadian journals are effective means of marketing.
- Site coordinators are necessary for extensive recruitment and communication strategies for multi-site intervention.
- Strategies to protect confidentiality and foster trust influence the impact of interventions.
- Commitment and attendance are critical to the development of group dynamics.
- Ongoing communication is necessary between leaders and the research team.

Future Directions in Research, Programs, and Policy

There is evidence that support mechanisms are needed for professional supporters. Canadian nurses are currently working in a climate of rapid changes, worklife issues, shortages of nurses, and cutbacks in health care. Given that the number of reported cases of PWA and the acute manifestations of AIDS are proliferating, and given that many nurses are 'hanging on' to their employment, both the number of nurses experiencing burnout and their level of burnout will continue to increase. This will have a serious impact on the quality of care delivered, and related sick time will significantly affect hospital and community budgets. Findings from our assessment study indicated that support interventions aimed at reducing stress, enhancing job satisfaction, and lowering turnover might enable nurses to provide quality care to PWA and also to reduce sick time. In our earlier study of community health nurses and the assessment study of nurses in HIV/AIDS care, lack of support from supervisors and inadequate contact with work associates outside work were considered stressful. This fact points to the need for peer and mentor support.

The tested intervention model, involving telephone support from peers (members) and mentors (experienced AIDS nurse facilitators), can be applied to nurses working in other regions and to other health professionals in HIV/AIDS care. Future research directions also include testing telephone interventions or other interventions (e.g., computer) in rural areas, so as to lower burnout and feelings of isolation. Participants in similar support interventions should have enhanced satisfaction with support and work and be better able to cope with the demands of HIV/AIDS care.

According to the AIDS Treatment Unit, Health Canada (Gerry Bally, personal communication, 1997), the health resource crisis in HIV/AIDS care in Canada will have a serious impact on the quality of care for people affected by and living with HIV/AIDS. Five indicators of this crisis are (1) the annual incidence of HIV is 3,000 to 4,000; (2) the age of seroconversion has dropped from thirty years old (1980s) to twenty-five years old (1990); (3) there is increasing seroconversion in women, intravenous drug users, Aboriginal people, and prisoners; (4) each health care provider can satisfactorily handle a caseload of thirty PWA; and (5) there are 900 self-identified HIV care providers in Canada, most of whom are located in three urban centres: Vancouver, Montreal, and Toronto. The increasing incidence of HIV, coupled with depletion of health provider resources, may result in substandard care to PWA if supportive policies and programs are not in place. It is imperative that formal mechanisms be created to support professional caregivers. Moreover, interdisciplinary educational opportunities designed to increase the number of health professionals competent to practise in HIV/AIDS care should be evaluated.

There are many policy issues yet to be faced in Canada. Recognition that HIV/AIDS is a spreading epidemic with a changing face and that the predominant formal supporters are nurses can inform programs and policies. Support mechanisms that focus on education and skill development, staffing, respite, and care for the caregiver are needed. Allocation of financial and human resources to support professional supporters is crucial, not only in AIDS care but in care of other chronic conditions.

References

AIDS Alert (1994a). AIDS support groups vary according to needs, expectations. *AIDS Alert*, February, 1–2.

AIDS Alert (1994b). Groups take different forms but address life/death issues. *AIDS Alert*, February, 30–32.

Barbour, R. (1994). The Impact of Working with People with HIV/AIDS: A Review of the Literature. *Social Science Medicine, 39*(2), 221–232.

Barrera, M. (1991). Social support interventions and the third law of ecology. *American Journal of Community Psychology, 19*(1), 133–138.

Bennett, L., Kelaher, M., & Ross, M. (1994). The impact of working with HIV/AIDS on health care professionals: Development of the AIDS impact scale. *Psychology and Health: An International Journal, 9*, 221–232.

Bennett, L., Milchie, P., & Kippox, S. (1991). Quantitative analysis of burnout and its associated factors in AIDS care. *AIDS Care, 3*(2), 181–192.

Bennett, L., Miller, D., & Ross, M. (1995). Review of the research to date on impact of HIV/AIDS on health workers. In L.L. Bennett, D. Miller, & M. Ross (Eds) *Health workers and AIDS research, interventions, and current issues in burnout and response* (14–33). Chur, Switzerland: Harwood Academic.

Blegen, M. (1993), Nurses' job satisfaction: A meta-analysis of related variables. *Nursing Research, 42*(1), 36–41.

Bolle, J. (1988). Supporting the deliverers of care: Strategies to support nurses and prevent burnout. *Nursing Clinics of North America, 23*(4), 843–850.

Brewington, J. (1994). The AIDS epidemic: Caring for caregivers. *Nursing Administration Quarterly, 18*(2), 22–29.

Cabaj, R. (1996). Management of anxiety and depression in HIV-infected patients. *Journal of the International Association of Physicians in AIDS Care, 2*(6), 11–16.

Canadian Association of Nurses in AIDS Care (1996). *A comprehensive guide for the care of persons with HIV disease.* Ottawa: Health Canada.

Canadian Hospital Association (1992). *Caring for HIV/AIDS caregivers.* Ottawa: Canadian Hospital Association.

Canadian Nurses Association (1992). *HIV/AIDS education for nurses: Practice issues and curriculum guidelines.* Ottawa: Canadian Nurses Association.

Carmack, B. (1992). Balancing engagement/detachment in AIDS-related multiple losses. *Image: Journal of Nursing Scholarship, 24*(1), 9–14.

Cormier-Daigle, M. & Stewart, M. (1997). Social support and coping of male hemodialysis patients. *International Journal of Nursing Studies, 34* (6), 420–430.

Crawford, K. (1991). National study on stress, vulnerability, and coping in HIV/AIDS counsellors. *National AIDS Bulletin*, November.

Cutrona, C.E. (1990). Stress and social support: In search of optimal matching. *Journal of Social and Clinical Psychology, 9*(1), 3–14.

Ferris, F., Flannery, J., McNeal, H., & Morissette, M. (1995). *A comprehensive guide for the care of persons with HIV disease: Module 4: Palliative care.* Toronto: Kirkpatrick & Associates.

Fisher, J.D., Goff, B.A., Nadler, A., & Chinsky, J.M. (1988). Social psychological influences on help seeking and support from peers. In B.H. Gottlieb (Ed.), *Marshaling social support: Formats, processes, and effects* (267–304). Newbury Park, CA: Sage.

Garmaise, D. (1997). *An overview of the role of complementary therapies and HIV/AIDS: Care, treatment and support issues.* Ottawa: Care, Treatment, and Support Program. HIV/AIDS Policy, Coordination and Program Division, Health Canada.

Garside, B. (1993). Physicians mutual aid group: A response to AIDS-related burnout. *Health and Social Work, 18*(4), 259–267.

Gottlieb, B. (1988). Marshaling social support: the state of the art in research and practice. In B.H. Gottlieb (Ed.), *Marshaling social support: Formats, processes, and effects* (11–51). Newbury Park, CA: Sage Publications.

Grady, C. (1989). Acquired immunodeficiency syndrome: The impact on professional nursing practice. *Cancer Nursing, 12*(1), 1–9.

Grossman, A., & Silverstein, C. (1993). Facilitating supports groups for professionals working with people with AIDS. *Social Work, 38*(2), 144–151.

Hearn, J., Nibill, P., & Ong, B. (1991). Stress in nurses caring for patients with AIDS. *Senior Nurse, 11*(5), 40–41.

Heller, K. (1990). Social and community intervention. *Annual Review of Psychology, 41*, 141–168.

Himle, D. , Jayaratne, S., & Thyness, P. (1991). Buffering effects of four social support types on burnout among social workers. *Social Work Research and Abstracts, 27*(1), 22–27.

Hinshaw, A., & Atwood, J. (1983). Staff turnover, stress and satisfaction: Models, measures and management. *Annual Review of Nursing Research*, 1, 133–153.

Holzemer, W. (1997). Post-Vancouver: Implications for nursing practice and nursing research. *Journal of the Association of Nurses in AIDS Care, 8*(4), 62–65.

House, J.S. (1981). *Work stress and social support.* Englewood Cliffs, NJ: Prentice-Hall.

Irvine, D., & Evans, M. (1992). Job Satisfaction and Turnover Among Nurses: A Review and Meta-Analysis. *University of Toronto Faculty of Nursing Monograph Series*. Toronto:

Jamieson, S. (1994). Developing staff support. *Nursing Standard, 8*(28), 44–46.

Kleiber, D., Enzmann, D., & Burkhard, G. (1992). Stress and burnout among health care personnel in the field of AIDS: Causes and prevalence (the ABBA Project). *International Conference on AIDS Care.* Amsterdam:

Knox, M., & Gages, J. (1990). The HIV clinical tutorial for community mental health professionals. *Community Mental Health Journal, 26*(6), 559–566.

Laboratory Centre for Disease Control. (1995). *1994 Annual Report of AIDS in Canada.* December 1995. Internet site: http://www.hwc.ca

Lazarus, R., & Folkman, S. (1984). *Stress, appraisal, and coping.* New York: Springer.

Lego, S. (1994). AIDS-related anxiety and coping methods in a support group for caregivers. *Archives of Psychiatric Nursing, 3*(6), 200–207.

Macks, J., & Abrams, D. (1992). Burnout among HIV/AIDS health care providers. In P. Volberling & M. Jacobson (Eds), *AIDS clinical review* (251–299). New York: Marcel Dekker.

Martin, D. (1990). Effects of ethical dilemmas on stress felt by nurses providing care to AIDS patients. *Critical Care Nursing Quarterly, 12*(4), 53–62.

Maslach, C. (1982). *The cost of caring*. Englewood Cliffs, NJ: Prentice-Hall.

Maslach, C., & Jackson, S. (1981). *Maslach burnout inventory: Research edition manual*. Palo Alto, CA: Consulting Psychologists Press.

Maslach, C., & Jackson, S. (1986). *Maslach burnout inventory manual*. (2nd ed.). Palo Alto, CA: Consulting Psychologists Press.

Maslach, C., & Ozer, E. (1995). Theoretical issues related to burnout in AIDS health workers. In L.L. Bennett, D. Miller, & M. Ross (Eds), *Health workers and AIDS research, intervention and current issues in burnout and response* (1–13). Chur, Switzerland: Harwood Academic.

McAbee, R. (1991). Occupational Stress and burnout in the nursing profession: A model for prevention. *AAOHN Journal, 39*(12), 568–575.

McEhany, G., Hughes, A., & Lee, K. (1996). Depression and HIV-AIDS nursing perspective on a complex relationship. *Nursing Clinics of North America, 31*(1), 57–59.

Meisenhelder, J. (1993). Contributing factors to fear of HIV contagion in registered nurses. *Journal of Nursing Scholarship, 26*(1), 65–69.

Miller, D. (1993). HIV/AIDS health worker stress and stress prevention. *AIDS Care, 5*, 517–521.

Miller, D. (1994). Models of management for occupational morbidity and burnout. In. L.L. Bennett, D. Miller, & M. Ross (Eds), *Health workers and AIDS research, intervention and current issues in burnout and response* (175–190). Chur, Switzerland: Harwood Academic.

Miller D. (1995). Occupational morbidity and burnout: Lessons and warnings for HIV/AIDS carers. *International Review of Psychiatry, 3*, 439–449.

Miller, L. (1991). The relationship between social support and burnout: clarification and simplification. *Social Work Research and Abstracts, 27*(1) 34–37.

Morrison, B. (1991). Identification of coping strategies among nurses who care for AIDS patients. Unpublished MN thesis. Spokane, WA.

Nodes, K. (1994). Educating advanced practice nurses to respond to the HIV pandemic. *Nursing Administration Quarterly, 18*(2), 81–87.

Oktay, J. (1992). Burnout in hospital social workers who work with AIDS patients. *Social Work, 37*(5), 432–439.

Pasacreta, J., & Jacobsen, P. (1989). Addressing the need for staff support among nurses caring for the AIDS population. *Oncology Nursing Forum, 16*(5), 659–663.

Pickhall, L. (1984). Caring for patients with AIDS. Unpublished MSc thesis. University of British Columbia, Vancouver.

Pines, A. & Maslach, C. (1977). The burnout syndrome in the day care setting. *Child Care Quarterly, 6*, 100–113.

Read, V. (1991). HIV/AIDS: Coping with the stressors. *Australian Nurses Journal, 20*(5), 15–16.

Ross, E. (1993). Preventing burnout among social workers employed in the field of AIDS/HIV. *Social Work in Health Care, 18*(2), 91–108.

Servellen, G., & Leake, B. (1994). Emotional exhaustion and distress among nurses: How important are AIDS-care related specific factors? *Journal of the Association of Nurses in AIDS Care, 5*(2), 11–20.

Silver, R.C., Wortman, C.B., & Crofton, C. (1990). The role of coping in support provision: The self-presentational dilemma of victims of life crises. In B.R. Sarason, I.G. Sarason, & G.R. Pierce (Eds), *Social support: An interactional view* (397–426). New York: John Wiley.

Silverman, D. (1993). Psychosocial impact of HIV-related caregiving on health providers: a review and recommendations for the role of psychiatry. *American Journal of Psychiatry, 150*(5), 705–712.

Simmons-Alling, S. (1984). AIDS: Psychosocial needs of the health care worker. *Topics in Clinical Nursing, 6*, 31–37.

Simpson, R. (1994). Computer networks show great promise in supporting AIDS patients. *Nursing Administration Quarterly, 18*(2), 92–95.

Stamps, P., Piedmont, E., Slavitt, D., & Hause, A. (1978). Measurement of work satisfaction among health professionals, *Medical Care, 16*, 337–352.

Stewart, M., & Arklie, M. (1994). Work satisfaction, stressors and support experienced by community health nurses. *Canadian Journal of Public Health, 85*(3), 180–183.

Stewart, M., Hart, G. & Mann, K. (1995). Living with haemophilia and HIV/AIDS: Support and coping. *Journal of Advanced Nursing, 22*, 1101–1111.

Strathdee, S., Flannery, J., & Graydon, D. (1994). Stressors in the AIDS hospice environment. *AIDS Patient Care, 8*(2), 11–21.

Topf, M. (1989). Personality hardiness, occupational stress, and burnout in critical care nurses. *Research in Nursing and Health, 12*, 179–186.

Tomblin Murphy, G., Stewart, M., Ritchie, J., & Johnson, A. (1995). Social support, work satisfaction and coping among Canadian Nurses in HIV/AIDS care. Manuscript in preparation, Dalhousie University at Halifax.

Ungvarski, P. (1997). HIV/AIDS: New knowledge, new treatments, and the challenges for nursing. *Journal of the Association of Nursing in AIDS Care, 8*(4), 5–6.

8

Relationships and Partnerships between Peers and Professionals in Mutual Aid Groups

Miriam J. Stewart, Sheila Banks, Doug Crossman, and Dale Poel

Abstract. The growth of self-help groups (SHG) in Canada and their relevance to health system reform point to the timeliness of partnerships between professionals and members and to the significance of professionals' attitudes, knowledge, skills, roles, and educational preparation. Accordingly, two assessment studies were focused on professionals' relationships with SHG. In the initial study, individual and group interviews were conducted with SHG members (n = 49) and professionals from five disciplines (n = 47). In the second study, questionnaires derived from findings in the initial project were administered to 474 professionals representing the same disciplines. Key themes emerged from these studies. Many professionals had never been involved with SHG. Only one-third had had actual experience with professional roles. The major roles identified by professionals were facilitator, referral resource, consultant, and educator. They tended to be more cognizant of SHG functions than of actual groups. In fact, most knew only two groups on average. The respondents typically had positive attitudes towards SHG, and more than 85 per cent desired a partnership relationship.

Given the knowledge deficiencies of these professionals, their inadequate educational preparation about SHG, and their desire for education, we developed a learning resource for professional programs and promotion of partnerships. The peer-professional partnership model was tested in intervention studies reported in this book. Furthermore, it was applied in two support group in-tervention studies involving seniors. The importance of training and of check-in sessions for peer and professional facilitators was evident in all studies.

Introduction

The mutual-aid self-help movement called attention to interpersonal aid; extolled the virtues of self-governing, self-reliant, consumer created and controlled small-group helping systems; and argued that these approaches were developed or evolved to meet needs not recognized by professionals or to fill professional service gaps (Gottlieb, in press). Typically, members of groups share a common condition or situation (Lieberman, 1990). Borkman (1982) distinguished a voluntary action perspective, marked by professional control, from a self-help perspective, in which participants create and control the helping structures and processes. Self-help groups are termed 'mutual aid self-help groups' in order to avoid the connotation that these groups are based on individual efforts rather than reciprocal aid exchanged among members (Gottlieb, in press).

Estimates of the number of Canadians participating in self-help groups (SHG) range from 299,000 (Romeder, 1993) to 420,000 (Gottlieb & Peters, 1991) to 900,000 (Guay, 1989). Information gleaned from self-help clearing houses, associations, and resource centres identify 3,349 SHG in Canada (Todres, 1995).The growth of SHG in Canada and their contribution to health system reform make it important to study the relationship between these lay groups and health professionals.

Traditional relationships between health professionals and laypersons can be conflictual and disempowering (Chesler, 1991; Wilson, 1993). To illustrate, family caregivers in one study were dissatisfied with most mental health professionals because they did not involve the caregivers or communicate with them (Biegel, Song, & Milligan, 1995). The professional's traditional direct service 'expert role' with individual clients differs greatly from the collegial consultant role (Borkman, 1990; Reissman, 1990) called for in working with SHG. Moving from expert provider to equal partner will require role modification and role preparation.

The *attitudes* and *knowledge* of professionals regarding SHG are key factors in role development. In U.K. studies, professionals were interested in working with SHG and held favourable attitudes about the benefits of such groups (Wilson, 1993; Woff, Toumbourou, Herlihy, Hamilton, & Wales, 1996). Similarly, psychology and social work students had positive beliefs and attitudes regarding self-help and intended to collaborate with SHG, yet they lacked understanding and knowledge about self-help (Meissen, Mason, & Gleason, 1991). Other studies of human service professionals (e.g., Stewart, 1990; Toseland & Hacker, 1985) have also pointed to knowledge deficiencies. Professionals should be aware of support groups in their area (Duncan, 1994), become familiar with SHG modalities, and facilitate referral (Murray, 1996). In this context, it is encouraging that in Toronto more professionals were aware of self-help clearing houses and their referral functions in 1991 than had been the case in an earlier (1988) survey (Todres & Hagarty, 1993).

The SHG literature is replete with discussion of appropriate professional *roles*. Professionals are involved typically in initiating, supporting, and maintaining mutual aid groups (Hildingh, Segesten, Bengtsson, & Fridlund, 1994). Most human service professionals (75 per cent) interviewed in a 1991 Canadian survey had referred clients to SHG (Todres & Hagarty, 1993). Although health professionals often act as educators in SHG, members of genetic support groups in one study wanted professionals to be more knowledgeable and to disseminate information (Duncan, 1994). Students ranked consultant and facilitator as the most appropriate professional roles (Meissen et al., 1991). Family members found attendance of professionals who were not in leadership roles helpful at support group meetings (Bouricius, Kersten, Nagy, McCartney, & Stein, 1994). Indeed, facilitative roles are often seen as more appropriate than leadership roles, unless leadership is shared with SHG members.

Partnerships and collaborative relationships between professionals and SHG members are emerging in research, practice, and education domains. Research partnerships between professionals and SHG members can yield understanding and information (Toumbourou & Hamilton, 1994): 'When support groups and health professionals enjoy a healthy partnership, support groups are more than willing to cooperate in ... research' (Duncan, 1994, 65). In practice, partnerships between professionals and family caregivers are also recommended (Biegel et al., 1995). In this context, SHG with the greatest longevity had shared leadership by parents of children with cancer and by professionals (Weiss, 1992). Yet partnerships can be faced with tensions between SHG and professionals (Wilson, 1993), derived in part from differences in experiential and professional knowledge (Borkman, 1990). Involving SHG and SHG members in professional training can produce partnerships based on mutual respect (Meissen et al., 1991). Although focused on partnerships with laypersons, not SHG, collaboration between faculty and family members as partners helped nursing students to view families as resources (Matteoli, Verhey, & Warda, 1994). Despite these embryonic efforts at partnership, 'We have yet to determine how to synergistically blend professionally delivered services with mutual aid activities in a way that capitalizes on and preserves the unique contributions of each sector, and makes the two sectors equally legitimate and accessible' (Gottlieb, 1995, 233).

Assessment Studies

Two studies in our research programs assessed professionals' attitudes, skills, knowledge and roles pertaining to SHG and their preparation for partnership.

The aim of the first study in the Social Support Research Program was to identify the 'meanings and mechanisms of partnership' between health professionals and SHG members. The partnership project sought to elicit the experiences and perceptions of professionals and members regarding the contribution that each makes to the self-help process, relationships between SHG and health professionals, characteristics of an effective partnership, barriers to partnership, and strategies for achieving partnership (Stewart, Banks, Crossman, & Poel, 1994).

Individual interviews were conducted with SHG members (n = 49) and professionals (n = 47) in Nova Scotia (phase 1), followed by separate focus group interviews of members and professionals (phase 2) and by a joint workshop (phase 3). Health professionals included psychologists (n = 8), social workers (n = 10), nurses (n = 7), physicians (n = 8), occupational therapists (n = 7), and 'counsellors' (n = 7). Health professionals' involvement with SHG ranged from two to twenty years (mean = 7). The members represented SHG for diverse stressful situations (e.g., addiction, lifestyle, caregiving, chronic conditions).

The semi-structured interview guide for the individual interviews included eleven questions and pertinent probes about the following topics: reasons for involvement with SHG, roles that health professionals played with respect to SHG, roles of SHG members, positive and negative interactions and relationships between health professionals and members, characteristics and perceived desirability of partnership, tensions or barriers to achieving partnership, and strategies for promoting partnership. The interviews were taped and transcribed and field notes were recorded. In phase 2, six focus group interviews were conducted separately with health professionals and SHG members (previously interviewed in phase 1) to clarify, explicate and validate themes from the individual interviews. In a subsequent workshop involving both professionals and members consensus was achieved on the diverse dimensions of a partnership model.

The second study was conducted as part of a larger research program entitled 'Self-help/mutual aid for seniors and their family caregivers.' The objectives of this particular project were to identify the knowledge, skills, attitudes, and roles of health professionals concerning self-help/support groups (SHG/SG) for seniors and their family caregivers; to determine the acceptability of a collaborative relationship or partnership with these SHG/SG; to compare health professionals who had involvement with SHG/SG and those who had no involvement according to skills, knowledge, roles, and attitudes; and to compare different health professions according to skills, knowledge, roles, attitudes, and involvement.

In the seniors study, professionals (n = 474) from the same five disciplines involved in the partnership project (i.e., nursing, psychology, occupational therapy, social work, medicine) completed a mail-out survey instrument. Health professionals from all five disciplines were recruited from Nova Scotia, Quebec, and Ontario. The recruitment strategy was similar to that employed in the partnership project; professional associations, self-help clearing houses, and health agencies and organizations were approached. The response rates by profession were as follows: social workers (22.1 per cent), nurses (21.5 per cent), occupational therapists (19.3 per cent), psychologists (21 per cent), and physicians (12 per cent). Respondents were employed primarily in urban areas (80 per cent). The largest group of professionals (46 per cent) worked in hospital settings, 12 per cent were employed in a community health centre / CLSC, and 11 per cent were in private practice.

The instrument was derived from the earlier partnership project. Items were amended and added to focus on SHG/SG for seniors and their family caregivers. This measure was modified according to feedback from experts in the United States and Canada and from a pilot test. The instrument items were predominantly closed-ended. Some qualitative information was elicited by open-ended items in each subscale. The subscales were focused on professionals' involvement, roles, knowledge, attitudes towards SHG/SG, previous experience, relationships with SHG/SG members, and pertinent educational preparation. The research design for the two assessment studies and the links to the intervention tool and intervention studies are summarized in table 8.1.

Involvement with Self-Help/Support Groups

Many health professionals in the seniors study (42 per cent) indicated that they had never had any involvement with any type of SHG/SG. Only 26 per cent had been involved with SHG/SG for seniors and only 23 per cent with SHG/SG for family caregivers of seniors. Few (16 per cent) had been a member of a group. The key barriers to involvement were lack of opportunity in the workplace (47 per cent) and time constraints (17 per cent). Type of profession was significantly associated with involvement. Nurses (60 per cent) were most likely to have had no involvement with SHG/SG, followed by physicians (53 per cent), occupational therapists (42 per cent), psychologists (39 per cent), and social workers (21 per cent).

In the seniors study, there were significant differences between professionals who had involvement with SHG/SG and those who did not. Involvement was linked to positive attitudes towards SHG. For example, health professionals who had been involved were more likely to agree that the public expects professionals and SHG to collaborate ($p = 0.02$). Professionals who had never been involved with SHG/SG more often believed that SHG spread misinformation ($p = 0.02$), have not been proved effective ($p = 0.001$), provide only temporary relief ($p = 0.01$), and compete with professionals ($p =$

TABLE 8.1
Research Design

	ASSESSMENT STUDIES	
	Partnership	Seniors
Sample	Purposive Health professionals ($n = 49$) SHG members ($n = 47$)	Convenience Health professionals ($n = 474$)
Design	Descriptive Phases: 1) Individual Interview 2) Group Interviews 3) Joint Workshop	Descriptive Survey
Measures	Phase 1: Interview guide Phase 2: Focus group guide	Questionnaire based on partnership project
Data analysis		
Qualitative	Thematic content analysis (phases 1 & 2) Model development (phase 3)	Thematic content analysis of open-ended items
Quantitative	Intervention Tool: Education Module for Health Professionals	MANOVA, chi square
	INTERVENTION STUDIES	
	Widows	Disabled Women
Sample	$n = 27$	$n = 25$
Design		Pre-test-post-test within subjects
Measures		
Support		*Arizona Social Support Interview Schedule*
Health		*Social Emotional Loneliness Inventory* *Positive Affect — Scale* *Negative Affect — Scale*
Data analysis		
Qualitative		Thematic Content Analysis
Quantitative		MANOVA

0.03). Involvement with SHG was also associated with more experience with professional roles/functions (e.g., consult, co-lead, refer, research, educate); greater knowledge of SHG and clearing houses; increased educational preparation regarding SHG, professional and member roles, group process, salient skills, and collaboration; more years in practice; practice in urban settings; and policies in the work environment pertaining to SHG/SG.

Given that the number of SHG is rapidly expanding and given health system reform initiatives, opportunities for professional participation are likely to increase. Professionals' attitudes and knowledge will influence their future involvement and roles, as described in the next three sections.

Professional Roles, Functions, and Skills

The top five professional roles identified in group interviews of health professionals in the partnership project (Stewart et al., 1994) were *referral source* (i.e., encourage individual clients to seek help from a SHG, reach out to potential members, advise SHG of potential members), empowerer, *educator* (i.e., informal/formal teaching, speaking, role modelling, interpret professional knowledge), helper, and *facilitator* (i.e., enable SHG start-up, progress towards goals, process, and interactions). The key professional roles identified as most important by SHG members included educator, counsellor, referral source, facilitator, and consultant. (Common themes among professionals and members are denoted in italics.)

The professional roles identified by respondents in the partnership project could be classified as indirect, 'partner' roles rather than direct, expert provider roles, with one exception – counsellor. This role seems to acknowledge the continuing needs of SHG members for supplementary professional support. Referral, educator, and facilitator roles were approved by both members and professionals in the second-stage group interviews, whereas leader roles were advocated by professionals more than by members in individual interviews (Stewart et al., 1994). Leader roles can reduce group autonomy and egalitarianism (Borkman, 1990). Consistent with our findings, professional roles identified in previous studies involved consultation, referral, education, liaison, facilitation, support (Chesler, 1991; Katz, 1993; Stewart, 1990; Wilson, 1993), and research (Hildingh et al., 1994). These roles reflect the professional knowledge base, which is distinct from the experiential knowledge base of mutual aid SHG.

In the seniors study, the participants' knowledge of potential professional roles emphasized consultation (72 per cent), initiation (64 per cent), facilitation (58 per cent), and co-leadership (49 per cent). Key professional roles assumed by participants were facilitator, referral resource, and consultant. Only one-third of these health professionals had actual experience with professional roles in SHG/SG. Very few had been members of SHG/SG. Professionals who are members of SHG have been labelled 'prosumers' (Fishbein, Manos, & Rotteveel, 1995).

In the study focused on SHG for seniors, participants' knowledge of functions and roles differed by profession. Social workers typically had the greatest understanding of potential professional roles, in contrast to physicians, who seemed to be least familiar with appropriate professional functions (e.g., initiate SHG: 83 per cent vs 42 per cent; develop leadership in SHG: 75 per cent vs 40 per cent; co-lead SHG: 64 per cent vs 33 per cent).

Only 35 per cent of professionals in the seniors study had been educated about professional roles with SHG. Less than two-thirds reported that they had received educational preparation for suitable skills: educating/teaching (64 per cent), referral (64 per cent), group facilitation (64 per cent), consultation (60 per cent), and group leadership (58 per cent).

Knowledge of Self-Help Group Functions

The SHG roles/functions most frequently identified by health professionals in the partnership project included reciprocity, destigmatization, emotional support, isolation reduction, and experiential knowledge. Those ranked highest by SHG members were *emotional support*, *experiential knowledge*, *destigmatization*, affirmational support, and *reciprocity* (italics indicate agreement between professionals and members). In other studies, professionals also identified support, reciprocity and enhanced self-identity as key benefits of support groups (Mitchell, 1996; Woff et al., 1996).

Both professionals and members in our study of partnership endorsed exchange of experiential knowledge as an important role for SHG. Dakof and Taylor (1990) contend that specific types of support are perceived to be most helpful when provided by specific network members. The partnership project suggests that peers are valued for both emotional and informational support.

It is noteworthy that the knowledge and skills deficiencies of professionals – which can be overcome in educational programs - were criticized by SHG members but were not well recognized by professionals in the partnership project (Stewart et al., 1994). Professionals' lack of information and knowledge concerning SHG and inadequate preparation for appropriate roles and skills are common barriers to collaboration (Fridinger, Goodwin, & Chang, 1992; Stewart, 1990; Wilson, 1993). Knowledge of members' experiences in SHG may increase professionals' attention to SHG (Hildingh et al., 1994).

In the seniors study, professionals were aware of only 2.7 SHG/SG, on average, in their area. There were significant differences in knowledge among professions. Social workers reported the highest mean number of groups (3.4), compared with a low of 2.3 groups identified by physicians. Fifty-six per cent of social workers were aware of the existence of SHG clearing houses, in contrast to 29 per cent of physicians. In this study, over 90 per cent of professionals knew the following SHG/SG functions and activities: foster sense of belonging, deal with concerns, provide emotional support, give and receive help, and validate and share feelings.

Attitudes

The vast majority (91 per cent) of health professionals in the seniors study rated the overall effectiveness of SHG/SG as high or very high. Ninety-seven per cent described their overall view of SHG/SG as positive or somewhat positive. Professionals were asked to indicate their level of agreement with statements describing attitudes towards SHG/SG. Some examples pertinent to relationships between professionals and SHG follow. Most participants agreed that SHG/SG members are capable of providing support to one another (90 per cent), that SHG/SG should make use of professional knowledge (85 per cent), and that SHG/SG serve as a viable alternative to professional help (48 per cent). Moreover, most disagreed that SHG compete with professionals (88 per cent), that SHG are more harmful than helpful (77 per cent), and that SHG spread misinformation (68 per cent).

Beliefs about the functions and activities of SHG/SG, in the seniors study, varied according to type of profession. Social workers were most likely to believe that SHG/SG share new ways of dealing with concerns/problems, lobby for health system reform, reduce stigma, build confidence, supplement professional services, seek help/advice from appropriate health resources, and provide emotional support.

Relationships and Partnerships

In the partnership project, positive relationships were characterized by professionals and SHG members as reciprocal, helpful, complementary, collaborative, understanding, and clear about group goals and respective roles. Both professionals and members perceived relationships as positive if they entailed understanding. Thus, knowledge and comprehension of the different perspectives of professionals and groups/members is a critical component of a successful relationship. In our study, the foremost features of a poor relationship between professionals and members were authoritarian, territorial, competitive, non-supportive, judgmental, and conflictual. In another study, positive relationships with professionals were depicted as supportive, respectful, and helpful, whereas negative relationships were described as distant and guarded (Warner, 1992). Although problematic relationships can professionalize and coopt SHG members (Wilson, 1993), groups can be empowered by positive relationships with professionals (Mitchell, 1996).

Eighty-three per cent of all participants in the partnership project believed that partnership between health professionals and SHG members was desirable. Effective partnerships were depicted as understanding, reciprocal, collaborative, egalitarian, and trusting. Participants believed that partnerships necessitate role clarification, shared goals, risk taking, flexibility, and diminished professional control. In this context, a coalition between SHG and professionals can result in a fundamental redefinition of the professional-client relationship (Chesler, 1991).

The findings from the seniors' study reinforced these results. The vast majority of professionals (89 per cent) indicated that a collaborative relationship between professionals and SHG/SG was desirable. The three most frequent open-ended responses to the question 'In your opinion, is a partnership or collaborative relationship between professionals and SHG desirable?' were affirmative: (1) 'complement each other/provide benefits to both,' (2) 'professionals should be a resource only,' and (3) 'collaboration is necessary.' There was a significant association between type of profession and desire for collaboration. Social workers (92 per cent) and occupational therapists (92 per cent) were most likely to want a collaborative relationship, followed by psychologists (88 per cent), physicians (85 per cent), and nurses (83 per cent). Despite their positive attitudes towards collaboration, however, most professionals (73-77 per cent) had little or no involvement with SHG/SG for seniors or for their family caregivers. Other research also highlights professionals' desire for collaboration and partnership (Wilson, 1993).

Education for Partnership

The foremost mechanisms for achieving partnership, according to health professionals in the partnership project, involved education, clearing houses, and role and goal clarification, whereas SHG participants maintained that the best strategies entailed trust building, communication, and *education* (italics denote agreement). There was a consensus about the need for professional education.

Most professionals in the seniors study (54 per cent) believed that they had been poorly prepared for partnership. The majority of the professionals (67 per cent) reported that their basic education provided no instruction about SHG/SG. Only 29 per cent had received some professional preparation regarding SHG/SG. The most common response to the open-ended question 'Did your basic education program offer any instruction on SHG/SG?' was 'very limited.' There were significant differences in educational preparation by profession. Social workers were most likely to report instruction on SHG/SG in their pre-professional programs (51 per cent), followed by occupational therapists (41 per cent), psychologists (24 per cent), nurses (12 per cent), and physicians (11 per cent).

Participants in the seniors study identified content themes germane to work with SHG/SG in their professional programs. Generic topics (I) were more prevalent than content specific to SHG/SG (II). Specific groups in the geographic locale (III) were rarely identified in educational programs.

Topics in Professional Education Programs

I • Group process and dynamics (76.3 per cent)
• Participation of individuals in caring for their health (68.7 per cent)
• Concepts and principles of primary health care (67.0 per cent)
II • Definitions of self-help / mutual aid (46.2 per cent)
• Principles of self-help / mutual aid (41.6 per cent)
• Roles of professionals in SHG/SG (34.7 per cent)
• Roles of SHG/SG members (32.9 per cent)
• Benefits and difficulties/challenges of SHG/SG (28.6 per cent)
• Ways for professionals and SHG/SG to work together (27.2 per cent)
• What SHG/SG can and cannot do (26.4 per cent)
III • SHG/SG in your area (17.5 per cent)

In this study, the most frequent response to the open-ended question 'What kinds of information would help you to be more comfortable working with / referring to SHG/SG?' was 'more education.' The top response to the query 'What strategies would help you to overcome barriers to the development of a relationship with SHGs?' reinforced this belief in the importance of professional education. Fifty-nine respondents confirmed that the most significant strategy was more education/information. Wilson (1993) points out that professional training for knowledge development and for change of practice regarding SHG has been neglected. Indeed, SHG/SG can help to educate health professionals (Duncan, 1994). In table 8.2 the key findings from these two assessment studies are summarized and compared.

Intervention and Intervention Studies

Education Module for Professional-Peer Partnership

Following the partnership project, we developed a learning resource, training tool, and education module entitled *Educating for partnership: Self-help/*

TABLE 8.2
Key Findings from the Assessment Studies

Partnership Project	Seniors Study
	Professional involvement • Only half involved • Involvement varied by profession • Key barrier = lack of workplace opportunity
Professional roles • Consultation, referral, education and facilitation roles	*Professional roles* • Consultation, referral, education and facilitation roles • Only one-third had actual experience or education re: roles
Professional knowledge • Knew few SHG in area • Knew SHG functions: emotional support, reciprocity, foster belonging, affirmational support (i.e., validation)	*Professional knowledge* • Knew few SHG in area • Knew SHG functions: emotional support, reciprocity, foster belonging, affirmational support (i.e., validation)
Professional attitudes • Very positive view of SHG	*Professional attitudes* • Very positive view of SHG • Rated effectiveness of SHG high
Partnership • Most (83%) believed partnership with SHG desirable • Key strategy for fostering partnership = professional education	*Partnership* • Most (89%) believed partnership desirable • Key strategy for fostering partnership = professional education
	Professional education • Most not educated about SHG in pre-professional programs

mutual aid learning resource manual and evaluation measure for health professionals (Banks, Stewart, Crossman, & Poel, 1993), to prepare students in health professional education programs and to pave the way for support intervention research. This strategy addressed the paramount need for professional education about SHG and preparation for partnership.

Part 1 of the education module focused on educational strategies, ordered according to faculty preferences. These twelve educational strategies were case studies; audiovisuals; building skills and perspectives for direct interaction with self-help / mutual aid groups; literature and other informational resources; self-helpers as educators; role playing; student projects, papers, or presentations; debates; lectures; simulated interactions; SHG for students;

and involvement of practising professionals. Each of the twelve sections began with feedback on the importance and application of these different strategies from health professional faculty who were interviewed during the development of the learning resources package. Each section also included a selection of relevant resources.

The remaining components of the education module were a general bibliography on self-help/mutual aid; a bibliography on teaching and learning; a list of further resources, such as self-help clearing houses; an evaluation measure; and an annotated bibliography. The annotated bibliography included citations on the following subjects: curriculum development regarding self-help/mutual aid, primary health care, consumer/client input and involvement, theoretical foundations of self-help/mutual aid, characteristics and types of SHG, role of SHG in health/health care, roles and perspectives of SHG members and health professionals, positive and negative relationships and interactions between SHG and health professionals, dimensions of positive relationships and interactions, barriers to positive relationships, self-help clearing houses in Canada; and research reports.

This module was distributed as an educational resource to some self-help clearing houses in the country and some university libraries and informed the intervention studies that tested peer-professional partnerships.

Peer-Professional Partnership in Support Intervention Studies

The partnership model, developed in the final stage of the partnership project, was tested in the intervention studies of the Social Support Research Program (described in previous chapters). The model was focused on findings pertaining to positive and negative relationships and to characteristics of, barriers to, and strategies for achieving partnership. The tenets of the peer-professional partnership model helped to guide the peer-professional relationships formed in each of the intervention studies. The training and check-in sessions and joint interviews were informed by these principles. In the interventions for parents of children with chronic conditions, hemophiliacs with HIV/AIDS and their family caregivers, family caregivers of stroke survivors, and couples coping with cardiac illness, the complementary roles of peer and professional intervention agents were emphasized. During training, particular attention was paid to the influence of professionals' and peers' beliefs on interaction with participants and to use of personal strengths to build capacity of members. The training sessions also addressed the purpose and intended outcomes of the support groups; the responsibilities of participants; the roles of peer and professional facilitators; and the nature, scope, and sequencing of discussion topics. Simulated situations and role playing were employed to practise group facilitation and co-leadership techniques. Strategies for handling process issues, documenting support processes, and assisting individuals who required more support than groups could offer were identified. Peer visitors and professionals were jointly trained for the dyadic intervention in the stroke study.

We also implemented check-in or booster sessions for peer and professional facilitators of these support group interventions. Every four weeks, leaders connected by phone with each other, the trainer, and the investigators to discuss progress, facilitator roles, process issues, and topics. During these sessions, facilitators exchanged feedback, provided reinforcement, and suggested strategies.

Peer and professional facilitators were interviewed jointly in some studies and individually in others to solicit their perceptions of the co-facilitator training session; leadership issues; facilitator roles, contributions, and communication; group processes; and partnership. (The lessons learned from these studies are summarized in chapters 3, 4, 5, and 6.)

The partnership model was also implemented in two intervention studies in the seniors research program.

Peer-Professional Partnership in Telephone Support for Disabled Seniors

The objectives of one intervention study were (1) to develop and evaluate an innovative and accessible support group intervention for seniors who have no access to face-to-face support groups; (2) to determine the impact of telephone support groups on loneliness / social isolation and social support experienced by senior women with limited mobility; and (3) to facilitate collaboration between support group members and health professionals by implementing and evaluating a partnership model of leadership.

Socially isolated women over the age of sixty-five (n = 25) with impaired mobility, which limited their access to face-to-face support groups, participated in telephone support groups. They ranged in age from sixty-six to ninety-three years (mean = 75.2). Most were widowed (64 per cent); and 80 per cent lived alone. Participants lived in both urban (52 per cent) and rural (48 per cent) settings. They were able to leave their homes only zero to three times a week. Indeed, 40 per cent never left their homes. The disabilities that limited their mobility included polio, spinal cord injury, cardiovascular disease, cancer, arthritis, visual impairment, osteoporosis, and stroke.

The four groups of six to seven women met weekly for twelve weeks via teleconference for approximately one hour and were co-facilitated by peer (i.e., elderly women with disability) and professional leaders. One peer facilitator was seventy-one and confined to a wheelchair because of polio; the other was sixty-eight and visually impaired. The professional leaders included a social worker and a physiotherapist who had worked with seniors and a health educator with SHG experience. Facilitators were trained jointly, using the partnership model. A facilitator guide included background information on potential topics for discussion, such as retirement issues, self-care, and grandparenting. The weekly discussions were audiotaped, transcribed, and subjected to content analysis to document group processes and discussion themes.

Facilitators and members were satisfied with the shared leadership of these seniors' support groups. As one elderly woman said: '*[The shared leadership] was very effective. They knew more than we did and were very knowledgeable about the topics. They were both really good, interesting people. They were able to stimulate conversation without making people feel imposed upon. A good blend of practical experience and professional knowledge.*'

All facilitators of the seniors support groups acknowledged the high level of member input into selection of topics and group processes. Sessions usually began with facilitators introducing potential topics and members taking over the direction of the discussion. Facilitators reported members' preference for free-flowing conversation rather than structured discussion. '*Leaders usually picked the topic. Usually it started that way, but something someone said would lead us off in other directions*' (senior). '*Everyone has input ... that was really nice about the group. Everyone felt part of the process. It wasn't a group run by two leaders. It was a collaborative effort*' (senior). '*The group became more peer led over time. [Professional leader] is very laid back and she let me try to organize the conversation within the group*' (peer leader).

Peer-Professional Partnership in Support Groups for Widowed Seniors

Since women, by virtue of their longer life expectancy, are more likely than men to suffer spousal bereavement, peer support groups can play a significant role in providing supplementary support. Widows over the age of fifty-five participated in a support group intervention co-facilitated by peer (i.e., widows) and professional leaders. The groups were conducted in Halifax and Toronto. The study had three major aims: (1) to examine the impact of a support group intervention on bereaved women's loneliness, negative affect, and perceived support; (2) to evaluate a peer and professional co-facilitated approach; and (3) to encourage the transition from a co-facilitated support group to a peer-facilitated SHG.

Twenty-seven widows ranging in age from fifty-five to seventy-six years (mean = 66.7) participated in the study. They had been married from six to sixty-three years (mean = 40.2). Fifty-two per cent were bereaved for less than one year; 21 per cent were bereaved for more than five years. Eighty-four per cent lived alone; only 16 per cent lived with someone else.

The groups met for approximately one hour weekly for a maximum of twenty weeks, depending on members' wishes and leaders' commitment (range: eight to twenty weeks). Peer and professional facilitators were trained together using a partnership model. The facilitator guide included background information on potential topics for discussion such as the grief process, loneliness, and discovering independence. The group discussions focused on practical concerns (e.g., personal health, finances, help seeking) and emotional stresses (e.g., grief, relationships, change, uncertainty regarding future, loneliness). Co-facilitators maintained weekly diaries, which documented discussion topics, support processes, group dynamics, and balance of leadership.

Participants' and facilitators' comments revealed predominantly positive group dynamics. Exemplar quotations of positive processes include '*forming a cohesive bond*'; '*members enjoyed the content of the group*'; '*looked forward to weekly meetings, felt they had made new friends*'; '*relaxed, comfortable*'; and '*members felt at ease with one another.*' Negative dynamics, however, in one group in particular, which ended after eight weeks, were illustrated by members' and leaders' observations: '*the group was small and discussions tended to get personal, and sometimes uncomfortable*'; '*two members who joined later changed the dynamics of the group*'; '*one member was very angry and tended to dominate the group*'; and '*the group dissolved when the leaders took a planned absence from the group*'. During the post-intervention interviews, participants recommended some changes in the group intervention. The lessons learned are outlined below.

Lessons Learned

- More structured topics versus members should identify topics for discussion (seniors expressed divergent views).
- There should be a flexible agenda versus professional speakers on specific topics (seniors expressed divergent views).
- There should be more participants within groups.

- Participants should be similar.
- Shorter duration versus group could run for up to twenty-four weeks (seniors expressed divergent views).
- Extend sessions to two hours.
- The training session was effective, but the following improvements should be made:
  - meet co-leader beforehand
  - make facilitator roles more explicit
  - have more role playing.
- The booster/check-in session was helpful.

Implications for Programs and Policies

Self-care and mutual aid programs and policies can reduce costs of health care and lost productivity associated with chronic conditions, caregiving, and other stressful life situations. Health system reform documents at the national and provincial levels emphasize empowerment of populations and expanded public participation (Angus, Auer, Cloutier, & Albert, 1995). Premises of primary health care and of health promotion, reflected in these documents, reinforce the importance of self-help and mutual aid as mechanisms for public participation. Trends related to the financing of health care rely on families and extended social networks to undertake caregiving roles; caregivers then turn to mutual aid groups and support groups for supplementary support (Stewart & Tilden, 1995). Self-help mutual aid groups are a mechanism by which consumers participate actively in their own health care and in policy issues related to their health (Lavoie & Stewart, 1995). Gottlieb contends that it is critical to keep self-help and mutual aid in the public eye 'and to remind policy makers that the fund of mutual aid cannot survive and replenish itself without a safety net of basic health, income security, and community services' (1995, 231). He also maintains that 'swings in the policy pendulum reflect the urgent need to enshrine mutual aid activities within every possible government funding program,' such as health, education, housing, and social services.

The National Forum on Health clarifies that resilience, so relevant to health, can pertain to communities as well as individuals. Resilient communities are characterized by 'successful leaders who work with a well developed and supported network of community development organizations, self help groups, and advisory groups' (1996, 17). Two pertinent policy recommendations issued by the Forum were 'invest in local community action' (43) and 'governments ... should provide support for local leadership and coordination of the various health-enhancing efforts and initiatives undertaken by public organizations, the private sector, families and community or volunteer groups' (49).

Almost all professionals in the two assessment studies affirmed their desire for a collaborative relationship. Yet despite this positive perspective, most had little or no involvement with SHG and limited awareness of actual SHG and of mutual aid mechanisms. There were important differences in educational preparation by profession; social workers were most likely to report instruction in their professional programs, whereas only 10 per cent of nurses and physicians reported educational preparation. Furthermore, professionals' knowledge deficiencies, particularly about SHG in their area, were consistent with the emphasis in education programs on generic topics more than on content specific to SHG and particular groups. Without a clear understanding of the nature, purpose, and function of SHG, health professionals may credit professional education in generic areas as adequate preparation for involvement. These educational programs, however, may not be directed sufficiently towards collaboration with SHG to prepare professionals for partnership.

Given the important differences among professions in awareness, attitudes, and orientations towards SHG, educational initiatives directed towards medicine and nursing could be important priorities. Accordingly, an interactive computer module, based on the education resource developed as a product of the partnership project, could be tested in schools of nursing and medicine. This module could focus on partnership with SHG, appropriate professional roles, benefits and challenges of self-help mutual aid, characteristics of SHG, their role in health and health care, positive and negative relationships and interactions between SHG and health professionals, and SHG in their geographic locale. The impact on knowledge, skills, attitudes, and assumption of future roles could be evaluated.

One key theme in a special issue of the *Canadian Journal of Community Mental Health* on mutual aid groups and support groups was the interface between formal (professional) and informal (lay) sectors (Lavoie & Stewart, 1995). Requisite role changes for professionals, ideological and control issues, mechanisms to expand interactions, and barriers posed by different knowledge bases were delineated in the four papers on this theme.

Programs that foster collaboration should incorporate training and check-in sessions for groups that are co-facilitated by both a peer and a professional. The perceived suitability of structure, the flow of leadership between peer and professional, and their unique and shared roles in SHG for different ages and stressful situations should continue to be distinguished and documented. Furthermore, national SHG organizations could help groups to develop collaborative relationships with professionals and professional associations (Wilson, 1993) and recommend pertinent programs and policies.

Acknowledgments

Both the partnership project and the three projects in the research program 'Self-help mutual aid for seniors and their family caregivers' discussed in this chapter were funded by NHRDP.

Note

A partial report of the results from the partnership project appeared in the publication Stewart, Banks, Crossman, & Poel (1994).

References

Angus, D., Auer, L., Cloutier, E., & Albert, T. (1995). *Sustainable health care for Canada: Synthesis report*. Ottawa: Ottawa Economic Projects.

Banks, S., Stewart, M., Crossman, D., & Poel, D. (1993). *Education for partnership: Self-help/mutual aid resource manual and evaluation measure for health promotion*. Report to National Health Research and Development Program, Health Canada. October.

Biegel, D., Song, L., & Milligan, S. (1995). A comparative analysis of family caregivers' perceived relationships with mental health professionals. *Psychiatric Services, 46*(5), 477–482.

Borkman, T. (1982). Where are older persons in mutual aid self help groups? In A. Kolker-Aliza & P. Ahmed (Eds), *Aging* (257–284). New York: Elsevier.

Borkman, T. (1990). Self-help groups at the turning point: Emerging egalitarian alliances with the formal health care system? *American Journal of Community Psychology, 18*(2), 321–332.

Bouricius, J., Kersten, E., Nagy, M., McCartney, P., & Stein, R. (1994). Family support groups: AMI of Western Mass. Style. *Innovations and Research in Clinical Services, Community Support, and Rehabilitation, 3*(3), 33–40.

Chesler M. (1991). Participatory action research with self-help groups: An alternative paradigm for inquiry and action. *American Journal of Community Psychology, 19*(5), 757–768.

Dakof, G.A. & Taylor, S.E. (1990). Victims' perceptions of social support: What is helpful from whom? *Journal of Personality and Social Psychology, 58*(1), 80–89.

Duncan, V. (1994). Partners in information: Genetic support groups, health care professionals, and the health sciences librarian. *Bibliotheca Medica Canadiana, 16*(2), 64–67.

Fishbein, S., Manos, E., & Rotteveel, J. (1995). Helping the helpers: A unique colleague support system for mental health professionals-consumers. *Journal of Psychosocial Nursing, 33*(11), 41–43.

Fridinger, F., Goodwin, G., & Chang, C. (1992). Physician and consumer attitudes and behaviours regarding self-help support groups as an adjunct to traditional medical care. *Journal of Health and Social Policy, 3*(3), 19–36.

Gottlieb, B. (1995). Research on mutual aid and social support: Progress and future directions. *Canadian Journal of Community Mental Health, 14*(2), 229–234.

Gottlieb, B. (In press). Self-help, mutual aid and support groups: A synthesis of the literature. *Canadian Journal of Aging*.

Gottlieb, B., & Peters, L. (1991). A national demographic portrait of mutual aid group participants in Canada. *American Journal of Community Psychology, 19*, 651–657.

Guay, J. (1989). *Self-help groups in Canada: A profile of volunteers based on the 1987 national survey on volunteer activity*. Ottawa: Secretary of State.

Hildingh, C., Segesten, K., Bengtsson, C., & Fridlund, B. (1994). Experiences of social support among participants in self-help groups related to coronary heart disease. *Journal of Clinical Nursing, 3*, 219–226.

Katz, A. (1993). *Self help in America: A social movement perspective*. New York: Twayne.

Lavoie, F., & Stewart, M. (1995). Mutual aid groups and support groups: The Canadian context. *Canadian Journal of Community Mental Health, 14*(2), 5–12.

Lieberman, M.A. (1990). Mutual aid groups: An underutilized resource among the elderly. In M. Lawton (Ed.), *Annual review of gerontology and geriatrics*, Vol. 9, 285–320. New York: Springer.

Matteoli, R., Verhey, M., & Warda, M. (1994). Collaboration between families and university faculty: A partnership in education. *Journal of Psychosocial Nursing, 32*(10), 17–20.

Meissen, G., Mason, W., & Gleason, D. (1991). Understanding the attitudes and intentions of future professionals toward self-help. *American Journal of Community Psychology, 19*(5), 699–714.

Mitchell, F. (1996). Carer support groups: The effects of organizational factors on the character of groups. *Health and Social Care in the Community, 4*(2), 113–121.

Murray, P. (1996). Recovery, Inc. as an adjunct to treatment in an era of managed care. *Psychiatric Services, 47*(12), 1378–1381.

National Forum on Health. (1996). *Canada health action: Building on the legacy.* Volume II. *Synthesis reports and issues papers.* Ottawa: National Forum on Health.

Reissman, F. (1990). Restructuring help: A human services paradigm for the 1990's. *American Journal of Community Psychology, 18*(2), 221–230.

Romeder, J. (1993). Of surveys and definitions of self-help and mutual aid. In M. Stewart & F. Lavoie (Eds), *Self-help / mutual aid for seniors: Research challenges* (5–11). Ottawa: Self-Help Canada.

Stewart, M. (1990). Expanding theoretical conceptualizations of mutual-aid self-help groups. *Social Science and Medicine, 31*(9), 1057–1066.

Stewart, M., & Tilden, V. (1995). The contributions of nursing science to social support. *International Journal of Nursing Studies, 32*(6), 535–544.

Stewart, M., Banks, S., Crossman, D., & Poel, D. (1994). Partnerships between health professionals and self-help groups: Meanings and mechanisms. *Prevention in Human Services, 11*(2), 199–240.

Todres, R. (1995). Self-help/mutual-aid clearinghouses and groups in Canada: Recent developments. *Canadian Journal of Community Mental Health, 14*(2), 123–130.

Todres, R., & Hagarty, S. (1993). An evaluation of a self-help clearinghouse: Awareness, knowledge, and utilization. *Canadian Journal of Community Mental Health, 12*(1), 211–223.

Toseland, R., & Hacker, L. (1985). Social workers: Use of self-help groups as a resource for clients. *Social Work, 30*(3), 232–237.

Toumbourou, J., & Hamilton, M. (1994). Researching self help drug treatment: Collaboration and conflict in the age of harm reduction. *Addiction, 89*, 151–156.

Warner, A. (1992). Participants' views on the impact of self-help on health. Unpublished manuscript. Halifax, NS: Self Help Connection.

Weiss, J. (1992). Support groups for patients with genetic disorders and their families. *Pediatric Clinical North America, 39*, 13–23.

Wilson, J. (1993). Vital yet problematic. Self-help groups and professionals: A review of the literature in the last decade. *Health & Social Care, 1*, 211–218.

Woff, I., Toumbourou, J., Herlihy, E., Hamilton, M., & Wales, S. (1996). Service providers' perceptions of substance use self-help groups. *Substance Use and Misuse, 31*(10), 1241–1258.

9

Mobilizing Support in Chronic Illness: A Relationship Perspective

Renee F. Lyons, Steve Duck, Lynn Langille, and Michael J.L. Sullivan

Abstract. In this chapter we focus on the conceptualization of social support needs in illness and call for increased attention to relationship processes as a key determinant of social support mobilization. We clarify key relationship and support issues that arise in coping with illness and influence the provision of needed support. The first part of the chapter is organized around four social support issues in illness and their impact on support mobilization: dealing with loss and change; dealing with conceptions of self; addressing adaptations in communication and companionate activity; and dealing with social support in the context of equity. Then we introduce four related dialectical tensions in relationships dealing with illness that also influence support mobilization. Finally, we provide recommendations to enhance support mobilization in chronic illness.

Introduction

Humans are essentially social creatures. Despite the North American orientation towards individualism and the irritations of relationship maintenance, we are used to communal living. Our need for membership in a collective becomes most obvious during serious illness, because illness presents enough threats to personal identity and performance that even the most individualistic of us shares this experience with others. Since illness is seen as countering contemporary values, such as prosperity, speed, independence, self-reliance, and production, it is not surprising that individuals and their relationships struggle to adapt. This struggle is reflected in the process of social support mobilization.

The chapters in the first portion of this book are evidence of the important discoveries researchers have made about social support processes and the value of interventions to increase support in chronic illness and caregiving.

There is still uncharted territory, however, surrounding the effective mobilization of support in real-life personal relationships. We know that there are problems in obtaining the support needed to cope effectively with the multidimensional impacts of chronic illness. Analysis of the most effective processes of support mobilization leads us to explore the deep and murky waters of relationship functioning; in particular, relationship processes in the context of chronic illness.

In this chapter we focus on the conceptualization of social support needs in illness and call for increased attention to relationship processes as a key determinant of social support mobilization. We clarify the key relationship and support issues that arise in coping with illness and that influence directly the provision of needed support.

Impact of Illness

What happens to individuals who experience chronic illness? Serious health problems, such as stroke, cancer, and multiple sclerosis, envelop their victims in loss (Gordon & Benishek, 1996). Decrease in physical function as a result of pain, paralysis, or treatment often leads to disruption or loss of roles in work, family, and community and to loss of financial resources. These changes contribute to increased dependence, loss of self-identity, and hopelessness (Brooks & Matson, 1982; Lyons, Sullivan, Ritvo, & Coyne, 1995).

There have been three major approaches to the study of losses associated with health problems (Lyons & Sullivan, 1998). The *individual perspective* has been focused on assessment of illness-related stressors and on helping individuals and distressed family members to cope more effectively with illness/disability in their lives (e.g., Thompson, 1996). The *social change perspective* attributes loss to the social construction of illness and disability and accentuates the need to change societal values and critical contextual factors such as poverty, and to develop policies and services that will lead to personal empowerment, social role valorization (Wolfensberger, 1983), and community access (e.g., Duval, 1984). The *relationship perspective* (the subject of this chapter) proposes that chronic illness is 'our' issue rather than an individual issue and that social support is a key factor in curbing and adapting to loss (e.g., Atkins, Kaplan, & Toshima, 1991) for the individual and the social unit (e.g., family).

Research from the relationship perspective has been focused largely on the provision of emotional and instrumental support to the persons with health problems. However, illness and disability do not happen in a social vacuum. They are embedded within the context of family and friendships. Studies of family caregiver distress, burden, and burnout show that losses due to illness or disability can have a substantive impact on family members (e.g., Gatz, Bengston, & Blum, 1990; Williamson & Shaffer, 1996).

Support Mobilization: Laying the Groundwork

A huge volume of research devoted to the social determinants of health has clearly identified the importance of social support (perceived, available, and provided) to general health and well-being, to buffering stress, and to coping with significant life stressors such as illness. It has been argued, however, that the piecemeal approach taken to study aspects of social support and caregiving has sidestepped key questions concerning the conditions that elicit necessary support provisions (Heller & Rook, 1997; Vaux, 1988).

The process of mobilizing the social network to provide members with support is a daunting task, particularly where illness is concerned. Unlike life challenges such as work or training for marathons, where extensive resources and energy are devoted to 'preparation,' illness evokes no conscious investment other than perhaps a disability pension. We believe that illness happens to someone else; that we will be untouched. A prime example of the denial of potential illness or disability is the construction of retirement homes and communities that are inaccessible to wheelchairs. Consequently, people are left on their own too often or with one overburdened caregiver to deal with illness, situations that exacerbate support needs. Clearly, disability pensions aren't enough of an investment to guarantee a good social support return.

Social support happens for three main reasons: because people care about the well-being of others, because they are obliged to provide support, and/or because the well-being of the social unit is affected by illness and social support mobilized to maintain that unit. It is surprising how much support is provided despite the paucity of preparation and knowledge about effective support provision. Effective mobilization of support means that needs are understood and communicated to others and that the social network is willing and able to respond. The challenge involves shared understandings of need and strengthening of social bonds to respond effectively to these needs.

Social Support Mobilization and Relationships

Just as illness arrives unexpectedly, so, too, does the social support for dealing with that illness. However, the support process occurs in the context of previous interactions. Thus, support is mobilized, not necessarily recruited, from an existing array of resources. Leatham and Duck (1990) argued that social support is derived from an everyday set of repeated interactions where parties have developed a history of interactions. Despite the fact that the interactions may be focused on something else, parties develop an understanding of the likelihood (and value) of the contributions of significant others during crises.

Unquestionably, many stressors in chronic illness are unresolved relationship issues about exactly what support is needed and who should provide it (Baxter, 1976; Cohen & Willis, 1985; Moos & Tsu, 1977; Russell, 1985). Effective mobilization of support is embedded within the nature of change and loss experienced as a result of illness (Bolger, Foster, Vinokurd, & Ng, 1996; Meyerowitz, Levin, & Harvey, 1997; Thompson, 1996) and within the conditions that contribute to the maintenance of quality relationships (Coyne & Fiske, 1992), the *primary determinant* of social support provision.

Although the perspectives given in this chapter have evolved from considerable research activity on relationships, illness, and disability (e.g., see Lyons et al., 1995, for a review), for the purpose of this chapter we draw on findings and personal accounts from a recent focus group study of relationship and support issues in chronic illness and disability. The study comprised sixteen three-hour focus group sessions in six locations in Canada and the United States. Eight sessions involved sixty-three adults with a range of acquired chronic health problems and disabilities (e.g., multiple sclerosis, cancer, spinal injury, and stroke). Another eight sessions included thirty-two researchers and clinicians (primarily clinical and social psychologists and social workers) who study relationships and/or work with persons with chronic health problems (Lyons, Langille, Coyne, Duck, Fitch, Gunter, Hood, Jackson, Miller, Ritvo, & Thompson, 1996).

The findings from this study are organized around four issues and their impact on support mobilization: dealing with loss and change; dealing with concepts of self, addressing adaptations in communication and companionate activity, and dealing with social support in the context of equity. Then we organize these findings conceptually into four dialectical tensions in relationships dealing with illness. Finally, we offer recommendations to enhance support mobilization in chronic illness.

Dealing with Loss and Change in Relationships

One key social support need in chronic illness is understanding the impact that illness has on people's lives and the loneliness that results. The enormous impact on functioning and lifestyle caused by illnesses such as multiple sclerosis, stroke, and environmental illness needs to be recognized and addressed, not glossed over or downplayed. For the individual, the stress of chronic illness is not restricted to the loss of physical abilities and function that ensue from symptoms. The stresses encompass changes in relationship systems. As one clinician in the study indicated: '*In terms of my practice, I guess one of the basic observations that I make is that once a family is touched significantly by illness and disability, their trajectories are altered perhaps for the full course of their family life. There is not really this question of being affected and then overcoming it, or adapting to it, and getting back to "normal." There isn't such a thing*' (clinician/researcher's group).

Illness and disability can change relationships substantively and the impacts on network structure, function, and quality are surprisingly similar across a broad range of disabling health problems (e.g., cancer, multiple sclerosis, spinal injury). Changes in *social network structure* typically include diminished size of network, decreased frequency of interaction, loss of friendships, and increased incidence of divorce in younger populations (Burman & Margolin, 1992; Coyne & Fiske, 1992; Janssen, Philipsen, & Halfens, 1990; Lyons, 1991). Changes in *relationship functioning* include reduction in the multidimensionality or range of 'companionate activity' (activities people engage in with others), decrease in social space (Brent, 1982), and discomfort in communication and support processes (Dunkel-Schetter & Wortman, 1982; Meyerowitz et al., 1997). Inevitably, *relationship quality* is affected by the absence of valued relationship provisions and difficulty of negotiating relationship constraints produced by illness and disability (Lyons, 1991; Burman & Margolin, 1992). The impact appears more substantial with degenerative or unpredictable health problems and/or with conditions involving severe chronic pain or cognitive functioning (Lyons, 1991). Nevertheless, the focus group participants agreed on the substantial impact of illness and disability on relationships across a broad range of chronic illnesses.

> *There is a lot of loss related to this condition (MS). A lot of people we talk to, talk about the social isolation, the loss, I think, of relationships.* (clinician/researcher's group)
>
> *I'm sure we've all had friends who just evaporated. Compatriots at work and partners in business and neighbors and what not who shared in the sort of trivialities of the community and they are all gone.* (prostate cancer group)
>
> *It (the divorce) was brought on by the MS, I think. It was beginning to be bad. But the MS, I was totally rejected and neglected at that time. I basically wasn't fed. I ruined his life, shattered his dreams.* (MS group)

Individuals are often confronted not only with relationship loss, but also with the prospect of being rejected: '*people are scared of being dumped, either by the medical profession or ... I think it's also very much with the couples. That they feel they are going to be dumped by the other person ... And there is a lot of talk about fear and anxiety about losing the loved one*' (clinician/researchers group).

Fears of relationship loss lead to actions that may have been contraindicated by the health problem in order to preserve the relationship. Needs for support may be concealed or obscured in the effort to show competence in order to preserve relationships: '*I think that [fear of marriage break-up] is a lot of the reason why I try to do more. Because as long as I can do, I will do, so he won't get tired of me real fast, real early*' (MS group).

Illness and resultant disability violate the implicit relationship 'contract,' the expectations and roles that were in place when both partners or friends were healthy and able-bodied. Individuals who are ill may perceive that they have changed the conditions of the contract, and as a result they fear relationship loss. Denial of the illness/disability by significant others, or resistance to the changes that are required to accommodate illness in the relationship, supports this belief, and unresolved relationship issues directly influence social support provision: '*It was with my family that I had the worst problem. It was so hard to get a ride even down here for treatment. Because if they brought me for treatment, they would have to acknowledge that I had a problem. That there was something wrong with me*' (breast cancer group).

The notion that illness and disability are inconveniences in our fast-paced, individualistic culture reinforces this fear of loss. Needs for support are interpreted as burdens: '*It's almost a matter of inconvenience ... People seem to be inconvenienced by you. And they take that, it seems to me in our conversation, quite personally*' (composite group comprising persons with a variety of health problems).

Teenagers, in particular, acted as if health problems in a parent were a personal inconvenience. Needs of the person with the health problem are obscured by the needs of children who 'suffer' from decreases in the support they are used to receiving. '*Teenagers are very selfish. So my cancer has been a total inconvenience to their lives*' (breast cancer group). '*I registered for school and I went back. And they all fought me every step of the way. And the teenagers ... They weren't teenagers. Actually, young adults by then. My son was 16 when I was diagnosed. And I would come home to sinks full of dirty dishes. This was my punishment for not being there*' (breast cancer group).

As indicated by these focus group accounts, the person with the disability may feel responsible for changing the rules of the relationship and for demanding more resources from the relationship.

Managing a network of friends, family, workmates, and the health care system takes tremendous energy, a scarce resource for persons devoting considerable effort to their health problem. The need for network shrinkage is exacerbated by relationship tensions that remain unaddressed. People with chronic illness must sometimes adjust their social network so that support provision is not overshadowed by stress provision: '*With chronic illness, one of the things that you have to do, with these types of disabilities, is that you have to pare down your friends. There is no sense spending time to save a relationship with someone who doesn't appreciate your strengths and weaknesses, what you can and cannot do. You'll put an enormous amount of effort into it and all they are going to do is lead you down the garden path into situations that are going to make your health worse*' (composite group 2).

It is ironic that relationship loss and change occur precisely at the time of heightened need for smooth functioning and supportive relationships. Well-functioning relationships are not a frill for persons with health problems. They can mean the difference between social isolation or social integration. Moreover, they will strongly influence whether the individual will be living at home or in an institution. With changes in health care and greater reliance on family, the need for family support has become even more critical.

> *I think family is so much more important to me today than it would have been if I hadn't had a stroke.* (stroke group)
>
> *Just for spinal cord injury, the presence of good relationships for somebody who is a quad is a key issue between being in the community or being in an institution ... I was just talking to some folks I work with about somebody who has been in the community for 10 years as a quad ... because the social support system has broken down, he's going to an institution. He has no other choice. I think the way health care is going, and we already know that the presence of a good support system is needed in the community. And how do we identify relationship problems early on? ... It is such an important issue.* (clinician/researcher's group)

Dealing with Adjustments to Self-Identity

Relationships are central to *self-identity*. Personal identity and self-esteem often have social origins, stemming from the reciprocal chaining of processes of personal performance and recognition (Heller & Rook, 1997). Typically, illness and disability result in the reassessment of personal identity (Charmaz, 1991; Hutchinson, 1996; Mathieson & Henderikus, 1995; Matson & Brooks,

1977). Individuals with chronic illness engage in a process of reformatting individual and relationship schema. Who am I? Who are we? What can I contribute to this relationship? What are realistic expectations for my relationships? Social support that gives rise to social validation and acceptance is directly provided by fulfilling relationships, love, and inclusion: '*I thought, well this is pretty scary, like who the hell am I and who is my wife and what is our relationship? Who are my children and what is our relationship?*' (prostate cancer group 2). '*It colors people's perceptions. Like if they get MS when they are single, "Can I ever marry? Can I have children? Can I follow through on those plans that I thought I had? Should I go to college? Should I buy a house?" You know, all of that kind of thing. So I think in that way it affects relationships, or even the expectation of having relationships*' (clinician/researcher's group).

Relationships with health professionals – in particular, physicians – dramatically influence self-appraisal: '*I think still there is a great deal of discomfort on the part of physicians and how they relate to persons with disabilities ... The only accessible examination table that I've ever seen in a doctor's office is the one in the Rehab. There's a message right there. If they can't examine you, it looks as if they don't want you. Or if there are stairs to the office, how do you get into their office?*' (composite group 2).

The belief that relationships define the self and that being on one's own is a sign of personal failure (Peplau & Perlman, 1982) adds pressure to be in relationships: '*Our culture puts so much emphasis on having a relationship that I feel that in order to be self-fulfilled, I must have one. I should have one. And my disability compounds that problem in a very significant way*' (composite group 3).

The strong desire for a partner may lead people with chronic conditions to rush the development of close relationships or to misperceive the willingness of others to have a close relationship and to provide social support: '*I feel that in order for me to feel complete, I want to be married. I want to date. I want to have an emotional and physical relationship ... You strive for that. You work towards that. And that creates problems for you because you put so much emphasis on it, you tend to overcompensate. You tend to try too hard. Or, you tend to misread situations from time to time as well*' (composite group 2).

These accounts demonstrate that the loss of self-identity is a key issue in coping with illness. Relationships play a strategic role in how people feel about themselves. Social validation is a central theme in emotional support provision. Paradoxically, we not only lose ourselves in relationships, we also find ourselves in relationships. Unfortunately, it is easy to miss cries for validation by persons with chronic illness, to perceive the need as consuming too much free time, to set up social barriers, or to attribute responsibility for support provision to another friend or family member.

Addressing Specific Relationship Challenges

The negotiation of stresses involves clarifying and addressing the relationship issues that were created by illness and disability. These issues are not pathologies or personal functional deficiencies, but are products of changed health circumstances.

Communication Challenges

Interactions with individuals with chronic illness and disability are often stressful, and people typically avoid them (Eisenberg, Griggens, & Duval, 1982). The scripts we learn in life to manage interpersonal situations may no longer be useful in interpersonal situations that are ambiguous and uncertain. We don't know how to approach people with chronic health problems and feel insecure about interpreting their responses. From the perspective of the person with the illness, relationship tensions stem from the need to disclose the health problem, educate others about their condition and its impact on functioning, and articulate their support needs. Communication issues surround whom to tell, how to tell, how much to tell about symptoms, prognoses, or changes in performance and, in particular, to explain how it feels. This process is particularly salient in circumstances where there are few visual cues to the disability. Everything needs explaining: '*For the last couple of years, I've been trying to think of a way to express to people what I feel. What it feels like. Because I guess that I feel that I want somebody who doesn't have MS to go through this for one day, or a couple of hours ... The actual sensation that your body has or does not have is hard to explain*' (MS group).

The task of informing, educating, and asking for assistance can become quite stressful and tedious, particularly for individuals who did not have a fluent interactional style prior to the illness. '*It's a big job to educate somebody every day, every day of your life. You get tired of it*' (composite group 1). '*I was never much of a talker, and my actions were louder than my words. I always rested on my laurels with that. It doesn't work any more. I have to explain so much and negotiate so much more*' (composite group 1).

For some individuals social withdrawal may be the least stressful adaptational option, which ends up being counter-productive to support seeking and provision: '*We avoid communication (with family) because of the misinterpretation and misunderstanding*' (composite group 2).

Some individuals in our society, particularly men, have difficulty in tolerating distress or illness in others. Their propensity for wanting to 'fix things' makes them feel helpless when confronted with another person's health problem. So individuals with chronic conditions are frequently urged to 'get on with it' or 'snap out of it' – anything except talk about it: '*My husband is having trouble dealing with the fact that I'm involved with the group (cancer support group) and very much involved with the group ... he thinks I should go into a severe depression. And this is really morbid stuff. You know, why do I have to talk to women with breast cancer? Like, 'Just get over it.' And this has been a long time for him to come to terms with*' (breast cancer group).

Insensitive comments relating to less fortunate circumstances are usually given in the name of support, but have the opposite effect. They reflect the 'downside' of social comparison: '*My pet peeve is that people are somehow compelled to tell you about their worst, worst, worst friend of a friend who was dying and suffering*' (breast cancer group). '*I don't like people to tell me how lucky I am. I know I'm lucky to be walking and everything but I just don't want people to tell me that*' (stroke group).

In the presence of chronic illness, communication becomes a risky venture, creating the opportunity to say the wrong thing even when the intention is support provision. Blows to a fragile identity are readily provided by people who have kind hearts but lack skill in communicating with persons with health problems.

Companionate Activity Adaptation

Family, Friends, and Leisure

Reducing relationship tension and finding mutually enjoyable activities were perceived as key factors in the maintenance of satisfying relationships with family, work colleagues, and friends. Efforts made at inclusion (versus avoidance) were seen as an important form of social support provision. Patience and flexibility were required to change traditional ways of performing in every social context, including family life, leisure, sexual intimacy, and work: '*In order to have a relationship with an ill or disabled person, flexibility is absolutely essential. You must be flexible*' (composite group 2).

Activities had to be organized to accommodate facility accessibility, transportation, increased support needs, and symptoms, including diminished energy. A major constraint was fatigue: '*There just comes a time when you say "Okay, I've seen enough of you people, go home." Your fatigue has hit a point where you don't want to be sociable any more. I don't want to put a strain on a relationship, but it [fatigue] will always affect a relationship with your family and spouse*' (MS group).

Loss of cherished companionate activity, the focal point of valued relationships, was difficult. The choice between sacrificing companionate leisure or exacerbating a health problem is stressful:

> *At first it was really tough getting used to what I could do physically and what I couldn't do. And I think my active lifestyle had a lot to do with that because I was involved in sports ... Like friends have asked me, 'Would you like to go snowmobiling?' Well, sure I would love to go snowmobiling. But I know if I hop on a snowmobile with friends of mine, that just the bumping is going to break my rearend. So I'm saying to myself, 'Well, I'm not going to do that because I'm not going to jeopardize my job and end up in bed for 3 months just for an hour's enjoyment going snowmobiling with some friends.' So these are some of the decisions that you make, that you have to make* (composite group 2).

There was also considerable tension regarding expectations that family and friends adapt their agenda and routines: '*We've all given up things. We know that we cannot do everything that we did pre-MS as far as entertainment and enjoying the family and all that. Those of us who are married, a lot of times our spouses will ... We're almost holding them back. My wife loves to dance and I'm not real good at the polka any more ... People would invite me somewhere, and I got so depressed because other people could dance and I couldn't. So I decided to stop going to those functions*' (MS group).

Intimacy

Many participants had relinquished or substantially reduced sexual activity because of their health problems: '*My sex life is "What is sex?"*' (prostate cancer group). They reported diminished feelings of sexual attractiveness, exacerbated by the perceived lack of interest from partners. Perceived rejection occurred at a time of increased need for love and social validation: '*We all need to be loved and cared for. When I was discharged and went home, I couldn't believe that my wife didn't want to have anything physical to do with me ... that is a real shock ... You're dying to be loved, and to love, and it isn't there. So that is a very difficult part of a relationship for people who have disabilities, I think*' (composite group 2).

The Workplace

The impact of relationship tensions on illness/disability was apparent in attributions for quitting work. Although some participants in the focus groups were employed, most had stopped working as a result of disability or illness. There was a strong desire among many participants to maintain meaningful activities but with reasonable performance expectations. Many work environments were not flexible enough to accommodate performance changes of people with chronic conditions who were now a 'burden' to the system. Support provision in the workplace was a key factor in the decision to continue working or to retire.

> *I worked in an extremely busy office where it's just go from the moment you step into the door until you walk out. And when you're not there, it puts stress on everyone else because everyone else has to fill your shoes. So you get guilt feelings as a result of not being there, and wanting to be there. And you get ... odd comments when you do return to work in relation to, 'Well, we were really busy while you were gone,' or, 'I had to do this and this for you while you were gone' ... So it did not help our relationships at work at all. I tended to withdraw from work more and more as time occurred, talking less to my peers, and interacting with them less.* (composite group 2)

Confronting Social Support and Equity Challenges

Social support is tied intimately to issues of reciprocity and equity (Antonucci & Jackson, 1990; Heller & Rook, 1997). Perceptions of fairness about social support expectations and role delegation in the process of support mobilization are influenced by individual, relational, contextual, and situational factors (e.g., gender). It is generally believed that women are more competent in dealing with illness than men and that dealing with illness is a woman's role. Women who are ill are often more concerned about the well-being of others than are men with the same illness. Women seem to put more effort into support mobilization for the benefit of others and their relationships than in meeting their own needs. Illness seems to push women towards more traditional 'service' roles (Lyons & Meade, 1995).

Participants described considerable awkwardness in giving and receiving support. They reported that although people could be helpful, the process of support provision often misfired. Issues that had to be negotiated in relationships included fairness and reciprocity, obligation versus desire, expectations regarding performance, overprotectiveness, and the stress of asking for help. There was an awareness that increased needs for support markedly altered the balance of power. Whereas before the illness the relationship may have enjoyed a comfortable give-and-take ratio, this balance had now been upset. Expressions of distress sometimes needed to be censored to avoid straining the relationship: '*Maybe before you weren't an individual who needed to depend on others. And now, because of your disability, you have to. And so in order for you to survive, you have to swallow your pride, and you ask for the help and the support of people who have always been around you*' (composite group 1). '*Having to ask makes you angry. And having to say "thank you." It's a funny role in life that I guess we're stuck with and can't do much about. But none of us like it*' (MS group).

Long-term needs for support require continuous negotiation around equity issues and support roles within friendships and family networks. The closest family member too often is left with overwhelming responsibilities for the well-being of the person who is ill. This circumstance also overwhelms the relationship, revealing the important links between support mobilization and relationship quality.

Respondents in the focus groups also expressed a desire to be useful to others, not identified solely as a person who is needy: '*Usually you go to a minister with your problems ... but I have a minister coming to me, and this minister has prostate cancer. And I was able to advise him. Like, "Tell me the fears that you have." He and his wife spent from 6:00 when they came until 10:00 when they left there talking about cancer, prostate cancer. And he was much more relieved when he left there. He had a living example of someone who had gone through it. So I did probably well advising him and listening. And I felt good after* (prostate cancer group).

As indicated by the four themes we have examined under social support mobilization and relationships, there is a strong interrelationship between these two concepts. Efforts to understand loss and change in illness and personal identity issues and to act on adaptations needed in communication, activity, and equity in relationships all will contribute to effective support mobilization regardless of the context. A new set of commonly accepted relationship rules around illness and increased competence in addressing the issues we have highlighted would facilitate support mobilization. Support mobilization requires time, flexibility, creativity, and a commitment to the maintenance of quality relationships. Another message in the accounts from this focus group study relate to the cognitive processes involved in mobilizing action on illness-related support needs. We frame these cognitive processes as dialectical tensions.

Dialectical Tensions in Support Mobilization

Relationships are not static. They are a combination of elements of stability and of change (Duck, 1994). Baxter speaks of relational maintenance dialectically as 'the process of coping with the ceaseless change that results from the struggle of contradictory tendencies inherent in relating' (1994, 233). The study of relationship dialectics is fairly new and has been focused on generic functions of relationships. Examples of relationship dialectical tensions include autonomy-connection (the most central), predictability-novelty, and openness-closeness.

Significant life changes like chronic illness create their own dialectical tensions; several have been introduced in the preceding discussion (e.g., whether or not to ask for help, looking after one's health versus relationship maintenance). Our data from this project and other studies (e.g., Lyons & Meade, 1995) suggests that there are four general relationship dialectical tensions related to illness and social support mobilization. They include illness impact, personal control, attachment, and coping style. The last three might be considered subsets of Baxter's (1990) autonomy-connection dialectic.

Illness Impact: Containing versus Globalizing Illness

People with illness and their intimates are chronically *in tension* with the illness state. How does this joint conflict with illness, which is issue oriented, become personalized and create conflict in relationships? Borrowing from the cognitive reformulation of learned helplessness theory (Abramson, Seligman, & Teasdale, 1978), we propose that conflict escalates and becomes increasingly *personalized* (it is something about you and me that is at the core of this conflict), *stabilized* (resolution or change is unlikely in the foreseeable future), and *globalized* (it is going to affect more and more contexts of living). For example, in the case of a serious illness, the conflict could become increasingly personalized if one or both parties are dissatisfied with the way the other is dealing with support provision. The conflict could become stabilized if a couple has exhausted all its resources to 'fight' the illness and to support each other, and the illness does not disappear. The conflict could become globalized as the illness interferes increasingly with relationship quality. The implications for support mobilization are obvious. It is exceedingly burdensome to provide support within the context of a deteriorating relationship.

Personal Control: Independence versus Reliance

The perceived ability to exert control over stressful situations is an important factor in coping (Bandura, 1986). Illness and loss of control associated with illness are threats to self-identity. The belief that health outcomes can be influenced will have an impact on efforts to resist the sometimes overwhelming presence of illness. Therefore, maintenance of identity and self-worth is tied to the perceived ability to control the illness and to minimize its intrusiveness. For instance, being forced by decreased mobility to use a wheelchair may be perceived as a symbol of defeat: 'I just didn't want to give in to this disease' (Russell, 1985, 34).

Similarly, the need to mobilize support can be interpreted as defeat (i.e., this illness is getting the best of me). The relevance of the independence versus reliance dialectic to social support mobilization is reflected in the following quotes from a study of mothers with multiple sclerosis: '*It takes a little pride to ask ... these things you used to be able to do, and now, you have to ask. And it just, oh that makes you so angry.*' '*And there are times when ... I'm not feeling well ... I really appreciate having the help. But I don't want the help forced on me when I'm capable of doing it myself. So I guess it's him assuming ... That bothers me, that he assumes that I ... can't do things sometimes, when I really could. So it's ... I guess he can't read my mind. Can't expect him to*' (Lyons & Meade, 1995, 203).

Attachment: Withdrawal versus Enmeshment

The withdrawal-enmeshment dialectic may be proposed to explain how experiential differences affect close relationships in which one person has an illness and the other is relatively healthy. The term 'withdrawal' is derived from Russell's (1985) work on the social implications of illness in which there is disengagement from social roles and responsibilities. At the other end of the dialectic is 'enmeshment,' Minuchin's (1974) term for overly attached individuals whose identities are too tightly connected to the relational unit. This dialectic identifies the movement away from relationships or towards relationships.

The experienced adversity of chronic illness can isolate the individual from close companions. The person who is ill manifests suffering in ways painful for companions to behold, and the companions may avoid this pain by decreasing contact. Reduced functional capacity also isolates and inhibits involvement in social events. A person fatigued or distracted by symptomatic distress may miss subtle interpersonal 'cues' or shades of meaning that previously contributed to shared intimacy and support provision. At the enmeshment end of the dialectic, individuals become more tightly connected, resulting in overprotectiveness, helplessness, and diminished individual freedom. A midpoint for explaining relationship effects emerges from the 'interdependence' orientation (Coyne, Ellard, & Smith, 1990), which emphasizes the needs and goals of both relational partners and the coordination of support mobilization. Both partners try to regain pre-illness satisfaction levels. Differences arising from the illness experience are no longer a source of separation, but become cues for compensatory acts of companionship and support. The illness no longer prevents participation in shared activities, since previously shared activities are adapted or new activities are initiated to ensure sustained involvement.

Coping Style: Individual versus Communal Coping Orientation

Coping traditionally has been conceptualized as the *individual* pursuit of *self-maintenance* through stress; that is, what do *I* do to deal with the emotional and instrumental stressors of *my* problem? People wish to enhance not only their own well-being, however, but the well-being of their family and friends, and they wish to decrease the illness burden on them. This orientation implies shared responsibility for dealing with illness.

Many aspects of coping and adaptation may be addressed communally, rather than individually, when couples, nuclear or extended family, or close friends adopt the position that illness is 'our problem' rather than 'my problem.' Jointly addressing the emotional (e.g., anger, frustration, disappointment) and instrumental (e.g. income, treatment, child care) aspects of a health problem substantially changes coping and adaptation processes (Lyons, 1993; Lyons, Mickelson, Coyne, & Sullivan, 1998).

The following account from the study of mothers with MS provides an example of the notion of communal coping:

> *I phoned up my close family and my close friends and thought I may as well do this all at once. So I sat down with Mother Bell just loving it. I did all the phone calls at once, just one after the other. 'The good news is I don't have a brain tumor. The bad news is, I have MS. We'll cope with this. You know, in a couple of weeks, two weeks from now, we'll cope with this ...' I think by giving the people closest to us this two-week*

> *hiatus ... then they don't feel obliged to say too much right away. And a number of them did say, one of my closest friends: 'I just don't know what to say to you.' 'Don't say anything. It's a bitch ... but better than a brain tumor.'* Lyons & Meade, 1995, 206

In this circumstance, the respondent is concerned with the emotional response of her friends to the diagnosis and how they will cope. Her language identifies the issue as 'our problem' versus 'her problem.' She has constructed the illness as a network issue, rather than isolating herself as the victim. In most close relationships, at least some aspects of coping will be addressed communally. Persons with an individualistic orientation, however, will resist accommodation and change for others. The individualistic coping style (which inhibits support mobilization) may be dominant if individuals want to avoid affecting others negatively, present a more stoic approach, or display personal competence in managing the illness, or if they believe that others are not capable of providing support. The individualistic style removes the necessity for asking for help and encourages non-interference from others (Heller and Rook, 1997; Sampson, 1977). In contrast, people with a communal orientation will feel less burdened or distressed by the relationship negotiation, adaptation, and support provision required of illness and disability. They should experience the stress of illness in others more strongly (Williamson & Schultz, 1995) and be more invested in support mobilization. Conversely, those with a weaker communal orientation may be left with the overriding responsibility for the stressor and for negotiating relationship and support issues. Researchers need to examine whether the communal coping perspective would be useful in understanding coping with illness and the nature and extent of support mobilization.

Illness creates such a plethora of personal and interpersonal issues at a time of resource depletion that negotiating how these issues will be addressed is extremely stressful. Illness invites tension and conflict in relationships, and through this lens we are expected, as good family members and citizens, to enact needed social support. No wonder support mobilization is so complex and sometimes difficult!

Key Findings from the Relationship Issues Study

Support challenges in chronic conditions

- Dealing with relationship loss and change
- Managing adjustments to self-identity
- Communication challenges

- Adaptation of companionate activities
- Intimacy issues
- Relationship tensions in workplace
- Confronting equity challenges in relationships

Dialectic tensions in support mobilization

- Containing versus globalizing illness
- Independence versus reliance on others
- Withdrawal versus enmeshment in relationships
- Individual versus communal coping orientation

Implications for Programs and Policies

Persons with chronic illnesses, researchers, and clinicians gave fairly straightforward, consistent messages about strategies to facilitate support mobilization in the context of illness. We summarize these strategies as follows.

- *Communicate the importance of relationships.* Inform the general public about illness and its impact on quality of life and increase awareness about the linkages among support mobilization, relational well-being, and the quality of life of persons with health problems. In other words, relationships play a key role in how people cope with illness. This dialogue should occur in the general population as part of investment in good support systems, through carefully designed illness and support education programs in schools, churches, and the media.
- *Pay attention to relationship issues.* Social support dialogue and education must also occur in the context of specific experience of illness as a part of the 'treatment' regime. This can occur in health care facilities through family education/counselling and specifically designed support sessions for patients and families and also in the community through support groups and conferences.
- *Pay attention to relationship roles.* Increase dialogue about changed personal and shared roles arising from the presence of illness in the family, workplace, and community. A key issue surrounding support mobilization is responsibility. How will this illness be managed and by whom? Equitable distribution and negotiation of support roles are extremely challenging, even in families or other social units where there is a communal approach to problems. Social workers and other health professionals can play a supportive role for families trying to

sort out these issues. Again, the question of role and responsibility (i.e., to which health professionals can a family turn?) needs to be clarified.

- *Increase relational competence around illness.* Individuals need to know how to communicate more effectively about illness. People in families, work settings, and communities need to know how to provide effective social support and to learn strategies for adaptation and inclusion. They need be able to negotiate adaptation and social support mobilization for various relational contexts, including work, family, leisure, community, and health care.
- *Communicate about social support and relationships.* Individuals with a chronic illness and family members need licence to discuss support issues and to share relationship stories and strategies. This process can occur in a variety of venues, including informal dialogue, individual and family counselling, and support groups. Models of successful support mobilization should be shared.
- *Examine public policy and its linkage to support mobilization in chronic illness.* Services such as home care, housing, transportation, work adjustment programs, and physical accessibility have a direct impact on support for families. In a recent study in Sweden it was demonstrated how supportive public policies for persons with chronic illness and their families directly influenced the quality of family relationships.

Two key factors will be very influential in implementing these actions: commitment and the place of support mobilization in the health services.

Commitment

What is the meaning of commitment when a family member, friend, or employee has a chronic illness? Commitment is a complex concept involving social obligation, relationship history, relationship rules and roles, degree of attachment, relationship expectations, and other roles and commitments. The nature of commitment to provide support in the context of illness is crucial. Concomitant with the relaxation of societal rules about commitment to relationships, people are left to negotiate their respective roles and methods for support mobilization in illness.

In a poignant 'letter to the editor' in response to an article on caregiving, Charlwood (1997) speaks of the time and effort required to understand his wife's capabilities (early-onset Alzheimer's) and the direct impact of his attention on her physical and emotional well-being. One is struck by the guilt he expresses when he reduced his involvement with his wife because of increased work demands. His letter highlights the meaning of commitment and the efforts required to be supportive when a partner has a chronic illness. What is a fair commitment for a family member or friend? This difficult question requires family and public debate.

Support Mobilization in Health Services

Although the quality of personal relationships is the key to social support mobilization, this subject has not received sufficient attention from those in the health system. The prevalent acute care model does not accommodate the stresses of chronic health problems, including social support issues. Relationship problems often fall through the cracks. Health professionals need to be more aware of the fact that chronic illness is a relationship issue and to examine how support mobilization features in their treatment and services. There were numerous accounts from both ill persons and clinicians about the lack of preparedness of health professionals to address the relationship and support challenges of illness and the importance of a family systems approach to illness: '*I had more instructions when I bought a toaster, in English and in French, than I did when I left the doctor*' (breast cancer group). '*What I noticed in my clinical experience, is that bringing people in from the family or from the significant others that help the patient, made a tremendous difference*' (clinician/researcher's group).

Health professionals can facilitate discussion of support mobilization in the social network and in support groups. Often members of support groups increase their general level of support through group involvement, but the level of support received from their family, friends, or workmates is deficient or diminished. Support groups could feature support mobilization more systematically in their discussions. Relationship and support protocols with tools for identifying and addressing relationship issues in illness are needed: '*But I just think, for a lot of people, they say, "Life isn't very good. And I'm not very happy in my relationships. But I'm not really sure what is going on." It's like they can identify the symptoms but they can't identify the underlying layer*' (clinician/researcher's group).

A Final Word on Support Mobilization

It is easy to be drawn into the compelling stories of the drama of illness, the active treatment phase, the near death stories, and so on. In a review of a recent book on coping with stroke, Drainie (1997) admits that 'the crisis portion' of stroke survival was a compulsively readable story, but that portion on living with a chronic illness, including the acceptance and meeting of support needs, was 'tougher slogging.' She realizes, however, that the latter portion is the primary story of chronic health problems: 'Even as the reader allows these negative reactions to surface, however, awareness dawns that this is what disabled people have to put up with everyday. As humans we are all fascinated by the high drama, the great tragedy that strikes someone low, but the long boring aftermath of a life of daily struggle is something we'd rather ignore.' (1997, D16)

For persons with chronic illness, everyday relationships and support processes are central to understanding the meaning of illness, but the particularly compelling portions of this story are the commitments and successes in renegotiating relationships and in support mobilization. With relief from unrelenting dependence and burden, one can experience the challenges and rewards of engaging in interdependence. Illness and support mobilization comprise not merely a sad story, but an opportunity for intimacy and collaboration.

References

Abramson, L.Y., Seligman, M.E.P., & Teasdale, J. (1978). Learned helplessness in humans: Critique and reformulation. *Journal of Abnormal Psychology, 87*, 49–74.

Antonucci, T.C., & Jackson, J.S. (1990). The role of reciprocity in social support. In B.R. Sarason, I.G. Sarason, & G.R. Pierce (Eds), *Social support: An interactional view* (173–198). New York: Wiley.

Atkins, C.J., Kaplan, R.M., & Toshima, M.T. (1991). Close relationships in the epidemiology of cardiovascular disease. In W.H. Jones & D. Perlman (Eds), *Advances in personal relationships*, Vol. 3 (207–231). London: Kingsley.

Bandura, I. (1986). *Social foundations of thought and action: A social cognitive theory*. Englewood Cliffs, NJ: Prentice-Hall.

Baxter, L.A. (1990). Dialectical contradictions in relationship development. *Journal of Social and Personal Relationships, 7*(1), 69–88.

Baxter, L.A. (1994). A dialogic approach to relational maintenance. In D.J. Canary & L. Stafford (Eds), *Communication and relational maintenance* (233–254). New York: Academic Press.

Baxter, L.A., & Dindia , K. (1990). Marital partner's perceptions of marital maintenance strategies. *Journal of Social and Personal Relationships, 7*, 187–208.

Blaxter, M. (1976). *The meaning of disability*. London: Heinemann Educational.

Bolger, N., Foster, M., Vinokur, A.D., & Ng, R. (1996). Close relationships and adjustment to a life crisis: The case of breast cancer. *Journal of Personality and Social Psychology, 70*, 283–294.

Brent, R.S. (1982). Community and institutional social spaces. *Therapeutic Recreation Journal, 16*(1), 41–48.

Brooks, N.A. & Matson, R.R. (1982). Social psychological adjustment to multiple sclerosis. *Social Science and Medicine, 16*, 2129–2135.

Burman, B., & Margolin, G. (1992). Analysis of the association between marital relationships and health problems: An interactional perspective. *Psychological Bulletin, 112*, 39–63.

Charmaz, K. (1991). *Good days, bad days: The self in chronic illness and disability.* New Brunswick, NJ: Rutgers University Press.

Charlwood, R.G. (1997). Caring for someone with Alzheimer's. Letters to the Editor. *Globe and Mail*, 25 January, D9. Toronto.

Cohen, S. & Wills, T.A. (1985). Stress, social support and the buffering hypothesis. A theoretical analysis. *Psychological Bulletin, 98*, 310–352.

Coyne, J.C., & Fiske, V. (1992). Couples coping with chronic illness. In T.J. Akamatsu, J.C. Crowther, S.C. Hobfoll, & M.A.P. Stevens, (Eds), *Family health psychology*. (129–149). Washington, DC: Hemisphere.

Coyne, J.C., Ellard, J., & Smith, D. (1990). Social support, interdependence, and the dilemmas of helping. In B.R. Sarason, I.G. Sarason, & G.R. Pierce (Eds), *Social support: An interactional view*. (129–149). New York: Wiley.

Drainie, P. (1997). Slowdance: A story of stroke, love, and disability by B. Sherr Klein. Book review. *Globe and Mail*, 8 February, D16. Toronto.

Duck, S.W. (1994). *Meaningful relationships: Talking, sense and relating*. Thousand Oaks, CA: Sage.

Dunkel-Schetter, C., & Wortman, C.B. (1982). The interpersonal dynamics of cancer: Problems in social relationships and their impact on the patient. In H.S. Friedman & M.R. DiMatteo (Eds), *Interpersonal issues in health care* (69–100). New York: Academic Press.

Duval, M.L. (1984). Psychosocial metaphors of physical distress among MS patients. *Social Science and Medicine, 19*, 635–638.

Eisenberg, M., Griggins, C., & Duval, R. (1982). *Disabled people as second class citizens*. New York: Springer-Verlag.

Gatz, M., Bengston, V.L., & Blum, M.J. (1990). Care-giving families. In J.E. Birren & K.W. Schail (Eds). *Handbook of psychology of aging*. (404–426). New York: Academic Press.

Gordon, P.A., & Benishek, L.A. (1996). The experience of chronic illness: Issues in loss and adjustment. *Journal of Personal and Interpersonal Loss, 1*, 299–307.

Heller, K., & Rook, K.S. (1997). Distinguishing the theoretive functions of social ties. In S. Duck (Ed.), *Handbook of personal relationships*, 2nd ed. (648–670). Chichester, England: Wiley.

Hutchinson, S.L. (1996). The altered self. An exploration of the process of self identity reconstruction by people who acquire a brain injury. MA thesis, Dalhousie University, Halifax, NS.

Janssen, M., Philipsen, H., & Halfens, R. (1990). Personal networks of chronically ill people. Paper presented at Fifth International Conference on Personal Relationships, Oxford University, Oxford, England.

Leatham, G., & Duck, S.W. (1990). Conversations with friends and the dynamic of social support. In S.W. Duck (Ed. with R. Silver), *Personal relationships and social support* (1–29). London: Sage.

Lyons, R. (1991). The effects of acquired illness and disability on friendships. In D. Perlman & W. Jones (Eds), *Advances in personal relationships*, Vol. 3 (223–277), London: Kingsley.

Lyons, R. (1993). The energy crunch: Relationship and support experiences of mothers with chronic illness. In *Studying human lived experience: Symbolic and ethnographic research '93*. University of Waterloo, Waterloo, ON.

Lyons, R. (1993). Research on relationships coping with stressful life events: An interview with Ben Gottlieb and James Coyne. *International Society for the Study of Personal Relationships Bulletin, 10*(1), 11–14.

Lyons, R., & Meade, D. (1995). Painting a new face on relationships: Relationship remodeling in response to chronic illness. In S. Duck & J.T. Wood (Eds), *Confronting relationship changes* (181–210). Thousand Oaks, CA: Sage.

Lyons, R., & Sullivan, M. (1998). Curbing loss in illness and disability: A relationship perspective. In J.H. Harvey (Ed.), *Perspectives on personal and interpersonal loss: A sourcebook* (137–152). Bristol, PA: Taylor & Francis.

Lyons, R.F., Sullivan, M.J.L., Ritvo, P.G., & Coyne, J.C. (1995). *Relationships in chronic illness and disability*. Thousand Oaks, CA: Sage.

Lyons, R., Mickelson, K., Coyne, J., & Sullivan, M. (1998). Coping as a communal process. *Journal of Social and Personal Relationships, 15*(5), 570–605.

Lyons, R., Langille, L., Coyne, J., Duck, S., Fitch, M., Gunter, A., Hood, C., Jackson, Z., Miller, D., Ritvo, P., & Thompsen, P. (1996). *Social integration and disability: Clarification of relationship challenges in work, family, and community*. Publication of research findings prepared for the Social Sciences and Humanities Research Council, Ottawa.

Mathieson, C.M., & Henderikus, S.J. (1995). Renegotiating identity: Cancer narratives. *Sociology of Health & Illness, 17*, 283–306.

Matson, R.R., & Brooks, N.S. (1977). Adjusting to multiple sclerosis: An exploratory study. *Social Science and Medicine, 11*, 245–250.

Meyerowitz, B.E., Levin, K., & Harvey, J.H. (1997). On the nature of cancer patient's social interactions. *Journal of Personal and Interpersonal Loss, 2*, 49–69.

Minuchin, S. (1974). *Families and family therapy*. Boston: Harvard University Press.

Moos, R.H., & Tsu, V.D. (1997). The crisis of physical illness. In R.H. Moos (Ed.), *Coping with physical illness* (3–21). New York: Plenum Press.

Peplau, L.A., & Perlman, D. (1982). Perspectives on loneliness. In L.A. Peplau & D. Perlman (Eds), *Loneliness: A source book of current theory, research, and therapy*. New York: Wiley.

Russell, S. (1985). *Social implications of multiple sclerosis*. Final report of a formulation apart from the National Health Research and Development Program, Department of Health and Welfare Canada, Ottawa.

Sampson, E.E. (1977). Psychology and the American ideal. *Journal of Personality and Social Psychology, 35*, 767–782.

Thompson, S.C. (1996). Barriers to maintaining a sense of meaning and control in the face of loss. *Journal of Personal and Interpersonal Loss, 1*, 333–357.

Vaux, A. (1988). *Social support: theory, research and intervention*. New York: Praeger.

Williamson, G.M., & Schulz, R. (1995). Caring for a family member with concern: Past communal behavior and affective reactions. *Journal of Applied Social Psychology, 25*, 93–116.

Williamson, G.M., & Shaffer, D.R. (1996). Interpersonal loss in the context of family care-giving: Implications of communal relationship theory. *Journal of Personal and Interpersonal Loss, 1*, 249–274.

Wolfensberger, W. (1983). Social role valorization: A proposed new term for the principle of normalization. *Mental Retardation, 21*(6), 235–239.

10

Family Caregiving: Issues in Gaining Access to Support

Anne Neufeld and Margaret J. Harrison

Abstract. The reduced resources associated with restructuring Canadian health systems have shortened hospital stays and increased expectations for family caregiving. Women outnumber men as family caregivers and experience caregiving demands throughout the lifespan. Support from others within the caregiver's social network may reduce the negative impact of caregiving. Two caregiving situations that create high demands and increased requirements for support are caring for an older person who is cognitively impaired and caring for an infant who was born prematurely. In this chapter we discuss issues in gaining access to support identified in longitudinal research involving women caregivers in these two situations. Barriers to access arose from social norms, characteristics of the woman's social network, and the personal costs of requesting support. Women caregivers employed two strategies to avoid direct requests for assistance - non-verbal distress cues and maintenance of relationships encompassing unsolicited support. Implications of these issues for development of policies and programs are addressed.

Introduction

As Canadian health system restructuring has reduced resources for health care services and shortened hospital stays, expectations for family caregiving have escalated. Recently, 2.8 million Canadian men and women were identified as caregivers of persons with chronic health problems (Statistics Canada, 1997). A large Canadian survey of men and women employees found that 46 per cent provided assistance to an elderly relative, 31 per cent had child care responsibilities, and 26 per cent combined child care with care of older relatives (Canadian Aging Research Network, 1993).

The impact on families of caring for children and adults with long-term chronic health problems is accentuated by trends to increased labour force participation by women (Baines, Evans, & Neysmith, 1993), smaller families, and more sole parent, blended, reconstituted, and dual career families (Tarman, 1994). One consequence of these trends is a diminished supply of unpaid family labour, despite increased social demands for family caregiving of people with chronic conditions.

Caregiving demands vary depending on the characteristics of the family member's condition as well as expectations within roles other than caregiving (Pearlin, Mullan, Semple, & Skaff, 1990). Examples of primary caregiving activities include assisting with activities of daily living, managing medical treatment requirements, dealing with difficult behaviours associated with illness, securing and coordinating health and related services, and making personal adaptations in other spheres of life, including employment and recreation (Gottlieb, 1996). In addition, many caregivers, particularly women, experience conflict between the demands of family caregiving and expectations within their work roles (Kramer & Kipnis, 1995). Among employed family caregivers in a Canadian survey, half experienced repercussions of caregiving in their work role (Statistics Canada, 1997). Family caregiving demands and roles are often associated with negative outcomes for the caregiver. One in five caregivers in Canada reported that caregiving had affected their health and over one-quarter reported altered sleep patterns (Statistics Canada, 1997).

In North American society, provision of unpaid health care is often labelled as women's work (Stoller, 1993) and is expected of wives and daughters in particular (Barr, Johnson, & Warshaw, 1992). This expectation has deflected responsibility for care from public institutions to families, and from families to women (Aronson, 1992). Women caregivers outnumber men by three to two (Statistics Canada, 1997), and women continue to spend significantly more time than men on the care of children and elderly relatives (National Forum on Health, 1996). The amount of time women spend in caring activities remains the same regardless of their employment status (Dowler, Jordon-Simpson, & Adams, 1992). For women, family caregiving is ongoing over the lifespan, from responsibility for parenting children to caring for senior family members. Sharing caregiving responsibility among family members is restricted by the separation of paid work from domestic work, the organization of the labour market, and gender-based expectations (Aronson, 1992).

The costs of caring are particularly high for women who experience the primary burden of care for both young children and older relatives. Caring for older family members has been associated with emotional, physical, and financial strains (Mui, 1995). Women with children consistently report more parental role strain and role demand than men (after single parent status, hours spent with children, number of children, employment status, and salience of parental role are controlled for) (Scott & Alwin, 1989), and they are at more risk of depression (Aneshensel, Frerichs, & Clark, 1981; McIntosh, 1993).

One factor that may influence the negative impact of caregiving is support from others within the social network (Palinkas, Wingard, & Barrett-Connor, 1990). In a Scandinavian study of family caregivers of adults with extensive care needs, women who shared responsibility for care with someone else in the informal network reported 30 per cent less stress than women who gave care alone (Johansson & Ahlfeldt, 1996). Employed mothers who had no difficulty in arranging child care and whose husbands shared child care reported lower depression levels (Ross & Mirowsky 1988). Conversely, higher levels of depression were reported by women with difficult-to-arrange child care and whose husbands did not share care.

In summary, in North American society, unpaid care of relatives is expected of women who outnumber men as family caregivers. Regardless of employment status, women spend more time than men in family caregiving and experience strain, high role demands, and often depression. Women who share caregiving responsibility with supportive others may experience less stress than those who lack such support.

Family caregiving demands are ongoing for women throughout the lifespan. Two specific situations in which women experience high caregiving demands involve (1) caring for an older person who is cognitively impaired and (2) caring for an infant who was born prematurely. These two caregiving situations are common in Canada. It is estimated that 252,600, or 8 per cent, of all Canadians aged sixty-five and over meet the criteria for some form of dementia. It is predicted that this figure will reach 592,000 by the year 2021 (Canadian Study of Health and Aging Working Group, 1994). In Canada, for 1993 alone, 18,977 infants were born at least three weeks before their expected due date and weighed less than 2500 grams.

Using these two caregiving situations as examples, our purpose in this chapter is to discuss issues that women caregivers encounter in accessing support. These issues were identified from a series of longitudinal qualitative studies. A brief discussion of the demands and outcomes of caregiving will be presented first, followed by an overview of the characteristics of social networks and relationships and issues in accessing support. The chapter ends with discussion of implications for policies and programs.

Caregiving Demands and Outcomes

Women caring for an older family member with cognitive impairment and mothers caring for infants born prematurely provide care for long periods of time. In these situations, care is given to a family member who has limited ability to be responsive or to provide emotional support to the caregiver. The disorientation of adults who are cognitively impaired limits their ability to communicate personal needs or to give feedback in response to the care they receive. They may be unable to recognize the caregiver or engage in meaningful interaction. Changes in affect and memory loss related to cognitive impairment further limit the care recipient's potential for reciprocity (Deimling & Bass, 1986). A recent review (Goldberg & DiVitto, 1995) indicates that premature infants, in comparison with term infants, are less responsive in non-verbal interactions with their mothers. They are less alert, less able to make eye contact, give less clear behavioural feedback, and spend less interaction time in face-to-face contact. Mothers of pre-term infants face a daunting task. Under stressful conditions, such as unexpected early birth and complex medical treatment, they care for infants who are behaviourally more difficult to manage (Goldberg & DiVitto, 1995).

For both groups of caregivers, the demands of caregiving make it difficult to sustain supportive relationships with family and friends. Although both of these situations involve high family caregiving demands, they differ in their expected outcome. Mothers of premature infants anticipate decreased caregiving demands over time, whereas women caring for an older adult with cognitive impairment expect increased demands as the older adult's condition deteriorates.

Most previous research with caregivers of older persons who are cognitively impaired has focused on the problems and negative health outcomes associated with caregiving (e.g., Canadian Study of Health and Aging Working Group, 1994; McDowell, 1994; Miller & McFall, 1992; Vitaliano, Russo, Young, Teri, & Maiuro, 1991; Zarit, Todd, & Zarit, 1986). Researchers have extensively examined burden as an outcome for caregivers (e.g., Barusch & Spaid, 1991; Canadian Study of Health and Aging Working Group, 1994; Jutras & Veilleux, 1991; Miller & McFall, 1992; Novak & Guest, 1992; Spaid & Barusch, 1994; Vitaliano, Russo, Young, Teri, & Maiuro, 1991; Zarit, Todd, & Zarit, 1986). Others have addressed a more general concept of wear and tear (Walker, Acock, Bowman, & Fuzhong, 1996) or caregiver strain (Bledin, MacCarthy, Kuipers, & Woods, 1990; Morycz, 1985).

The experience of heavy demands over an extended time may negatively affect family caregivers' health (Wright, Clipp, & George, 1993). Caregivers of the cognitively impaired are at risk for negative mental and physical health outcomes. For example, depression has frequently been associated with caregiving (Fitting, Rabins, Lucas, & Eastham, 1986; Palinkas et al., 1990; Pruchno, Kleban, Michaels, & Dempsey, 1990; Williamson & Schulz, 1990).

Others have found that upsetting social interactions, reactions to behaviours of the care recipient, negative life events, and perceived stress were related to recurrent syndromal depression, although positive support mitigated negative events (Redinbaugh, MacCallum, & Kiecolt-Glaser, 1995). In contrast, negative relationships characterized by conflict are associated with depression, although the caregiver's response may vary with the type of conflict experienced. In one study, conflict directed towards the caregiver's performance was associated with depression, whereas conflict over others' interactions with the care recipient was associated with anger (Semple, 1992). A review of the literature on morbidity among dementia caregivers shows that the strength of association for caregiving and physical morbidity outcomes is weaker than the association for depression (Schulz, O'Brien, Bookwala, & Fleissner, 1995). Nevertheless, across studies, physical morbidity was associated with care recipients' problem behaviours and degree of impairment and with perceived lack of social support. Physical morbidity was measured in different ways, such as self-rated health, number of illnesses, symptomatology, health care utilization, and preventive health behaviours.

Mothers of infants born prematurely report disturbances in support from their extended family (Wereszczak, Miles, & Holditch-Davis, 1997), alienation from the child (Pederson, Bento, Chance, Evans, & Fox, 1987), and initial anxiety and depression (Gennaro, 1988). For those mothers who experience longer periods of depression, maternal depression has been related to less satisfactory development of the child (Dodge, 1990; Rutter, 1990; Webster-Stratton, 1990). Support and lack of conflict in relationships, especially with the father of the infant, are important, since continued maternal stress is related to less satisfactory development of the child (Tobey & Schraeder, 1990). Mothers who have support from their husband and a close friend experience increased satisfaction in their parenting role (Crinic, Greenberg, Ragozin, Robinson, & Basham, 1983), less resentment and despair, and a closer attachment to the infant (Hodnapp & Young, 1992). Heinicke's (1995) review of research on the transition to parenting concluded that support from a partner is an important factor in a mother's ability to function effectively as a parent. The role of support in decreasing the impact of stressful parenting demands on maternal psychological well-being was reported in a study of mothers of deaf children (Quittner, Glueckauf, & Jackson, 1990).

In summary, support from family and friends is an important resource in sustaining health while caring for a family member. Caregivers rely on multiple, interrelated sources of support that may include formal sources such as health care, income support, and employment agencies.

Issues in Gaining Access to Support

Barriers that may inhibit a woman caregiver's ability to access adequate support were identified from a series of longitudinal qualitative studies of caregivers of older persons who were cognitively impaired or infants born prematurely (Fudge, Neufeld, & Harrison, 1997; Harrison & Neufeld, 1997; Hibbard, Neufeld, & Harrison, 1996; Neufeld & Harrison, 1995). As the women described the support that they used while giving care, they also related the impediments they experienced to obtaining support.

The women were recruited through advertisement and referrals from other women participating in the study. All were English speaking from middle-income and working-class families. The mean age of the women caring for an older person with cognitive impairment (n = 20) was 58.4 years; thirteen were the wife of the care recipient. Over half had some education beyond grade 12. The number of years devoted to caregiving ranged from one to twenty (M = 7.4). Some care recipients resided with the caregiver, while others resided in a long-term care facility. The mean age of the mothers of premature infants (n = 20) was 29.8 years. Fifteen mothers had some post-secondary education. All were living with the infant's father at the beginning of the study. For thirteen mothers, the infant was their first child. Twelve infants had major health problems and seven weighed less than 1500 grams at birth.

In order to obtain in-depth information about support from the women's perspective, we primarily used qualitative research methods. The women's descriptions of support over time were obtained in a series of three or four guided interactive interviews over eighteen months. We asked the women to tell the story of how they came to be the caregiver, what support they had for their caregiving, and how they decided to use support from family and friends. These qualitative data were supplemented by a profile, based on the *Arizona Social Support Interview Schedule* (Barrera, 1981), of their social network size, composition, and sources of conflict. The research design is summarized in table 10.1.

To create a unique and holistic perspective of each caregiver's situation, a detailed summary was constructed for each woman. We then used a process of constant comparative analysis to identify key categories and the relationships among categories in the interview data (Strauss & Corbin, 1990). The interviews were analysed separately for each group of women and the analyses for the two groups were compared. The size of each caregiver's network and the number of persons with whom she had conflict were also computed.

TABLE 10.1
Research design

Sample	Purposive Women caring for an older person over 60 years of age with cognitive impairment ($n = 20$) Mothers of an infant 35 or fewer weeks gestational age at birth ($n = 20$)
Design	Descriptive
Instruments	*Arizona Social Support Interview Schedule* Interview guide focused on caregiving experiences, support for caregiving, and use of support
Data collection	3–4 guided interactive interviews over 18 months
Data analyses	
Qualitative	Constant comparative analysis of interview data
Quantitative	Descriptive analysis of characteristics of support networks (ASSIS)

The women identified numerous issues or impediments in gaining access to support. Our analysis showed that influence of social norms, characteristics of the women's social networks, and their evaluation of concerns in personal relationships were obstacles to obtaining support. We also identified two strategies that the women used to gain access to support.

Influence of Social Norms

Responsibility for caring for family members is frequently labelled 'women's work' (Aronson, 1992; Thompson, 1991), and social norms and expectations reward women for being family caregivers. Consequently, many women believe that they have an obligation to provide care. In our study (Harrison & Neufeld, 1997), both mothers and women caring for cognitively impaired elders described their obligation to give care: '*I wouldn't let someone else take over what I do because I need to*' (caregiver of an older adult). '*I'm the one that had the children, so I should be the one that takes care of them*' (mother of a premature infant). In addition, women sometimes excused potential supporters, such as household help or substitute care, from providing assistance. For example, one woman explained why she would not ask her daughter to help: '*I wouldn't want to damage the relationship between her and her father because when he was in the early stages* [of decreased cognitive functioning] *she was still at home and it was difficult.*' Mothers of premature infants frequently excused their husbands from providing help with household duties, since they (mothers) accepted the primary responsibility: '*If he's lying on the couch with a very sleepy look on his face and says "don't worry, dear, I'll clean it up," I'll say "no, don't worry about it" because I know his heart is not in it.*'

Other women did not ask for support because they thought that they were responsible for the care and that their request would place a burden on family members or friends. These women described the degree of burden their request for assistance would likely impose, but they had not verified this assessment. This approach resulted in inadequate support, because many individuals who could potentially provide support were never approached. Women chose to delay seeking support until they were in a crisis or an extreme situation: '*It has to be something that I need to do really, really badly before I would ask anybody else to help because I realize that everybody is busy with their own problems and nearly everybody has somebody sick or some reason that they can't do it*' (caregiver of an older adult). When a family member or friend was excused or deemed too busy to provide support, although the women recognized that those individuals were potential sources of support, they did not want to approach them. As caregiving is viewed as women's work, women believed that they should be able to provide care. When they asked for support, it was because they were not able to provide care, not because they expected others to share in family caregiving. In this context, one consequence of acknowledging the need for support was loss of self-esteem. As one mother of a premature infant said, '*When you can't manage on your own, you feel like somehow you've failed and so if you're a failure, you hate to point this out to someone else and ask for help.*' Those women who viewed a request for support as an indication of inadequacy as caregivers chose not to ask for assistance.

When both women and their families accept the social expectation that women do the 'lion's share' of family work like caregiving and that others help, necessary family work is attributed to women's personal need to provide care, and others' contributions are seen as a sacrifice or as care for the woman (Thompson, 1991). Further, women may consider excusing other family members in order to reduce the strains on family relationships that arise when societal expectations for women's role in caregiving are challenged (Abel, 1989; Hochschild, 1989; Smith, Smith, & Toseland, 1991). In a study of sister-brother dyads, siblings' descriptions of the rationale for their division of labour in caring for elderly parents were analysed qualitatively (Matthews, 1995). Family members adopted cultural assumptions about gender-appropriate behaviour in which both brothers and sisters described the sister as the one who assumed the responsibility. Although some brothers described several contributions to care of their parents, including tasks usually performed by women, (e.g., checking on mother's safety in cooking), these contributions were downplayed. Sisters acknowledged their brothers' contributions only when they shared tasks usually assumed by women or gave assistance in the way desired by the sister (Matthews, 1995).

In summary, women accept social norms that define family caregiving as women's work and excuse other family members from providing support. Consequently, family work becomes defined as women's personal need, and cultural assumptions about gender-appropriate behaviour are reinforced.

Characteristics of the Social Network

The nature of the woman caregiver's social network, or ties to family members, friends, and others in their community (Berkman, 1984), influenced their opportunity to choose an acceptable source of support. A detailed analysis of the social network described by the women caring for an older person with cognitive impairment revealed three types of networks: diverse, semi-diverse, and kin focused (Fudge et al., 1997). Diverse networks consisted of different types of relationships, including relatives, friends, professionals, support groups, and social groups and organizations. Semi-diverse networks had fewer variations in the type and number of members, and kin-focused networks were composed primarily of family members and a small number of friends. Women in diverse networks were satisfied with support, whereas satisfaction was limited among caregivers with semi-diverse networks, and none of the women in kin-focused networks expressed satisfaction with support received.

Diversity of relationships within the network may be an asset, since different people may provide different types of support, thus expanding the range of resources available (Litwak, Jessop, & Moulton, 1994). A study of rural elderly persons in Wales revealed an association of diverse networks with higher life satisfaction and lower service demands (Wenger, 1991). Studies of social network composition have expanded to include contact with churches, support groups, or support programs. For example, frequency of contact with a church had both direct and indirect positive effects on psychological distress reported by caregivers of a relative with Alzheimer's disease (Cohen, Teresi, & Blum, 1994).

Although women had sources of support who were kin or close friends, sometimes they were not able to obtain support, particularly when family members lived in distant areas, could not offer financial help or information needed by the women, or lacked the skills to assist them with caregiving tasks. Even staff from community agencies could lack requisite skills. The need to coach others to provide assistance, particularly when staff changes were frequent, was another impediment to gaining access to support. For example, women caring for an older adult sometimes refused assistance from homemakers because of the time and effort required to show them how to provide care. Mothers of premature infants on supplemental oxygen at home reported that the energy required to train babysitters exceeded the benefits of respite from child care.

In general, the women preferred to receive support from members of their social network who had close kinship or emotional ties. Women were disappointed when these close family members and friends did not volunteer assistance. This perception is congruent with the distinction others have made between unsolicited and solicited support (Eckenrode & Wethington, 1990). Unsolicited support may have fewer implications for threat to self-esteem, since it avoids the psychological costs of acknowledging weakness. When the need for assistance is publicly known (e.g., in the case of a car accident or death), unsolicited offers of support are more likely.

Women expected that those who were close emotionally would respond positively to their request for assistance. As one woman said, '*I was really disappointed with them [friends] because I thought they were really close*' (mother of a premature infant). Alternative sources of support, however, were less acceptable because the women were not as close to them emotionally. The women's desire for support from those with whom they had a close relationship is consistent with other research on families with a premature infant (Prudhoe & Peters, 1995) and our study of women in different life transitions (Harrison, Neufeld, & Kushner 1995). Other research suggests that network members may be differentiated as core or periphery: core members are those with whom close ties remain stable over time, whereas those on the periphery are less likely to be named repeatedly as network members (Morgan, Neal, & Carder, 1997). Antonucci (1991) proposes a 'convoy' model of social relations within a lifespan developmental perspective to represent the stability of relationships and the hierarchical differentiation of close relationships from those that are less intimate.

In some situations, because of the need for specialized skills, professional sources of support are used – often referred to as the formal support network. The interrelationship between the 'informal network' of family and friends and the 'formal network' has been conceptualized in three ways: different sources contribute different types of support; informal sources are preferred, but formal sources are used when they are unavailable; and demands for support are shared in a complementary or supplementary fashion by both formal and informal networks (Chappell & Blandford, 1991; Litwak et al., 1994).

In summary, the women described several characteristics of the social network that were beneficial for securing acceptable sources of support. These features included diversity in the types of relationships within the network, geographic accessibility, possession of required skills or resources, and a close relationship.

Obstacles within Personal Relationships

In deciding whether to request support, the women carefully considered the obstacles to obtaining support from their friends and family. These obstacles included difficulty in reciprocating support that was provided, presence of non-support concurrent with support in personal relationships, and fear of personal exposure.

Inability to Sustain Reciprocity

One dimension of social support that may influence caregiving is reciprocity (i.e., the bidirectional exchange of valued resources between individuals) (Tilden & Gaylen, 1987). Women caregivers indicated that reciprocity, or give and take, was important for the continuation of relationships that were sources of support (Neufeld & Harrison, 1995). The women wanted to be able to reciprocate support provided by friends and family. In their relationship with the care recipient, the women experienced a lack of reciprocity, since the care recipient was unable to respond to their care, although mothers of infants anticipated future reciprocity as the baby matured.

The women were reluctant to seek support if they thought that they might be unable to return the favour. As one woman said of her relationships, '*I feel better when I can reciprocate the help than [when it is] a one-sided affair.*' In their view, inability to reciprocate would leave them obligated to their friend or family member and open to the censure of others. When caregivers gave support to family and friends, their contribution allowed them to accept and use support from others when the need arose: '*You're not strong all the time. And when you are strong, you can give to the one who's not as strong at that time and it bounces back and forth. Then, when you need some support, whether it's with your job or your child, you can take from the other person*' (mother of a premature infant).

The women assessed the reciprocal exchange of support within a flexible time period. Some noted that it was not always necessary to return the same kind of assistance as one received. As a mother of a pre-term infant said, '*It's not always fifty-fifty. Sometimes it's going to be ninety-ten. But you know it always comes out in the long run.*'

Mothers of premature infants used support from people whom they believed they could assist in the future, whereas caregivers of older persons accepted assistance from friends and kin whom they had helped in the past. This perspective is congruent with the concept of a 'support bank,' which recognizes that assessments of reciprocity in relationships may be long term throughout the lifespan (Antonucci & Jackson, 1990). People maintain an ongoing account of the benefits they have received and given to others.

Non-reciprocal relationships with friends and family members created an obstacle to gaining access to support. When there was an imbalance in reciprocity, the caregivers often ended the relationship. As one mother stated, '*If someone is doing all the giving and somebody is doing all the taking, there is no relationship. That's like a parasite ... a normal, well-balanced person who recognizes their own needs – they're not going to stay in a relationship like that for long*' (mother of a premature infant).

In many caregiving situations, there is reciprocity and exchange of support in the relationship with the care recipient. Research has shown that some types of support, such as companionship and positive feedback in appreciation for care received, are given by the recipient (Cohen, Gold, Shulman, & Zucchero, 1994). In relationships with adults with cognitive impairment or premature infants who are unable to communicate verbally, however, communication may be confused or ambiguous. In our studies, confused and ambiguous communication was a barrier to receiving affirmation and emotional support from the care recipient.

In the presence of this barrier to give and take, some caregivers developed a different form of reciprocity, 'constructed reciprocity' (Neufeld & Harrison, 1995). Constructed reciprocity was based on observations of non-verbal responses of the care recipient that were interpreted as meaningful interaction and feedback. An infant's smiles or the recognition perceived in an older parent's eyes were seen as positive feedback: '*I take her somewhere [and] it seems to me, she really is looking around and she knows more about what is going on than she'll let on. I guess that gives me some satisfaction. It is worth doing this*' (caregiver of an older person). '*He'd [baby] give you a real sappy look and I didn't realize that that small of a baby was that expressive as far as their emotions. That's pretty rewarding*' (mother of a premature infant). Such feedback from the care recipient gave the caregiver a sense of satisfaction and reward and fostered a closer relationship with the care recipient. This form of support, which includes affirmation, has been named 'appraisal support' (House & Kahn, 1985).

In spousal relationships, the care recipient may have been the primary source of support for the caregiver. The inability of many caregivers of older persons with cognitive impairment to perceive a meaningful response from the care recipient reduces support that was formerly available to them, at a time when they experience increased demands. Consequently, their requirement for support from other sources may increase. The quality of the prior relationship with the care recipient, particularly with the spouse, can influence the experience of caregiving (Morgan & Laing, 1991; Ory, Williams, Emr, Lebowitz, Rabins, Salloway, Sluss-Radbaugh, Wolff, & Zarit, 1985; Wright, 1993). Wright found that, in spite of their spouse's cognitive impairment, caregivers who had experienced marital happiness in the past valued the uniqueness of their spouse and their loving relationship in the present.

The infant's responsiveness provides rewarding feedback and affirmation, which is important for mothers of infants born prematurely, who often report initial anxiety and depression (Gennaro, 1988). The mothers' ability to interpret infant behavioural cues and to respond contingently is related to optimal development of the child (Barnard, 1997).

Several caregivers of older persons and mothers of premature infants who did not develop this constructed reciprocity with the care recipient expressed negative feelings of being overwhelmed, or having to make sacrifices, or that they 'can't stand much more.' For these women, absence of reciprocity in the caregiving relationship precluded access to a valued source of affirmation support.

In summary, the women were reluctant to ask for support unless they could reciprocate in an acceptable time period. Their ability to reciprocate was restricted by limitations on their time and resources as a consequence of the demands of caregiving. Non-reciprocal relationships with friends were often ended, while non-reciprocal relationships with family were viewed more tolerantly. The inability to reciprocate support may leave the caregiver with feelings of indebtedness and discomfort (Greenberg & Westcott, 1983) that inhibit requests for aid. Some caregivers, however, were able to develop a constructed reciprocity with the care recipient, which provided affirmation.

Presence of Non-support in Relationships

In addition to assessing reciprocity in seeking support, women weighed the potential for experiencing non-supportive interactions in the process of receiving support. The women described many types of 'non-support' in interactions with members of their social network. Consistent with the findings of others (Barrera, 1981; Brody, Hoffman, Kleban, & Schoonover, 1989), support and non-support often co-existed in these relationships. Non-support refers to unhelpful comments or actions, indifference, or conflict with someone who is supportive in other ways. To illustrate, one mother described the unhelpful and upsetting actions of her mother-in-law, who was willing to babysit her premature infant, but while doing so, cut the infant's hair without prior discussion. She decided not to ask for further assistance from her mother-in-law.

In another study (Fudge et al., 1997), a caregiver for a person with cognitive impairment described indifference by her family: '*And to me, I've got non-support in what I've asked for. I feel that they are not involved at all.*' Other examples of negative interactions experienced by women caring for a cognitively impaired older adult (Fudge et al., 1997) included dissatisfaction with support given to either the care recipient or the caregiver, and disagreements with family members over the care provided to the care recipient. For example, a granddaughter who cared for her grandfather disliked the way her grandmother was treating her grandfather. '*She [her grandmother] could afford to give him any lifestyle he wanted, [but she did not] ... and made me really angry.*' Siblings sometimes disagreed about decisions to admit the care recipient to long-term care. '*I know that my brother was very upset at me putting her in [the long-term care facility].*' Negative interactions among siblings in relation to care of a parent have been well documented (Brody et al., 1989; Cicirelli, Coward, & Dwyer, 1992; Matthews, 1995; Merrill, 1996; Suitor & Pillemer, 1993). Sisters usually assume the primary responsibility for parent care, and daughters who were the primary caregiver were most distressed or rewarded by actions of siblings (Brody et al., 1989).

The non-supportive interactions in our study were more commonly described by the women in kin-focused networks that primarily comprised family members. In another study (Hibbard et al., 1996), we found that women, in comparison with men, reported a significantly larger number of people with whom they had conflict and more family sources of conflict.

Other researchers also have found conflict and non-support in the relationships of women caring for an older person with cognitive impairment. For example, Semple (1992) described three dimensions of conflict: disagreements over the level or type of care required, over family members' ways of interacting with the care recipient, and over their assessment of the care provided by the caregiver. In other research, another source of conflict was the denial of siblings' requests for assistance (Merrill, 1996). Most caregivers whose requests were denied experienced conflict as they continued to seek assistance from their siblings.

Fear of Exposure

Another barrier that women in both groups experienced in requesting support was the fear of exposure if a request was made. These women were reluctant to provide explanations to others about why support was needed. '*When you're asking for it [support] a lot of times you've got to tell them the reason why and go into great depths about it. You can't just say, would you do this for me*' (mother of a premature infant). In providing explanations, the women experienced a loss of privacy that made them more vulnerable if their request for support was refused.

Women in both groups of caregivers described fear of exposure as another obstacle to requesting support. We know of no other studies that address this issue specifically. It is noteworthy, however, that the fear of others' reactions to their situation prevented cancer patients from seeking support (Dunkel-Schetter, 1984). Similarly, hemophiliacs with HIV/AIDS described fears of loss of confidentiality if they disclosed their condition, which prevented many from revealing their condition to anyone other than immediate family (Stewart, Hart, & Mann, 1995).

Strategies for Obtaining Support

Because of the complex and challenging issues associated with requests for support, the women caregivers expressed a preference for support that was volunteered. When support was offered, the women were able to avoid many barriers associated with asking for assistance. Support was offered infrequently, however, or was offered at times when the women did not need it.

The women described two strategies to avoid some challenges associated with requesting support: use of non-verbal behavioural cues to indicate a need for support and maintenance of relationships in which support was offered without a request (Harrison & Neufeld, 1997). An example is given for each of these strategies.

One mother of a premature infant used behavioural cues to communicate her need for support without having to ask for it. Her frequent reliance on non-verbal cues during the period of the infant's hospitalization, however, became limited once her child was home. '*I'm not giving them signs that I need help. Before they could hear it in my voice, they could see it in my face when Amy was in hospital. Now Amy is six months old and I don't let it show ... because I don't want to get hurt.*' The mother perceived that explicit forms of expressing support needs would result in personal pain if other friends and family members believed that she should be able to manage without support.

The strategy of maintaining relationships with individuals who would offer support without a request was described less frequently by the caregivers. One woman caring for her husband who was cognitively impaired described this approach. '*I've learned if someone phones on a cold day and says "do you need something at the store?" whether I need bread or not, I always say, "Oh, I'd sure like a loaf of brown bread." Whereas, perhaps two or three years ago, I would have said, "Oh, I'm fine. I don't need anything, thank you." But now if somebody does offer a specific thing I try really hard to say, "yes I need it." Because then I think they might do it again.*' This woman had learned to maintain relationships in which support was offered as insurance for times when she would need help. Her approach is acknowledged by others (Eckenrode & Wethington, 1990), who suggest that maintenance of relationships that have inherent expectations for support provides an established source of unsolicited offers of assistance.

The support mobilization process includes both unsolicited offers of support and help-seeking components (Eckenrode & Wethington, 1990). The type of relationship between caregivers and others may influence the way that support is mobilized, since individuals in intimate relationships are more likely to offer support without requests for assistance, whereas professional support will almost always be preceded by specific requests. Intimate relationships may also facilitate detection of 'distress signals' that lead to support without verbal requests, as described by the mother who relied on behavioural cues. The quality of social skills may influence ability to request support effectively. Among caregivers of older persons with dementia, Robinson (1990) found a significant positive relationship between better social skills and available support.

Mobilization of support may also reflect different perspectives on relationships: some individuals hold a 'communal' or collective perspective, which is based on the needs and concerns of the other, whereas others are more 'individualistic' or 'exchange' oriented and focus on the comparability of specific benefits available to each individual in the relationship (Clark, Powell, & Mills, 1986; Jones & Vaughan, 1990; Williamson & Schulz, 1990). A communal perspective is more likely to be associated with offers of assistance and acceptance of unsolicited help, whereas an exchange perspective is more likely to involve concern with whether assistance can be repaid, perhaps relying more extensively on professional sources of assistance (Pyke & Bengston, 1996).

Key Findings

Barriers to gaining access to support

Influence of social norms

- Women view themselves as the expected caregiver.
- Women excuse others from providing support.

Characteristics of the social network

- Network members are absent, unavailable, or lack resources.
- Support is not available from close personal ties, the preferred source.

Personal costs in requesting support

- Women need to reciprocate support, but are not able to do so.
- Women experience non-supportive interactions such as conflict and indifference.
- Women lose privacy and fear exposure.

Strategies for Obtaining Support

- Women use non-verbal distress cues.
- Women maintain relationships in which support is volunteered.

Implications for Programs and Policy

The issues women caregivers experience in gaining access to support encompass several levels of social relations: social norms that influence expectations for women's caregiving work, the characteristics of caregivers' social networks, and the obstacles present within interpersonal relationships. Strategies to address these issues are also required at multiple levels.

Public policy changes are needed to achieve shared responsibility for care and challenge the social norms that sustain expectations of caregiving as women's work (Bridges & Lyman, 1993). To reduce the economic burden of caregiving, change is required both in taxation policies to acknowledge the economic demand of all types of family caregiving and in workplace policies to accommodate pension contributions for caregivers who work part time or have interrupted careers (National Forum on Health, 1996). Flexible work hours and access to information and support services can reduce the stress experienced by employed caregivers and improve morale. High-quality, low-cost, accessible care for children and older adults can provide ongoing complementary assistance as well as respite (Canadian Aging Research Network, 1993; Gottlieb, 1996). These policy initiatives are particularly important for women who are dual caregivers, with responsibility for care of both children and parents or for care of more than one adult relative (Canadian Aging Research Network, 1993).

Much of the public debate about recent health system restructuring has been focused narrowly on costs of government funding for insured health services. Little attention has been given to the hidden costs for women and families who have assumed demanding responsibilities for care of relatives in the home setting. Some critics have questioned whether the espoused shift to community health care is a euphemism for a shift to family responsibility (Rosenthal, 1994; Tarman, 1994). Sole-parent families, in which the caregiver is responsible for children and parents as well as for financial support, are particularly vulnerable. The long-term health and social consequences of these increased demands on both caregivers and ill family members are unknown (Strawbridge & Wallhagen, 1991; Tarman, 1994), but they need to be documented and addressed in public discussion.

Public discussion of mechanisms to facilitate shared responsibility can generate support for new arrangements. As indicated in our studies, women often accept caregiving responsibilities and excuse other family members from assisting. Better public understanding of the scope and demands of caregiving could foster family sharing of responsibility, support for the primary caregiver, and support for appropriate community programs. For example, respite programs can provide temporary relief for the primary caregiver and an opportunity to fulfil other commitments. Existing respite and adult day care programs are not utilized extensively (Kosloski & Montgomery, 1993). Variations in the requirements of different groups of caregivers, the characteristics valued by caregivers, and convenience to the caregiver (Strang & Neufeld, 1992) should be assessed in development of respite and adult day care programs.

Women's existing social networks are a key resource and an important focus for support interventions. In view of the women's descriptions of the criteria for acceptable sources of support, it is important to recognize that the presence of individuals within a caregiver's social network is not necessarily an indication of support that the women may utilize. For example, close emotional ties may be a prerequisite for accepting support, or negative interactions may eliminate an individual as a source of support. Important characteristics of social networks for assessment include type of social network (i.e., diverse, semi-diverse, kin focused) and size of the available and utilized social network. Assessment of these characteristics can identify caregivers who may be at risk for inadequate support or vulnerable to the impact of negative interactions. When caregivers describe an extensive available network but a limited utilized network, it may be possible to assist them to gain access to additional sources of support that they currently do not use. Intervention can assist caregivers to acquire specific skills useful in mobilizing support, such as assertiveness, social skills (e.g., initiating conversation, speaking fluently on the telephone, understanding non-verbal communication), and network building (Robinson, 1988). Thus, professional intervention can help caregivers to gain access to their social networks in different ways, to expand their networks if necessary, and to develop social skills to foster a more effective network (Clipp & George, 1990; George & Gwyther, 1986; Gwyther, 1992; Wilson, 1989). Education of the public and the caregivers' family and friends about the importance of volunteering assistance to family caregivers may also foster increased access to support by reducing the personal costs associated with requests for help.

Although referrals to community resources, such as day care programs, respite programs, or sitter programs, can provide additional sources of assistance for caregivers with small available networks, there is a need for improved linkages between the formal and informal care systems (LeNavenec & Vonhof, 1996). In most communities, a directory of local agencies and programs provides information about community services. Health professionals can share with the family caregiver the perspectives of other caregivers in similar situations. Support groups that enable caregivers to interact with others whose experience is similar can also be helpful (Boukydis, & Moses, 1995; Roman, Lindsay, Boger, DeWys, Beaumont, Jones, & Haas, 1995; Toseland, 1990), but some participants may benefit more than others (Cuijpers, Hosman, & Munnichs, 1992). A range of self-help or peer-led support groups has been developed, and the question of the comparative contributions of peers and professionals has been explored (Lapierre, Perreault, & Goulet, 1995; Stewart, 1990; Toseland, 1990). Evidence indicates that the contribution of professionals and peers may differ and that peers may make a unique contribution that overcomes some limitations of professional intervention. A shared leadership role for peers and professionals may be one way to facilitate access to the strengths of both peers and professionals (Stewart, Banks, Crossman, & Poel, 1994).

The obstacles to obtaining support within the women's personal relationships included inability to sustain reciprocity, the presence of non-support, and fear of exposure of their situation. Family caregivers can be assisted to address these interpersonal issues through individual counselling or specific education and support group interventions. For example, encouraging caregivers to employ a long-term perspective in assessing reciprocity can expand the number of perceived reciprocal relationships. Some women may reframe their perspective of reciprocity by recognizing that assistance need not necessarily be returned in kind. In addition, professionals may assist women to recognize and respond to non-verbal cues of care recipients with limited or impaired non-verbal abilities. By role modelling recognition of these cues and subsequent responses to the care recipient, professionals may facilitate the caregivers' establishing constructed reciprocity with care recipients. Intervention programs that teach mothers how to recognize and interpret non-verbal cues from their infant, such as the 'Keys to Caregiving Program' (developed by Kathryn Barnard and colleagues at the University of Washington, Seattle), could be a model for similar types of intervention for women caring for dependent adults who are unable to communicate verbally. In support groups, the experiential knowledge of others in similar situations may encourage new perspectives on reciprocity. Further research is needed to identify effective support mobilization strategies that could be shared with other women and men in caregiving situations. As this research was limited to Caucasian women of primarily middle-income and working-class families, it is particularly important that future research include low-income women, women of different cultural backgrounds, and men.

Program and Policy Implications

Public

- Increased public discussion of issues for family caregivers

Workplace

- Policies to support pension contributions if work is interrupted by caregiving
- Flexible work hours
- Support services, such as day care, in the workplace
- Access to information on community resources

Community agencies

- Identification of family caregivers with inadequate support networks
- Programs that increase caregivers' skills for maintaining or creating support networks
- Support services such as day care, respite, peer support groups
- Individual counselling or education to manage non-supportive interactions or maintain reciprocal relationships
- Programs that assist caregivers to maintain or establish reciprocity with care recipients

Note

Portions of this chapter were published in Neufeld & Harrison (1995) and Harrison & Neufeld (1997).

References

Abel, E.K. (1989). The ambiguities of social support: Adult daughters caring for frail elderly parents. *Journal of Aging Studies, 3*, 211–230.

Aneshensel, C., Frerichs, R., & Clark, V. (1981). Family roles and sex differences in depression. *Journal of Health and Social Behaviour 22*, 379–393.

Antonucci, T. (1991). Attachment, social support and coping with negative life events in mature adulthood. In E.M. Cummings, A. Greene, & K. Karraker (Eds), *Life-span developmental psychology: Perspectives on stress and coping* (261–176). Hillsdale, CA: Lawrence Erlbaum.

Antonucci, T., & Jackson, J. (1990). The role of reciprocity in social support. In B.R. Sarason, I.G. Sarason, & G.R. Pierce, (Eds), *Social support: An interactional view* (173–198). New York: Wiley.

Aronson, J. (1992). Women's sense of responsibility for the care of old people: But who else is going to do it? *Gender and Society, 6*, 8–29.

Baines, C., Evans, P., & Neysmith, S. (1993). Caring: Its impact on the lives of women. In C. Baines, P. Evans & S. Neysmith (Eds), *Women's caring: Feminist perspectives on social welfare* (11–33). Toronto: McClelland & Stewart.

Barnard, K.E. (1997). Influencing parent-child interactions for children at risk. In M.J. Guralnick (Ed.), *The effectiveness of early intervention* (249–268). Baltimore: Paul Brooks.

Barr, J.K., Johnson, K.W., Warshaw, L.J. (1992). Supporting the elderly: Workplace programs for employed caregivers. *Millbank Quarterly, 70*(3), 509–533.

Barrera, M. (1981). Social support in the adjustment of pregnant adolescents. In B. Gottlieb (Ed.), *Social networks and social support* (69–96). Beverly Hills, CA: Sage.

Barusch, A., & Spaid, W. (1991). Reducing caregiver burden through short-term training: Evaluation from a caregiver support project. *Journal of Gerontological Social Work, 17*(1/2), 7–33.

Berkman, L. (1984). Assessing the physical health effects of social networks and social support. *Annual Review of Public Health, 5*, 413–432.

Bledin, K., MacCarthy, L., Kuipers, L., & Woods, R. (1990). Daughters of people with dementia: Expressed emotion, strain and coping. *British Journal of Psychiatry, 157*, 221–227.

Boukydis, C.F.Z., & Moses, L. (1995). Establishing and maintaining a parenting network for parents of premature/high risk infants. *Infants and Young Children, 7*(4), 77–87.

Bridges, J.M., & Lyman, M.J. (1993). Informal carers: A marxist analysis of social, political, and economic forces underpinning the role. *Advances in Nursing Science, 15*(3), 33–48.

Brody, E., Hoffman, C., Kleban, M., & Schoonover, C. (1989). Caregiving daughters and their local siblings: Perceptions, strains, and interactions. *Gerontologist, 29*(4), 529–538.

Canadian Aging Research Network (1993). *Work and family: The survey*. Guelph, ON: Work and Elder Care Research Group.

Canadian Study of Health and Aging Working Group (1994). Canadian study of health and aging: Study methods and prevalence of dementia. *Canadian Medical Association Journal, 150*(6), 899–913.

Chappell, N., & Blandford, A. (1991). Informal and formal care: Exploring the complementarity. *Ageing and Society, 11*(3), 299–317.

Cicirelli, V., Coward, R., & Dwyer, J. (1992). Siblings as caregivers for impaired elders. *Research on Aging, 14*(3), 331–350.

Clark, M.S., Powell, M.C., & Mills, J. (1986). Keeping track of needs in communal and exchange relationships. *Journal of Personality and Social Psychology, 51*(2), 333–338.

Clipp, E.C., & George, L.K. (1990). Caregiver needs and patterns of social support. *Journal of Gerontology, 45*(3), 102–111.

Cohen, C., Gold, D., Shulman, K., & Zucchero, C. (1994). Positive aspects in caregiving: An overlooked variable in research. *Canadian Journal of Aging, 13*(3), 378–391.

Cohen, C., Teresi, J., & Blum, C. (1994). The role of caregiver social networks in Alzheimer's disease. *Social Science and Medicine, 38*(11), 1483–1490.

Crinic, K.A., Greenberg, M.T., Ragozin, A.S., Robinson, N.M., & Basham, R. (1983). Effects of stress and social support on mothers and premature and full-term infants. *Child Development, 54*, 209–217.

Cuijpers, P., Hosman, C., & Munnichs, J. (1992). Carer support groups: Change mechanisms and preventive effects. In B.M.L. Miesen & G.M.M. Jones (Eds), *Care-giving in dementia: Research and applications*, Vol. 2 (233–248). New York: Routledge.

Deimling, G.T. & Bass, D.M. (1986). Symptoms of mental impairment among elderly adults and their effects on family caregivers. *Journal of Gerontology, 41*, 778–784.

Dodge, K. A. (1990). Developmental psychopathology in children of depressed mothers. *Developmental Psychology, 26*, 3–6.

Dowler, J., Jordon-Simpson, D., & Adams, O. (1992). *Health Reports, 4*(2), 125–136.

Dunkel-Schetter, C. (1984). Social support and cancer: Findings based on patient interviews and their implications. *Journal of Social Issues, 40*(4), 77–98.

Eckenrode, J., & Wethington, E. (1990). The process and outcome of mobilizing social support. In S. Duck (Ed.), *Personal relationships and social support* (83–103). Newbury Park, NY: Sage.

Fitting, M., Rabins, P., Lucas, M. L., Eastham, J. (1986). Caregivers for dementia patients: A comparison of husbands and wives. *Gerontologist, 26*(3), 248–252.

Fudge, H., Neufeld, A., & Harrison, M.J. (1997). Social networks of women caregivers. *Public Health Nursing, 14*(1), 20–27.

Gennaro, S. (1988). Postpartal anxiety and depression in mothers of term and preterm infants. *Nursing Research, 37*(2), 82–85.

George, L.K., & Gwyther, L.P. (1986). Caregiver well-being: A multidimensional examination of family caregivers of demented adults. *Gerontologist, 6*, 253–259.

Goldberg, S., & DiVitto, B. (1995). Parenting children born preterm. In M. Bornstein (Ed.), *Handbook of parenting.* Vol. 1 *Children and parenting* (209–231). Mahwah, NJ: Lawrence Erlbaum.

Gottlieb, B. (1996). Summary of protecting and promoting the well-being of family caregivers. In National Forum on Health (Ed.), *What determines health?* (115–118). Ottawa: National Forum on Health.

Greenberg, M.S., & Westcott, D.R. (1983). Indebtedness as a mediator of reactions to aid. In J.D. Fisher, A. Nadler, & B.M. DePaulo (Eds), *New directions in helping.* Vol. 1, *Recipient reactions to aid* (85–111). New York: Academic Press.

Gwyther, L. (1992). Research on gender and family caregiving: Implications for clinical practice. In J.W. Dwyer & R.T. Coward (Eds), *Gender, families and elder care* (202–218). Thousand Oaks, CA: Sage.

Harrison, M.J., & Neufeld, A. (1997). Barriers to mobilizing support while caregiving. *Health Care for Women International, 18*, 591–602.

Harrison, M. J., Neufeld, A., & Kushner, K. (1995). Women in transition: Access and barriers to social support. *Journal of Advanced Nursing, 21*, 858–864.

Heinicke, C.H. (1995). Determinants of the transition to parenting. In M. Bornstein (Ed.), *Handbook of parenting.* Vol. 1, *Children and parenting* (277–303). Mahwah, NJ: Lawrence Erlbaum.

Hibbard, J., Neufeld, A., & Harrison, M.J. (1996). Gender differences in the support networks of caregivers. *Journal of Gerontological Nursing, 22*(9), 15–23.

Hodnapp, R.M., & Young, K.T. (1992). Maternal emotional reactions to the premature infant in the family context. *Canadian Journal of Behavioural Science, 24*, 29–40.

Hochschild, A. (1989). *The second shift.* New York: Avon.

House, J.S., & Kahn, R.L. (1985). Measures and concepts of social support. In S. Cohen & L. Syme (Eds), *Social support and health* (83–108). Orlando, FL: Academic Press.

Johansson, S., & Ahlfeldt, J. (1996). Stress experienced by informal caregivers. *Scandinavian Journal of Social Welfare, 5*, 83–96.

Jones, D.C., & Vaughn, K. (1990). Close friendships among senior adults. *Psychology and Aging, 5*(3), 451–457.

Jutras, S., & Veilleux, F.(1991). Informal caregiving: Correlates of perceived burden. *Canadian Journal of Aging, 10*(1), 40–55.

Kosloski, K., & Montgomery, R. (1993). Perceptions of respite services as predictors of utilization. *Research on Aging, 15*(4), 399–413.

Kramer, B., & Kipnis, S. (1995). Eldercare and work-role conflict: Toward an understanding of gender differences in caregiver burden. *Gerontologist, 35*(3), 340–348.

Lapierre, J., Perreault, M., & Goulet, C. (1995). Prenatal peer counseling: An answer to the peristent difficulties with prenatal care for low-income women. *Public Health Nursing, 12*(1), 53–60.

Le Navenec, C.L., & Vonhof, T. (1996). *One day at a time: How families manage the experience of dementia.* Westport, CT: Auburn House.

Litwak, E., Jessop, J., & Moulton, H. (1994). Optimal use of formal and informal systems over the life course. In E. Kahana, D. Biegel, & M. Wykle (Eds), *Family caregiving across the lifespan* (96–130). Thousand Oaks, CA: Sage.

McDowell, I. (1994). Caregiving patterns. *Chronic Diseases in Canada, 15*(2), S11–S12.

McIntosh, J. (1993). Postpartum depression: Women's help seeking behaviours and perceptions. *Journal of Advanced Nursing, 18*, 178–184.

Matthews, S. (1995). Gender and the division of filial responsibility between lone sisters and their brothers. *Journal of Gerontology: Social Sciences, 50B*(5), S312–S320.

Merrill, D. (1996). Conflict and cooperation among adult siblings during the transition to role of filial caregiver. *Journal of Social and Personal Relationships, 13*(3), 399–413.

Miller, B., & McFall, S. (1992). Caregiver burden and the continuum of care. *Research on Aging, 14*(3), 376–398.

Morgan, D., & Laing, G. (1991). The diagnosis of Alzheimer's disease: Spouse's perspective. *Qualitative Health Research, 1*, 370–387.

Morgan, D.L., Neal, M.B., & Carder, P. (1997). The stability of core and peripheral networks over time. *Social Networks, 19*, 9–25.

Morycz, R. (1985). Caregiving strain and the desire to institutionalize family members with Alzheimer's disease. *Research on Aging, 7*(3), 326–361.

Mui, A. (1995). Multidimensional predictors of caregivers strain among older persons caring for frail spouses. *Journal of Marriage and the Family, 57*, 733–740.

National Forum on Health (1996). *Canada health action: Building on the legacy.* Vol. II, *Synthesis reports and issues papers*. Ottawa: Minister of Public Works and Government Services.

Neufeld, A., & Harrison, M.J. (1995). Reciprocity and social support in caregivers' relationships: Variations and consequences. *Qualitative Health Research, 5*, 349–366.

Novak, M., & Guest, C. (1992). A comparison of impact of institutionalization on spouse and nonspouse caregivers. *Journal of Applied Gerontology, 11*(4), 379–394.

Ory, M.G., Williams, T.F., Emr, M., Lebowitz, B., Rabins, P., Salloway, J., Sluss-Radbaugh, T., Wolff, E., & Zarit, S. (1985). Families, informal supports, and Alzheimer's disease. *Research on Aging, 7*, 623–644.

Palinkas, L.A., Wingard, D.L. & Barrett-Connor, E. (1990). The biocultural context of social networks and depression among the elderly. *Social Science and Medicine, 30*, 441–447.

Pearlin, L., Mullan, J., Semple, S., & Skaff, M. (1990). Caregiving and the stress process: An overview of concepts and their measures. *Gerontologist, 30*(5), 583–594.

Pederson, D.R., Bento, S., Chance, G.W., Evans, B., & Fox, A.M. (1987). Maternal emotional responses to preterm birth. *American Journal of Orthopsychiatry, 57*(1), 15–21.

Pruchno, R.A., Kleban, M.H., Michaels, J.E., & Dempsey, N.P. (1990). Mental and physical health of caregiving spouses: Development of a causal model. *Journal of Gerontology: Psychological Sciences, 45*(5), 192–199.

Prudhoe, C.M., & Peters, D.L. (1995). Social support of parents and grandparents in the neonatal intensive care unit. *Pediatric Nursing, 21*, 140–146.

Pyke, K., & Bengston, V. (1996). Caring more or less: Individualistic and collectivist systems of family eldercare. *Journal of Marriage and the Family, 58*, 379–392.

Quittner, A.L., Glueckauf, R.L., & Jackson, D.N. (1990). Chronic stress: Moderating versus mediating effects of social support. *Journal of Personality and Social Psychology, 59*, 1266–1278.

Redinbaugh, E., MacCallum, R., & Kiecolt-Glaser, J. (1995). Recurrent syndromal depression in caregivers. *Psychology and Aging, 10*(3), 358–368.

Robinson, K.M. (1988). A social skills training program for adult caregivers. *Advanced Nursing Science, 10*(2), 59–72.

Robinson, K.M. (1990). The relationships between social skills, social support, self-esteem and burden in adult caregivers. *Journal of Advanced Nursing, 15*, 788–795.

Roman, L.A., Lindsay, J.K., Boger, R.P, DeWys, M., Beaumont, E.J., Jones, A.S., & Haas, B. (1995). Parent-to-parent support initiated in the neonatal intensive care unit. *Research in Nursing and Health, 18*, 385–394.

Rosenthal, C. (1994). Long-term care reform and 'family' care: A worrisome combination. *Canadian Journal on Aging, 13*(4), 419–422.

Ross, C., & Mirowsky, J. (1988). Child care and emotional adjustment to wife's employment. *Journal of Health and Social Behaviour, 29*, 127–138.

Rutter, M. (1990). Commentary: Some focus and process considerations regarding effects of parental depression on children. *Developmental Psychology, 26*, 60–67.

Schulz, R., O'Brien, A., Bookwala, J., & Fleissner, K. (1995). Psychiatric and physical morbidity effects of dementia caregiving: Prevalence, correlates, and causes. *Gerontologist, 35*(6), 771–791.

Scott, J., & Alwin, D. (1989). Gender differences in parental strain: Parental role or gender role? *Journal of Family Issues, 10*(4), 482–503.

Semple, S. (1992). Conflict in Alzheimer's caregiving families: Its dimensions and consequences. *Gerontologist, 32*(5), 648–655.

Smith, G.C., Smith, M.F., & Toseland, R.W. (1991). Problems identified by family caregivers in counselling. *Gerontologist, 31*, 15–22.

Spaid, W., & Barusch, A. (1994). Emotional closeness and caregiver burden in the marital relationship. *Journal of Gerontological Social Work, 21*(3/4), 197–211.

Statistics Canada (1997). Who cares? Caregiving in the 1990's. *Daily*, 19 August, 5–6, Ottawa.

Stewart, M.J. (1990). Professional interface with mutual-aid self-help groups. *Social Science and Medicine, 31*(10), 1143–1158.

Stewart, M.J., Banks, S., Crossman, D., & Poel, D. (1994). Partnerships between health professionals and self-help groups: Meanings and mechanisms. *Prevention and Human Services, 11*(2), 199–240.

Stewart, M.J., Hart, G., & Mann, K. (1995). Living with hemophilia and HIV/AIDS: Support and coping. *Journal of Advanced Nursing, 22*(6), 1101–1111.

Stoller, E.P. (1993). Gender and the organization of lay health care: A socialist-feminist perspective. *Journal of Aging Studies, 7*(2), 151–170.

Strang, V., & Neufeld, A. (1992). Issues in the evaluation of small-scale adult day care programs. *International Journal of Nursing Studies, 29*(3), 261–273.

Strauss, A., & Corbin, J. (1990). *Basics of qualitative research.* Newbury Park, NY: Sage.

Strawbridge, W., & Wallhagen, M. (1991). Impact of family conflict on adult child caregivers. *Gerontologist, 31*(6), 770–777.

Suitor, J., & Pillemer, K. (1993). Support and interpersonal stress in the social networks of married daughters caring for parents with Dementia. *Journal of Gerontology: Social Sciences, 48*(1), S1–S8.

Tarman, V. (1994). Age and gender: The missing analysis in long term care reform. In B. Bolaria & R. Bolaria (Eds), *Women, medicine and health* (366–373). Halifax, NS: Fernwood.

Thompson, L. (1991). Family work: Women's sense of fairness. *Journal of Family Issues, 12*, 181–196.

Tilden, V.P., & Gaylen, R.D. (1987). Cost and conflict: The darker side of social support. *Western Journal of Nursing Research, 9*, 9–18.

Tobey, G.Y., & Schraeder, B.D. (1990). Impact of caretaker stress on behavioural adjustment in very low birthweight school children. *Nursing Research, 39*, 84–89.

Toseland, R. (1990). Long-term effectiveness of peer-led and professionally led support groups for caregivers. *Social Service Review, 62*(2), 308–327.

Vitaliano, P., Russo, J., Young, H., Teri, L., & Maiuro, R. (1991). Predictors of burden in spouse caregivers of individuals with Alzheimer's disease. *Psychology and Aging, 6*(3), 392–402.

Walker, A., Acock, A., Bowman, S., & Fuzhong, L. (1996). Amount of care given and caregiving satisfaction: A latent growth curve analysis. *Journal of Gerontology, 51B*(3), 130–142.

Webster-Stratton, C. (1990). Support systems for spouses of chronically ill persons in rural areas. *Family and Community Health, 16*(1), 46–54.

Wenger, G.C. (1991). A network typology: From theory to practice. *Journal of Aging Studies, 5*(2), 147–162.

Wereszczak, J., Miles, M.S., & Holditch-Davis, D. (1997). Maternal recall of the neonatal intensive care unit. *Neonatal Network, 16*(4), 33–40.

Williamson, G., & Schulz, R. (1990). Relationship orientation, quality of prior relationship, and distress among caregivers of Alzheimer's patients. *Gerontologist, 5*, 502–509.

Wilson, H.S. (1989). Family caregiving for a relative with Alzheimer's dementia: Coping with negative choices. *Nursing Research, 38*(2), 94–98.

Wright, L.K., Clipp, E.C., & George, L. (1993). Consequences of caregiver stress. *Medicine, Exercise, Nutrition and Health, 2*, 181–195.

Wright, L.K. (1993). *Alzheimer's disease and marriage.* Newbury Park, NY: Sage.

Zarit, S., Todd, P., & Zarit, J. (1986). Subjective burden of husbands and wives as caregivers. *Gerontologist, 26*(3), 260–266.

11

Common Themes and Lessons Learned

Miriam J. Stewart

Abstract. Common themes emerging from the assessment and intervention studies in the Social Support Research Program generated conceptual insights. Themes from assessment studies reveal the significance of support from peers and professionals, diminishing support in chronic stressful situations, negative interactions and deficient support, relationship-focused coping, and the influence of support on health behaviour and health status. Themes from intervention studies include the elements of successful peer-professional partnerships, the need for different interventions for people in different circumstances, and the impact of support interventions on support need and satisfaction and on health outcomes. Furthermore, support provided to family caregivers had an impact on the use of health services by care recipients with chronic conditions. The intervention projects highlighted the importance of participatory approaches and interdisciplinary collaboration.

There is a continuing need for longitudinal research, theory-testing research, qualitative approaches that document processes of interpersonal interactions and support interventions, and careful selection of situation-specific health outcomes. Practical lessons emerging from intervention studies point to the importance of (1) guides, training, monitoring, and reinforcement for peer and professional intervenors; (2) similarity of peers and participants; and (3) an intervention dose of sufficient duration. Policy directions – reflected in the renewed interest in health promotion, population health strategies, and the National Forum on Health's recommendations – reinforce the role of social support as a social determinant of health, a health promotion mechanism, and a protective factor in resilience.

Conceptual Insights

Sources of Support

Consistent with other research on support providers (e.g., Dakof & Taylor, 1990), the studies in the research program reported in this book revealed that most support is provided by family members and within close relationships. Mothers of children with chronic conditions and persons with ischaemic heart disease (IHD) indicated that most support came from spouse/partners, family members, and friends. Children with chronic conditions identified parents and family members as their key supporters. Sources of support for professionals (formal caregivers) were similar to those for lay caregivers with one exception – work associates were named frequently by Canadian nurses in HIV/AIDS care.

[Two other research programs, focused on persons with chronic conditions (chapter 9) and family caregivers (chapter 10), reinforce and supplement the studies in our social support research program. Salient findings are integrated throughout this chapter.]

Women caregivers in diverse networks were more satisfied with support than women in kin-focused networks; diversity of relationships expanded the range of their available resources. Furthermore, these family caregivers of premature infants and cognitively impaired elders preferred support from those with whom they had close personal ties (chapter 10). Similarly, desire for intimate relationships, such as that with a spouse/partner, was paramount among persons with chronic conditions (chapter 9).

The support provided by or desired from professionals and peers emerged as a common theme in several studies. Young children, observed during venipuncture, received support from nurses. Although some mothers of children with chronic conditions referred to health professionals as support providers, others reported inadequate support from professionals. In this context, health professionals were identified infrequently as sources of support in the studies of persons with cardiac conditions and their family caregivers, stroke survivors and their family caregivers, and hemophiliacs with HIV/AIDS and their family caregivers. Women caregivers of infants and seniors required support from professionals, primarily when family and friends were geographically dispersed or lacked requisite resources to provide assistance (chapter 10). They preferred support from core (i.e., close relationship) rather than peripheral (e.g., professional) members of the network or convoy (Antonucci, 1991). In contrast, relationships with health professionals had an important impact on self-appraisal, according to accounts of people with chronic conditions (chapter 9).

These studies revealed that it is important for peer supporters to be as similar as possible to support recipients. Thus, persons with hemophilia and AIDS desired support from identical peers – hemophiliacs with AIDS, *not* persons with AIDS contracted from other causes – and mothers of young children with cystic fibrosis wanted support groups composed of other mothers of young children with cystic fibrosis, *not* mothers of children of any age with any chronic illness. In the peer visitor intervention, family caregivers of stroke survivors contended that similarity of peers, in terms of relationship with survivor, age, personality, and lifestyle, contributed to the success of the intervention.

Functions of Support

Mothers of children with chronic conditions reported informational support from health professionals; however, they wanted, but did not typically receive, feedback (affirmational support), reassurance, and understanding (emotional support) from these professionals. Informational support for hemophiliacs with AIDS and their family caregivers was offered by health professionals, practical aid was provided by relatives, and spouse/partners and close family members were primary sources of emotional support. The investigation of self-help groups revealed that professionals were consultants, educators, and referral resources (i.e., informational support providers), while peers were valued for both emotional support and affirmational support. The findings from this study and the assessment study of hemophiliacs with AIDS indicated that participants preferred joint leadership of mutual aid/support groups by peers and professionals. Therefore, the telephone support groups for hemophiliacs with AIDS and their caregivers, for parents of children with chronic conditions, and for seniors with limited mobility and the face-to-face support groups for couples coping with MI were co-facilitated by a peer and a professional. In these intervention studies, professionals primarily provided informational support, while peers predominantly offered affirmational and emotional support, although blending and blurring of functions occurred.

Appraisal of Support

Direction/Reciprocity

Elderly persons with severe heart disease or stroke and their family caregivers were hampered by illness-imposed limitations from reciprocating support to others in their network. Furthermore, they reported diminished reciprocity in spousal support as the illness progressed. Family caregivers of hemophiliacs with AIDS and mothers of children with chronic conditions did not express negative feelings of burden typically associated with inequitable relationships between caregivers and care recipients. It seemed that their commitment to long-term intimate relationships with their ill relatives overshadowed their need for immediate reciprocation, reflecting lifespan reciprocity (Antonucci

& Jackson, 1990). Similarly, caregivers of seniors and infants engaged in assessment of reciprocity within the context of long-term relationships (chapter 10).

Reciprocity emerged as a key characteristic of partnership and positive relationships between health professionals and self-help group members (peers). Furthermore, the assumption that interventions that involve peers can promote reciprocity (Katz, 1993) informed the design of support group interventions. Indeed, reciprocity with peers and mutual exchange of information and support were cited as key benefits of face-to-face support groups for couples coping with MI and of telephone support groups for persons living with HIV/AIDS and for parents of children with chronic conditions.

Negotiation around equity and reciprocity (i.e., giving and receiving support) emerged as a key theme in focus groups of people with chronic illness (chap. 9). Women caring for infants and cognitively impaired elders articulated their obligation to provide care and excused others from providing support. They revealed their inability to sustain reciprocity with network members and their resultant reluctance to seek support. Moreover, they constructed reciprocity from non-verbal responses of infants and seniors (chapter 10). Women with chronic conditions (chapter 9) and caregiving responsibilities (chapter 10) emphasized support mobilization for others more than for themselves, reflecting the public perception that dealing with illness and caregiving is women's work.

Drawbacks

Negative relationships in our study of health professionals and self-help group members entailed conflict, competitiveness, dominance, territoriality, and judgmental interactions. Hemophiliacs with AIDS experienced prejudice and insensitivity from health professionals and avoidance by friends. Mothers of children with chronic conditions encountered conflictual support, involving critical or condescending interactions, predominantly from health professionals. Nevertheless, these mothers were most concerned about absent spousal support and miscarried helping. Their partners' failure to enforce children's care regimens and positive health behaviours reflected miscarried support efforts.

In the intervention studies, the men with AIDS and their family caregivers and the couples coping with cardiac conditions expressed concerns about lack of information and inadequate attention from health professionals, and caregivers of stroke survivors contended that absent support from family, friends, and health professionals was stressful.

Individuals with stroke, breast cancer, and other chronic conditions reported insensitive comments, despite other people's intent to provide support. They also suffered from others' denial of their illness and from relationship tensions (chapter 9). Similarly, mothers of premature infants and women caring for cognitively impaired older adults encountered unhelpful comments and actions, indifference, conflict with otherwise supportive people, and disagreements over care. They were disappointed when support from family and friends did not materialize because of distance or lack of resources (chapter 10).

Duration of Support

Persons with varied chronic conditions expressed concerns about relationship loss with the passage of time (chapter 9). Readmitted persons with cardiac disease experienced less support from neighbours after more than one admission to hospital. Some mothers of children with chronic conditions revealed that support provided initially by others did not endure. This finding points to the costs of providing support over time.

The timing of support is also critical. Although mothers needed support at the time of diagnosis of their child's illness, it frequently was not available when they were overwhelmed by new caregiving demands. Therefore, our follow-up telephone support intervention trial was focused on parents of children with chronic conditions under seven years of age. Furthermore, other support interventions were directed at new family caregivers of first-time stroke survivors recently discharged from hospital and at first-time MI survivors and their spouses.

The intervention studies revealed the importance of duration of support, in terms of intervention 'dose' and the stability of outcomes. Peers visited the homes of new family caregivers of stroke survivors twice weekly over a period of twelve weeks. In the delayed post-test interviews, after six months had elapsed, caregivers contended that they missed the peers when the visits terminated. Similarly, although the telephone support groups for hemophiliacs with HIV/AIDS and their family caregivers lasted twelve weeks – longer than most telephone interventions reported in the literature – both affected men and their caregivers maintained that they would have liked the groups to continue longer. Likewise, many parents felt a sense of loss when the telephone sessions ended.

Relationship between Stress and Social Support

Relationships with social networks sometimes generate stress. Conflict with spouses over the ill child's care and the absence of anticipated support were perceived to be stressful by mothers of children with chronic conditions. The investigation of the support needs of hemophiliacs with AIDS and their family caregivers revealed that insensitivity, prejudice, and avoidance were particularly stressful. Caregivers of stroke survivors considered stressful the demands associated with interactions with health professionals and with changes in the reactions of and their relationship with their ill relative. The children with chronic conditions identified peer relationships as a major everyday life stressor and restrictions that inhibited social activities and relationships as a key illness-related stressor.

The findings across studies revealed instructive linkages between stress appraisal and social support. Persons admitted for the first time appraised the stress associated with their cardiac condition as less central and threatening and described less emotional and affirmational support from health professionals than those with multiple admissions reported. Mothers of children with chronic conditions described specific types of support from specific sources with respect to specific caregiving stressors. In the investigation of the resources that influence young children's coping with a stressful procedure, supportive nursing interventions were associated with reports of less pain. Support was also related to diminished stress experienced by community health nurses. All intervention studies were based on the premise that support has a moderating effect on appraisal of the stressfulness of chronic illness and caregiving. To illustrate, it was predicted that telephone support groups for parents of children with chronic conditions would decrease parental perceived stress.

Social Support and Coping

The links between coping and support were explored in several studies. In the study of children's support, healthy children sought support from friends more often as a coping strategy and had more supporters than children with a chronic condition. The investigation of nurses in HIV/AIDS care revealed that the coping strategies 'seeking support' and 'positive reappraisal' were related to receipt of work-related social support. Moreover, as social support increased, their distancing coping decreased. The key coping strategy used by men with hemophilia and AIDS and their family caregivers was 'seeking support,' in particular, informational support. In contrast, hemophiliacs with AIDS who coped by avoiding others did so because of fear of negative reactions, concern about confidentiality, and associated reluctance to seek support. 'Seeking social support' was also the most common coping strategy used by persons admitted to hospital for IHD. These studies seemed to reinforce the view that persons skilled at seeking support are more effective in obtaining social support (Silver, Wortman, & Crofton, 1990). Barriers to seeking support were recounted by family caregivers who were reluctant to request support for fear of exposure and vulnerability. Accordingly, they used non-verbal behavioural cues to seek support and maintained relationships in which unsolicited support was offered (chapter 10).

In contrast to the strategies used by adults and older healthy children in these studies, most coping behaviours used by young children experiencing a painful procedure were primarily directed at self-protection and less often included support seeking. Coping skills may be learned in later developmental stages. Nevertheless, the coping behaviours of these young children were influenced by supportive interactions with nurses, and their preparation for the procedure was positively related to their ability to seek informational support, again suggesting links between coping and social support. The proposed computer support intervention for older children with physical disabilities is hypothesized to increase support-seeking coping behaviours.

According to post-intervention interviews, all the support interventions for hemophiliacs with AIDS and their family caregivers, for MI survivors and their spouses, for family caregivers of stroke survivors, and for parents of children with chronic illness enhanced coping with the demands of a chronic health condition and caregiving. People living with HIV/AIDS reported increased use of problem-focused coping strategies, in particular, seeking informational support and advocacy. Peers provided explanations about coping to caregivers of stroke survivors; participants noted improved information seeking and distraction from caregiving stress. Couples coping with MI described enhanced problem-focused coping and relationship-focused coping following the support group intervention.

Evidence of 'relationship coping' was revealed in the mothers' appraisal of interactions with their spouses/partners. Mothers described their efforts to maintain their marriage and to cope with their spouses' lack of support for and involvement in caregiving by using 'active engagement' and 'protective buffering' (Coyne & Downey, 1991). Couples coping with MI reported less protective buffering following the support intervention. Hemophiliacs with AIDS and their family caregivers primarily used coping strategies aimed at keeping their 'personal relationships normal,' attributable perhaps to the absent and conflicted support in their relationships. In contrast, elderly participants with heart failure and stroke, who had been married for forty years on average, experienced stressors and support as a couple and expressed satisfaction with their spousal relationship, despite decreasing reciprocity. This finding may reflect a mastery of relationship coping in long-term, stable relationships.

People with multiple sclerosis and other chronic conditions exhibited both individualistic and communal coping orientations. The individualistic style inhibits support-seeking coping strategies, in contrast to those with communal approaches, who adapt their relationships to illness (chapter 9). Some family caregivers of relatives at vulnerable life stages (i.e., infants and seniors) reflected communal/collective perspectives towards support mobilization in their relationships, whereas others had individualistic or exchange-oriented views (chap. 10).

Impact of Social Support on Health Status, Health Behaviour, and Use of Health Services

Consistent with the buffering model (Quittner, Glueckouf, & Jackson, 1990), our intervention studies hypothesized that support has a moderating impact on health and functioning outcomes in the context of chronic stress. To illustrate, face-to-face support groups for persons coping with MI decreased negative affect experienced by spouses. A pilot study suggested that telephone support groups for persons living with AIDS can enhance psychological health by decreasing social and emotional loneliness. Similarly, we predict that computer support for older disabled children will decrease their loneliness. Finally, the telephone support groups for parents of young children with chronic conditions enhanced some aspects of parents' health (e.g., resistance and susceptibility) and functioning (e.g., valuing and comfort components of competence).

In two assessment studies, support was associated with health outcomes of professionals. Total support and work-related support were linked to diminished burnout among community health nurses, and emotional support was associated with less emotional exhaustion (i.e., a component of burnout) experienced by nurses in AIDS care. In this assessment study, as affirmational and informational support increased, burnout of these nurses decreased. As hypothesized, the follow-up telephone support group intervention for nurses in HIV/AIDS care influenced burnout (i.e., increased personal accomplishment).

Conversely, the impact of chronic health conditions on support was revealed in several studies. Hemophiliacs with AIDS and their family caregivers reported isolation and avoidance by friends who formerly had been supportive. Mothers of children with chronic conditions experienced inadequate support from persons in their social network. These mothers and family caregivers of stroke survivors seemed to suffer from the negative impact of caregiving on their health and well-being; they reported fatigue and emotional and physical health problems. In another study, support from neighbours deteriorated for persons with a history of prior hospital admission for IHD.

The positive influence of social support on health behaviours emerged as another theme. Following face-to-face support groups for couples coping with MI, spouses and survivors reported increased confidence to make requisite lifestyle and health behaviour changes. Negative outcomes may also result from interactions with network members, however, such as reinforcement of poor health behaviours or diminished self-care. For instance, mothers expressed concern about the negative impact of peers on health regimen adherence and self-care by their adolescents with diabetes or cystic fibrosis. In a related study, disadvantaged women's smoking was linked to the social influence of smoking peers and spouses (Stewart, Gillis, Brosky, Johnston, Kirkland, Leigh, Persaud, Rootman, Jackson, & Pawlin, 1996a).

Social support was also related to health services use. For example, significant decreases were noted in hospital admissions and visits to hospital outpatient departments, indicating that family caregivers of stroke survivors who received peer support were less likely to seek expensive professional intervention for their relative. In another study, mothers discussed their need for support pertaining to the caregiving demands associated with their child's health care, clinic appointments, and use of health services. Following the telephone intervention, parents reported changes in their use of the health system and altered behaviours in health care encounters.

Themes from the Assessment Studies

- Different types of providers are valued for different types of support.
- Support from both professionals and peers is important.
- Support can dissipate over time in chronic stressful situations.
- Delayed or altered reciprocity may be acceptable in close relationships.
- Persons in chronic stressful situations experience problems with support from partners, family, friends, and professionals (e.g., miscarried helping, conflict).
- The coping strategy 'seeking support' is positively related to receipt of social support. Relationship-focused coping strategies can help to maintain relationships with network members.
- Social network members may have a positive or negative impact on health behaviours.
- Selected types of support are associated with diminished professional burnout.

Support Processes

Across the interventions at both dyadic and group levels, social comparison, social exchange, and social learning predominated.

Social Comparison

All participants identified social comparison as a benefit of the face-to-face support groups for couples coping with MI. Similarity of life circumstances played an important role in group development. Perceived lack of similarity with peers hindered comparisons and depth of discussion in some groups. The tone of the group discussions was often set by the peer leaders' describing situations similar to those experienced by members. Participants found solace in the realization that they were not the only ones in that situation.

Parents compared demands of caregiving, ways of coping, ages of children, and severity of children's conditions in the telephone support groups. In this study, as in the cardiac study, dissimilar circumstances constrained the process of social comparison and the effectiveness of group interactions.

Similarities in caregiving experience, personality, age, and interests contributed to the success of the match between family caregivers and peer visitors. Caregivers recommended that in future projects the peer visitor should be matched as closely as possible to the family caregiver, in terms of the relationship between the caregiver and the stroke survivor as well as the specific stroke disability.

Nurses in HIV/AIDS care who participated in telephone support groups were impressed with the benefits of social comparison. They felt validated and connected with others in similar circumstances.

Social Learning

In the cardiac support groups, the process of social learning encompassed information based on both experiential and professional knowledge. Participants gained insight into their reactions and behaviours through role modelling by other members and exchange of experiential knowledge. Some participants learned about themselves by observing the behaviour of other group members and peer leaders (i.e., vicarious learning). During the post-intervention interviews, participants referred to the positive impact of the informational support provided by the intervention on their coping, confidence, and spousal relationship.

In the telephone support groups for parents of children with chronic conditions, peer facilitators and other parents were role models. For instance, one women claimed that she 'looked up to' the other mothers and wanted to be more like them. Experiential knowledge was often solicited by the facilitators in the initial sessions and was exchanged more spontaneously among members as the support group developed.

Nurses in HIV/AIDS care reported learning coping strategies, relationship skills, harm-reduction techniques, and stress identification and management from peers in telephone support groups. They also learned how to say 'no' and 'I don't know.'

Social Exchange

There was a strong sense of mutuality and equality among group members in the support interventions. Most participants indicated that they contributed to and received benefits from the group. Some peer facilitators reported that although they provided support, they also learned from members.

Most supportive interactions in the dyadic intervention involving the peer visitor were considered reciprocal. Indeed, participants valued mutuality in their relationships with peer visitors.

Themes from the Intervention Studies

Support intervention: social comparison, social exchange, social learning

Satisfaction with interventions: peers, professionals, participants

- Peer-professional partnership successful
- Different support modes suitable for different people

Support intervention outcomes (quantitative)

- Loneliness ↓
- Negative affect ↓
- Parenting competence ↑
- Resistance and susceptibility in health ↑
- Child ego strength ↑
- Stigma/discrimination ↓
- Seeking support ↑
- Personal accomplishment ↑
- Job satisfaction ↑
- Health services use ↓
- Social support need ↓
- Social support satisfaction ↑

Perceived impact of interventions (qualitative)

- Improved ability to make health behaviour changes
- Increased confidence, competence, and empowerment
- Enhanced communication
- Satisfaction of emotional support needs
- Satisfaction of information support needs
- Expanded coping repertoire (e.g., moved to action)
- Improved interactions with natural network

Research Insights

The trends in Canada towards creation of research centres, units, institutes, and programmatic research involve interdisciplinary and intersectoral teams and partnership with consumers and community groups. The latter reflects participatory approaches.

Participatory elements in our research projects are illustrated in several features of the intervention for parents of children with chronic conditions: (1) a parent of children with cystic fibrosis was an investigator, (2) key issues for discussion were identified by mothers in the earlier assessment study, (3) parents provided ongoing input into the content of group discussions, and (4) a professional and a parent shared the group leadership. The research program, which was focused on seniors and their family caregivers, had an advisory committee composed of a senior who was former director of Self-Help Canada, two seniors in self-help groups in Toronto, seniors in Nova Scotia associated with One Voice Seniors and Canadian Pensioners Concerned, family caregivers of seniors in Nova Scotia and Quebec, and self-help clearing house directors.

Interdisciplinary investigators and staff in the project teams represented community health and epidemiology, health education, medicine, nursing, occupational therapy, physiology, physiotherapy, psychology, public administration, social work, and sociology. Interdisciplinary collaboration is congruent with the important principle of intersectoral collaboration in primary health care and health promotion. We found that collaboration of disciplines yielded a comprehensive combination of diverse perspectives in our assessment and intervention research.

Design issues illuminated by this research program pertain to the continuing need for (1) longitudinal research, (2) theory-testing research, (3) qualitative approaches that document processes of interpersonal interactions and support interventions, and (4) intervention research. Several queries posed by Gottlieb and Feeley (1995) have direct relevance to the intervention projects in our program: 'How does change come about? How can we determine that change can be attributed in part to the intervention? Does the intervention seek to develop the phenomenon, change it, or maintain it? When should the intervention begin? At what time would the intervention be most effective in bringing about the desired outcomes? How long does an intervention have to be in effect for long-term change? How frequent should it be?'

The impact of interventions on situation-specific health and functioning outcomes and the mechanisms by which determinants of health, such as social support, exert their effect have often been neglected in previous investigations. This research program has begun to bridge these gaps.

Finally, there is a need to communicate results of this research to varied audiences (i.e., academics, consumers, participants, practitioners, and policy makers). In this context, there is increasing recognition that research should inform practice, programs, and policy.

Practical Insights

Implications for Programs and Interventions

Respondents' preferences for meeting with similar peers were revealed in assessment studies that illustrated the importance of personal and illness dimensions (e.g., sex, age, marital status, length of time since diagnosis, how illness was contracted, impact of illness). The completed intervention studies for family caregivers of stroke survivors, for couples coping with MI, for parents of children with chronic conditions, and for hemophiliacs with HIV/AIDS and their family caregivers reinforced the significance of similarity of peers.

An apparent pattern of specialization in support functions emerged across the assessment studies: family members were perceived to specialize primarily in practical support, health professionals in informational support, intimates such as spouses/partners in emotional support, and peers in affirmational support. Blending of functions also occurred. To illustrate, the key source of emotional support and affirmational support in the intervention for caregivers of stroke survivors was peers, whereas professionals and peers provided informational support and family members were the sole providers of instrumental support. This finding suggests that support figures may not readily substitute for one another in interventions.

The facilitator guides used in these intervention studies summarized relevant and current information and were modified according to participant feedback. Although most participants were satisfied with the information received from support group interventions, some cardiac group members wanted more information about diet, exercise, stress, communication skills, and sexual intimacy. In the AIDS study, one caregiver suggested that death and bereavement could be explored in greater depth. Some parents wanted more information about the chronic condition or treatment than the telephone support groups provided.

Group sessions often lasted longer than the originally scheduled duration, reflecting the members' needs for support and for discussion with others in similar circumstances. In the AIDS, cardiac, and parent support group interventions, some participants wanted the support groups to continue beyond the predetermined twelve weeks, indicating their need for this type of support and their positive perceptions of the intervention. A few nurses in HIV/AIDS care reported a sense of disappointment, and even of abandonment, when the telephone support groups terminated.

The success of the face-to-face and telephone support groups and the dyadic intervention can be attributed in part to the fact that the content of discussions could be controlled by participants. Leadership was another critical factor in the optimum functioning of the support groups. In general, participants were very satisfied with the model of co-peer and professional leadership.

Lessons Learned

- There are recruitment challenges with small, geographically dispersed populations.
- The telephone mode is appropriate for socially isolated participants.
- The facilitator guides were helpful; they were updated and modified for use in future interventions.
- The training session anticipated issues that arose during support interventions.
- A consistent balance between peer and professional facilitators is important.
- Booster/check-in sessions for facilitators are effective.
- Sessions and support groups should be of longer duration to increase intervention dose.
- Information is important to caregivers and people with chronic conditions.
- Similarity of participants in age, life circumstances, and condition is important.

The results of the intervention studies involving caregivers of stroke survivors and parents of children with chronic conditions suggest that support for family caregivers may influence health services use by persons with chronic conditions. This indirect influence can be taken into account in planning support interventions.

Successful Interventions Involving Social Support

Many efficacious interventions involving social support were depicted in the Canadian success stories elicited by the Determinants of Health Working Group of the National Forum on Health. Some supportive interventions were targeted at families and workplaces. For example, in the *Family Matters Program*, home visiting, cluster groups that connected families with neighbourhoods, and child care resulted in decreased stressors, improved parent-child relations and activities, and enhanced child performance. When interventions were focused on work-related determinants of health, such as control over work, work pressures, and support from colleagues, the pace of work decreased, and supportive, flexible family policies, job security, and social support increased (National Forum on Health, 1996b).

Support interventions emphasized all stages of the lifespan – children, youth, adults, and seniors. In the *Prenatal Early Infancy Project*, first-time parents at risk for child abuse were visited at home by nurses throughout the pregnancy and for the initial two years of the child's life. Substance abuse, child maltreatment, chronic welfare dependence, child injuries, and subsequent pregnancies decreased; mothers' involvement with their children and social networks improved; and their workforce participation increased following this professional support intervention. In the *Alexandria Park Project*, (Toronto) community partners and the residents' association provided support to youth within an economically disadvantaged community. Social support and networking increased, personal health practices and coping skills improved, job opportunities and career training expanded, and drug traffic diminished. In an intervention focused on adult women immigrants (London, Ontario), encompassing support, counselling, and employment and life-skills training, a 92 per cent success rate in placing graduates was reported (National Forum on Health, 1996b). The *Tenderloin Seniors Organizing Project* in the United States involved social support, health education, and empowerment for isolated elderly residents of low-income hostels. Seniors created a health resource centre and a tenants' association. Impressive outcomes included decreased rent; enhanced transportation, safety, and living conditions; increased social contacts; and improved morale (Minkler, Frantz, & Wechsler, 1982–83).

Implications for Policies and Reform

The social, economic, and employment challenges in the changing context in Canada point to the significance of social support (National Forum on Health, 1996a, b; Stewart, 1996).

Challenges of the Changing Context

- Aging population ↑
- Cost of chronic conditions ↑
- Economic and social inequalities ↑ → health status ↓
- Socio-economic environment influences personal health practices
- High rates of unemployment affect health
- Work patterns changed and barriers to healthy work environments → psychological and social well-being ↓
- Economic cutbacks → social programs ↓
- Family structure and function undergoing profound changes
- Cuts in social supports affect men and women differently
  - Poverty among women in lone-parent households and elderly women ↑
  - Family caregiver burden ↑ → adverse effects on women's health
- Family and neighbourhood violence is widespread social problem
- Life transitions more challenging (e.g., family to school, school to work, work to retirement)

Health System Reform and Renewal

Provincial and national documents reflect the shift to a balanced emphasis on social, economic, and environmental determinants of health; empowerment of populations; and individualistic lifestyle/health behaviours. The recent interest in health promotion, population health, new public health, and determinants of health will pave the path for programs and policies involving social support, coping, and self-care.

The renewed interest in health promotion is due to five factors: (1) individuals' and communities' desire to exercise control over their situations, (2) shifts in power distribution created by self-care and women's movements, (3) evidence that increased investment in health care has not improved health status, (4) pressures imposed on social programs and 'high-tech' care by deteriorating economic and environmental conditions, and (5) epidemiological research documenting the powerful influence of broader determinants on health (Rootman & Goodstadt, 1996).

The 1994 document *Strategies for population health: Investing in the health of Canadians* recommended strengthening public understanding about the broad determinants of health and supporting actions that improve the health of populations. This document identified important determinants of health, such as social support/networks, social environments, and coping.

The 'New Public Health' emphasized social-political-economic determinants of health; social, mental, and spiritual dimensions of health; and an ecological approach to health (i.e., health is a product of interactions between individuals and their social-economic-physical environments).

The National Forum on Health (1996a, b) concluded that the emerging knowledge about health-enhancing non-medical interventions demands action at all levels of society. Key non-medical interventions involved social support networks (e.g., family, volunteer organizations, communities) and early stimulation and support of children. These themes were reflected in the following recommendations relevant to social support: (1) *Support families with children*: broad, integrated child and family strategy of programs and income support; targeted, community-based programs with a home visiting component; child care and early childhood education services; supportive workplace policies favourable to families. (2) *Support communities* to enhance the security and resiliency of citizens/members. (3) *Support youth* in transitions to employment and create 'bridge jobs' for *older workers*. (4) *Support research* on the *social*, economic, cultural, and gender determinants of health.

These recent health policy documents reflect the five important premises of primary health care: accessibility, health promotion and illness/injury prevention, public participation, interdisciplinary and intersectoral collaboration, and appropriate technology. These principles were also implemented in the projects within the Social Support Research Program.

Primary Health Care Premises Reflected in the Research Program

Promotion and prevention

- Enhanced health outcomes (health status, health behaviour, health services use)
- Focus on groups and populations at risk

Interdisciplinary and intersectoral collaboration

- Research teams composed of diverse disciplines in health and other sectors
- Intersectoral-agency involvement in recruitment

Public participation
- Peer involvement in projects
- Consumers/consumer groups as partners
- Consultation with participants

Appropriate technology and accessibility
- Telephone and computers
- Home visits
- Community-based interventions

Resilience was a common theme in the National Forum on Health (1996a, b) documents and success stories. Social support is a key factor in resilience at the individual (Stewart et al., 1996a), family (Mangham, Reid, & Stewart, 1996), and community (Stewart, Reid, Jackson, Buckles, Edgar, Mangham, & Tilley, 1996b) levels. Our telephone support intervention improved indicators of individual and family resilience, specifically parents' competence and the perceived ego strength of their children with chronic conditions. In our recent study of community resilience, social isolation was a major risk factor, and social support and communal coping were primary protective factors (Stewart et al., 1996b). Social isolation appeared to be a key risk for newcomers, arising from perceived lack of belonging and hostility from long-term residents. Although participants referred to family and friends as sources of support, consistent with research on protective factors at the individual level, aggregate and community-level support was also evident. The community itself seemed to offer support for specific populations at risk and for stressful situations and crises. Voluntary organizations played a key supportive role in all communities, as did churches and service organizations. Thus, at the community level, lay sources of support were much more prominent than professional sources of support. Indeed, formal agencies were rarely mentioned. Instances of communal coping, in which people collectively found solutions to shared problems, were evident in all communities. Relevant recommendations for programs and policies were (1) formal and informal social support mechanisms should be strengthened and expanded, and (2) programs that foster social integration of new members into the community should be developed.

These national initiatives reinforce the significance of social support and of the strategies employed in the Social Support Research Program for the future.

References

Antonucci, T.C. (1991). Attachment, social support and coping with negative life events in mature adulthood. In E.M. Cummings, A. Greene, & K. Kamaker (Eds),

Life-span developmental psychology: Perspectives on stress and coping (261–276). Hillsdale, CA: Lawrence Erlbaum.

Antonucci, T.C., & Jackson, J.S. (1990). The role of reciprocity in social support. In B.R. Sarason, I.G. Sarason, & G.R. Pierce (Eds), *Social support: An interactional view* (173–198). New York: Wiley.

Coyne, J.C., & Downey, G. (1991). Social factors and psychopathology: Stress, social support and coping processes. *Annual Review of Psychology, 42*, 401–425.

Dakof, G.A., & Taylor, S.E. (1990). Victims' perceptions of social support: What is helpful from whom? *Journal of Personality and Social Psychology, 58*(1), 80–89.

Gottlieb, L., & Feeley, N. (1995). Nursing intervention studies: Issues related to change and timing. In M. Stewart (Ed.), *Community nursing: Promoting Canadians' health* (618–639). Toronto: Saunders.

Katz, A. (1993). *Self help in America: A social movement perspective.* New York: Twayne.

Mangham, C., Reid, G., & Stewart, M. (1996). Resilience in families: Challenges for health promotion. *Canadian Journal of Public Health, 87*(6), 373–374.

Minkler, M., Frantz, S. & Wechsler, R. (1982–83). Social support and social action organizing in a 'gray ghetto': The Tenderloin experience. *International Journal of Community Health and Education, 3*(1): 3–15.

National Forum on Health. (1996a). *Canada health action: Building on the legacy.* Vol. I, *Final report of the National Forum on Health.* Ottawa: Minister of Public Works and Government Services.

National Forum on Health. (1996b). *Canada health action: Building on the legacy.* Vol. II, *Synthesis reports and issues papers.* Ottawa: Minister of Public Works and Government Services.

Quittner, A.L., Glueckouf, R.L., & Jackson, D.N. (1990). Chronic parenting stress: Moderating versus mediating effects of social support. *Journal of Personality and Social Psychology, 56*(6), 1266–1278.

Rootman, I., & Goodstadt, M. (1996). Health promotion and health reform in Canada. A position paper prepared on behalf of the Canadian Consortium for Health Promotion Research.

Silver, R., Wortman, C., & Crofton, C. (1990). The role of coping in support provision: The self-presentational dilemma of victims of life crises. In B.R. Sarason, I.B. Sarason, and G.R. Pierce (Eds), *Social support: An interactional view* (397–426), New York: Wiley.

Stewart, M. (1996). Keynote presentation on Future of Community Health Nursing for International Community Health Nursing Educators Conference. Vancouver, BC, June.

Stewart, M., Gillis, A., Brosky, G., Johnston, G., Kirkland, S., Leigh, G., Persaud, V., Rootman, I., Jackson, S., & Pawliw-Fry, B. (1996a). Disadvantaged women and smoking. *Canadian Journal of Public Health, 87*(4), 257–260.

Stewart, M., Reid, G., Jackson, S., Buckles, L., Edgar, W., Mangham, C., & Tilley, N. (1996b). Community resilience: Strengths and challenges. *Health and Canadian Society, 4*(1), 53–81.

12

Accomplishments and Challenges of Social Support Intervention Research

Benjamin H. Gottlieb

Abstract. When people experience unremitting adaptive challenges, they are more in need of effective support because of how difficult it is to maintain long-term support from the social network. It is a daunting task to design a support intervention that is both appealing to its intended beneficiaries and relevant to their needs, life stage, and social contexts. We know little about how to create the social conditions that are likely to animate the support process and even less about how to maintain this delicate process over an extended period of time. The dilemma faced by program planners and evaluators is to determine how to be responsive to feedback about the process while also maintaining high fidelity to the original blueprint of the intervention. When planning support interventions and selecting potential participants, we need to carefully consider people's stage of coping, their stage in the lifespan, and cohort differences in the acceptability of different types of interventions. In measuring the outcomes of social interventions, we have tended not only to reserve to the 'experts' decisions about the outcomes that are most meaningful, but also to over-rely on indicators of emotional ill health without sufficient recognition of their contextual relativity. The end points that matter to consumers should be evaluated. Moreover, the distinction between viewing social support as a means to an end and viewing it as an end in itself should be considered. Accordingly, when researchers aim to generate support as a way of increasing a protective factor, they should take the participants' reports of increased support as evidence that they have achieved the desired outcome without looking for any more distal effects. The helping professions can engage in the work of prevention, treatment, and rehabilitation by spurring or strengthening social bonds. Non-medical interventions that optimize interpersonal support can effect significant reductions in morbidity and even mortality.

Introduction

In this chapter, I touch on some of the accomplishments of the Social Support

Research Program described in this volume and identify certain features of the research that make it truly unique. In addition, I address several daunting challenges entailed in conducting and evaluating social support intervention research.

Four aspects of the Social Support Research Program testify to its intellectual vigour, breadth, and originality. The first is that each of the fourteen projects named in the original program proposal to National Health Research Development Program (NHRDP) and Medical Research Council of Canada (MRC) received funding. This in itself is impressive testimony of the relevance, originality, and scientific merit of the work that has been accomplished. It also speaks to the creativity and problem-solving skills of the researchers who zealously and convincingly demonstrated that social support could ameliorate the quality of life for persons diagnosed with a range of chronic disorders and their caregivers. In these times of funding famine, it is truly remarkable that all these projects were supported. Moreover, the list of funding sources and the total dollars committed to date are equally impressive.

The second impressive feat of the Social Support Research Program has been its ability to deliver on the promise of interdisciplinary and community collaboration. Most of the projects have been conducted by teams of investigators from several disciplines, including nursing, medicine, psychology, physiotherapy, nutrition, public administration, and occupational therapy. Equally laudatory, ordinary citizens have been included in the research teams and accorded great respect for the experiential knowledge they bring to the team's planning. The chapters in this volume reveal that the design is driven and enriched by a highly participative process, involving close consultation with members of the target population, discussion of the intervention plans with collaborating institutions and agencies, and revisions based on the input of key informants and participants in focus groups and pilot studies. For example, the mother of a child with cystic fibrosis played a key role in guiding the intervention plans in a project designed to mobilize support on behalf of parents of children with chronic illnesses. In the projects that involve creating support groups, one of the group leaders is usually a lay person who has the disease or disability or caregiving responsibility in common with the group members. The message is clear! If you want to strengthen social ties and mobilize their informal support, you have to listen to and learn from the people who know what support means and what support is needed in their particular circumstances.

Virtually every aspect of the teams' decision making reflects the spirit of partnership. It comes through in the shared lay and professional leadership of the intervention activities, in the breadth of the consultative relationships formed with agencies and institutions, and in the multiple authorships of the publications that have issued from the research. Partnership not only is exemplified in the research process, but also represents a paramount goal of the research. For example, one group of investigators has thoroughly researched ways of promoting mutually advantageous partnerships between self-help groups and professional practitioners in the health field. Several of the assessment and intervention projects that are reported in this volume are focused on understanding and promoting the social and psychological forces that yield responsive and durable informal helping partnerships among people with common life difficulties.

Third, this team of investigators has done more than any other to push forward the frontiers of knowledge regarding the conduct and evaluation of support interventions among diverse community and clinical populations. The list of beneficiaries spans the entire life course, including parents of children with chronic health conditions, children with chronic conditions themselves, couples coping in the aftermath of a myocardial infarction, family caregivers of hemophiliacs who are seropositive or who have AIDS, family caregivers of stroke survivors, recent widows, elderly women with impaired mobility, and even nursing professionals who work with individuals and families affected by AIDS. Moreover, these and other populations have been the beneficiaries of varied strategies for mobilizing support, including the introduction of new social ties through one-to-one peer support and through creating support and self-help groups, as well as initiatives directed to strengthening natural support systems in the family and the community. In order to serve populations that are typically bypassed or underserved by agencies and practitioners, such as people who live in rural areas and those plagued by the stigma of their illness, the investigators have pioneered novel outreach strategies of marshalling support, such as creating telephone and computer-based support networks. This work is on the cutting edge of our knowledge about how to deliver cost-effective programs to culturally and geographically isolated populations.

The fourth and final aspect that distinguishes this research is its emphasis on chronic illnesses and caregiving. Past work has focused mainly on marshalling support on behalf of populations affected by acute life events and time-limited role transitions (Gottlieb, 1983). Chronic illness and, for that matter, chronic stressors call for more sustained intervention and therefore require more of support providers by way of commitment and reasonable expectations for change in the recipient's health and well-being. By definition, chronic stressors are open ended, if not enduring in nature, and therefore intervention goals are more likely to revolve around accommodation to rather than resolution or termination of the stressor. For people facing continuous stressors that do not promise resolution, it is a matter of making compromises, learning to live with one's lot, and making certain adjustments that may enhance quality of life despite persistent stressful demands.

Indeed, when people experience unremitting adaptive challenges, they are even more in need of effective support because of the difficultly of sustaining long-term support from the social network. Hence, the goals of support interventions are to keep distress within manageable limits, preserve or restore a sense of self-worth, develop a personally meaningful understanding of one's situation, and gain a sense of confidence that progress is being made towards a more desirable future despite persistent stress. Although support interventions may focus to some extent on techniques of managing stressful demands and reducing distress, it may be more important to concentrate on ways of promoting positive emotions despite adversity. That is, the group's support should help its members to face continuing threat with a greater measure of confidence and equanimity. Instead of looking only for stress-buffering effects of social support, we should also look for its direct or main effect on emotional functioning. Simply stated, when people are in circumstances defined by the continuing possibility of harm or threat, the support of their peers can make it possible for them to experience positive emotions, such as hope and pleasure, even though it may not moderate their distress. After all, coping is not always in the service of stress reduction; it can also contribute to positive affect. This point is illustrated in the following observation by Register in her account of the adjustments made by people who live with a chronic illness: 'The first day I ever realized you could be happy and still be sick was a real red-letter day' (1987, xiv–xv). It is also illustrated in several chapters of this volume, documenting the greater confidence, optimism, and hopefulness that were experienced by the participants in the support groups. Group members displayed humour in managing life affected by HIV/AIDS, and spouses of MI survivors reported enhanced positive affect following the support group intervention.

Assessing Group Process and Prospective Members' Coping Styles

The work entailed in planning, pilot testing, implementing, and evaluating support programs is enormously taxing, both intellectually and logistically. It is a daunting task to design a support intervention that is both appealing to its intended beneficiaries and relevant to their needs, life stage, and social contexts. Much can go awry in the implementation of support interventions, especially when the intervention's success depends on the formation of new personal relationships or the modification of existing relationships with key network members. In virtually every chapter in this volume the authors address the dilemmas that surround decisions about ways of arranging social conditions so as to foster supportive interactions.

Although the support process can be understood in terms of social-psychological theories of small group dynamics, such as social learning, social comparison, and social exchange, there are few guidelines on ways of creating social contexts that optimize these processes. What are the most important criteria for selecting the membership of a support group composed of parents of children who have a chronic illness? Is it sufficient to ensure that their children have the same chronic disease, or should the stage and severity of the disease or the child's age and sex figure in decisions about the group's composition? Similarly, questions arise regarding the importance of the caregivers' characteristics, in terms of their age and sex, their mastery of the stressful demands they face, and even their support needs. Indeed, there are so many potential bases for determining group composition and so many ways in which the composition may not be conducive to a climate of support that it is almost miraculous that any group achieves cohesion and satisfactory levels of mutual aid. Moreover, in the context of chronic stress, the challenges of animating the support process are even more daunting, because stressful demands may change over time, ebbing and flowing with the changing course of the disease and with the changing life circumstances and coping strengths of the caregiver.

The point is that we know precious little about how to create the social conditions that are likely to animate the support process and even less about how to maintain this delicate process over an extended period of time. On the latter score, one should not minimize the practical problems associated with maintaining the steady participation of people in interventions that last for two to three months and then following them up six to twelve months later. For example, in creating support groups for men with prostate cancer and women with breast cancer, Helgeson and Lepore (1997) have observed that once time, cost, and transportation difficulties are overcome, there still may be people who miss group meetings, those who refuse to be interviewed about the group process or outcomes, or those who simply decide to drop out of the intervention because they are not getting what they want or else have received as much as they want from it. To prevent these problems, Helgeson and Lepore suggest assigning the same person to gather all the data from each participant, offering financial incentives to participants who might otherwise refuse to schedule follow-up interviews and maintaining close contact with participants who miss meetings so that they can be brought back into the fold before they lose interest entirely and are forgotten by the remaining group members. Friendly reminders by telephone and visually appealing updates of participants and the status of the study were attempted strategies for sustaining parents' involvement in the telephone support group intervention.

At the same time, since ethical standards dictate that participants can terminate their involvement at any point, it is highly desirable to gain information from those who have decided to drop out about why they chose to discontinue. Without making them defensive and in the spirit of contributing to the improvement of future interventions, questions should probe aspects of the group's process and composition that may have been implicated and aspects of the respondent's own personality make-up or coping style that may have conflicted with the group's culture of managing stress. In addition, any changes in the nature or intensity of the stressful demands faced by the respondent should be assessed, including additional stress created by the intervention itself. For example, the group may recommend health behaviours that are not sanctioned by the participant's physician or call attention to certain attitudes or behaviours of household members that group members feel should be challenged or encouraged; in either case, such intervention likely would upset the existing pattern of social relations.

In several chapters in this volume the program planners' struggles with decisions about whether and how to capture the group process are also recorded. On the one hand, the best way of testing theoretical postulates regarding the mechanisms through which social support affects health and morale is by dipping into the unfolding interpersonal dynamics. Through observation or the use of structured diaries, investigators can determine whether certain types of supportive communications, verbalized social comparisons, or information exchanges occur, and how actively participants are involved in these processes. For support groups, they can also use such information to modify the activities or emphases of the facilitators within the limits of the original program design, adjust the balance between the educational and the experience swapping components, and revise the order or detail in which certain topics are addressed. On the other hand, concerns have been raised about both the burden and the reactive effects of these techniques of sampling the group process. The burden associated with the use of diaries is indeed onerous when it is added to the burden entailed in completing the baseline and outcome measures. For the research team, diaries also create the extra work of chasing after respondents to ensure that they complete their entries and then analysing the diary data. Moreover, the existence of diaries may lead participants to expect that the investigators will take remedial action on unsatisfactory aspects of the group process, resulting in a negative rebound effect if such action is not forthcoming.

The dilemma faced by program planners and evaluators is to determine how to be responsive to feedback about the process while also maintaining high fidelity to the original blueprint of the intervention. Of course, even minor tinkering with a program's design could backfire if it were initiated to accommodate one member's feedback but caused dismay to other program participants. One solution is to eschew diaries and other self-report tools and rely on audio and/or video recording devices to capture the process. Although this strategy still requires labour-intensive coding and analysis of the recordings for research purposes, its virtues are that it minimizes reactive effects while still allowing the group planners and facilitators to monitor and introduce changes to the unfolding intervention process. When recording devices are used, it is essential that the confidentiality of recorded material is emphasized. If possible, permission should be sought from those whose voices and/or faces are recorded to use the tapes as a tool to train future group facilitators and as a vehicle for prospective support group participants to preview the experience they are being asked to consider.

The last point raises a broader issue that concerns people's suitability for an intervention that depends on the disclosure of their feelings, worries, and uncertainties. Specifically, it may be useful to examine the relationship between the ways people normally cope with adversity and the culture of the support group. In my consultations with people who are trying to implement support groups, I have learned that many individuals who are invited to join a group decline, and an additional proportion drop out of the group after a short time. Information about refusals and attrition is rarely reported in the literature. Aside from the standard psychological (e.g., stigma and fear of disapproval or rejection) and logistical (e.g., access, scheduling, and coverage of competing demands such as childcare) impediments to participation in any social program, support groups pose some unique threats and offer a particular way of coping with one's difficulties that does not have universal appeal or benefit.

The threats posed by support groups include a fear of becoming overwhelmed by attending to and disclosing one's difficulties and by exposing oneself to the more severe difficulties faced by other group members, especially if those difficulties preview one's own possible fate. Although some members may benefit because of the anticipatory coping and sense of control such advance information may promote, others may cope most effectively by keeping such information out of conscious awareness. In short, differences in people's coping styles may powerfully affect their interest in and the value they gain from participating in support groups. Specifically, differences in people's information- and help-seeking propensities and, more generally, avoidant versus approach-oriented coping styles under threat may distinguish those who are attracted to and make good use of the group experience from those who do not (Miller, 1987). In plain language, some people deal with threat by seeking as much information about it as they can and by venting their fears and emotional distress, whereas others maintain their equilibrium best by avoiding threatening information and blunting their emotions.

Depending on how they are marketed and actually conducted, support groups may be more or less threatening or attractive to people with contrasting information- and support-seeking coping styles. People who are 'blunters' (i.e., avoidance coping style) may fare better with more structured, task-centred, behavioural intervention protocols, whereas those referred to as 'monitors' (i.e., approach coping) may respond best to formats that provide plentiful details about the stressful context and allow them to discuss their feelings and experiences and to ask questions. If support groups are introduced in a way that suggests group therapy, with its emotional and disclosure norms, or if they promise to deliver detailed information about the more threatening aspects of the present and future, then they are likely to be shunned by and unsuitable for those who tend to regulate their emotions by avoidance and distraction. Indeed, the combination of unbridled emotional expression among peers and abundant information from experts is likely to drive the blunters away while appealing to the monitors, whose emotional self-regulation and sense of control are augmented by these two components. It follows that, in both advertising and implementing groups, the format, emotional climate, and type of information supplied should be pitched differently, depending on the prospective participants' coping styles. Where feasible, a measure of their information processing style can be used as a screening and group placement tool (Miller, 1987). If this is not possible and people with different styles are assigned to the same group, then potential moderating effects of these coping styles can be statistically tested to determine whether they have influenced intervention outcomes.

Assessment-Intervention Nexus

A distinctive feature of this volume is the contributors' commitment to a two-stage intervention planning process, which commences with a systematic assessment of the target population's support sources, needs, and deficiencies, coping resources, and stress appraisals and then proceeds to the intervention design. This is a highly laudable approach, which compares favourably with the multitude of support interventions that are reported in the literature without any justification based on the participants' current social and personal resources. The link from assessment to intervention is not always transparent, however, and some aspects of assessment may have been overlooked despite their bearing on the program's design.

With respect to the assessment tools used by the contributors, a certain degree of information overload may have complicated the planning process, along with some uncertainty about how to weight the various findings in terms of their relevance to the intervention design. The former problem is reflected in the authors' greater reliance on the respondents' expressed preferences for certain kinds of support interventions than on the voluminous data gathered about the respondents' support needs, coping efforts, and appraisals of stress. Moreover, when the latter data were invoked to inform the intervention plan, they were not always drawn upon in a systematic and composite way. For example, in the chapter on spousal support for coping with cardiac conditions, the authors used a stress appraisal measure, along with social support and coping measures, to determine how people who had multiple hospital admissions for IHD differed from those who were not readmitted. The idea was to prevent multiple readmissions by identifying and then remediating the support or coping deficiencies experienced by the relapsers. The investigators spotlighted three principal findings that had relevance for guiding their intervention plans, namely, the fact that persons with multiple admissions received more support from health professionals and less support from neighbours and sought support more as a coping strategy. The fact that readmitted persons also made significantly less use of the coping strategy called 'accepting responsibility' and appraised their admission as less controllable than those who were not readmitted during the study period was acknowledged only implicitly in the emphasis on education, as well as support, in the group discussions and exercises, in outcome measures focused on perceptions of control and self-efficacy, and in documentation of role modelling of these characteristics by peer leaders and other group members. However, the coping strategies and stress appraisals identified during the assessment study could have guided the group composition in the intervention. Enhanced control and confidence emerged as important indicators of the perceived success of these support groups for MI survivors and their spouses.

The intervention planning process may also have suffered from insufficient information related to the prospective participants' stage of coping with their stressful demands and their life stage. The relevance of these two considerations for the group's composition can be illustrated by an example taken from my own research on the impact of centre-based respite programs on family caregivers of persons with dementia (Gottlieb & Johnson, 1995). In a study of 103 caregivers attending sixteen different centre-based respite programs, one of the outcomes I adopted was a measure of 'institutional readiness' that ranged from ever having discussed long-term placement with anyone to placing one's relative's name on an active waiting list, meaning that the caregiver would take the next bed that came up. I postulated that, by easing the caregivers' burden and reducing their captivity in the role, a respite program would either avert or slow down preparations for institutional placement. I had not counted on the fact that, at the time they enrolled their relative in the day program, over half of my sample of caregivers had already placed their relative's name on a waiting list. Within only five months, 27 per cent had moved their relative into long-term care. Furthermore, of the fifty-eight caregivers who remained in the study after about five months, one-third had shifted their relative's status towards institutional placement by activating their name or applying for placement for the first time.

The point is that, if plans were being made to offer support groups to these caregivers as a supplement to the respite service they were using, it would be of utmost importance to take into account their stage of coping with their caregiving responsibilities. One-third of my sample was made up of people who were looking for resources to help them shore up their role as caregiver, and two-thirds were looking for a way of testing the institutional waters and smoothing their relative's entry to long-term care and their own emotional adjustment to role exit. In short, the sample could be divided into people who were psychologically already on the road to placement and those who were not. If these two different groups of caregivers were to be placed together in one support group, they would bring different expectations to their involvement and would find different outcomes relevant to their respective stages of coping.

These observations imply that more carefully targeted marketing has to be done for respite programs, so that those who want to relinquish the caregiving role can get what they need, and those who want support to continue get what they need. The same logic applies to the selection of people for participation in support groups. People join at different stages of their caregiving careers, and they therefore expect the group to address the issues that are most pertinent to their career stage and expect the investigators to gauge outcomes that are relevant to the psychological and emotional needs that are aroused at this stage. The fact that they share the caregiving role rarely levels these differences. After all, what does a forty-five-year-old employed daughter whose father has mild dementia and still lives independently have in common with a seventy-five-year-old wife of a man with severe dementia? It is unlikely that they will view each other as appropriate targets of comparison or that they will share similar goals and trajectories or relate to the same criteria for judging a support group's benefit to them. The significance of similarity of peers in dyadic and group interventions is a recurrent theme in the lessons learned from intervention studies with parents, family caregivers of stroke survivors, and couples coping with cardiac conditions.

In addition to carefully considering people's stage of coping, we also need to consider their stage in the lifespan. It is almost a truism that the meaning, significance, and stressfulness of caregiving will differ depending on when such responsibilities must be borne in the life course. There are people who have the role thrust upon them at a time when they had not expected it, when their peers do not have it, and when the role is unwanted and interferes with other life domains. Other people assume caregiving responsibilities at a time that is normative for themselves and their peers and view this role as the most valued and the most important aspect of their identity. For those who experience role entry as an off-time crisis-like event that forces other psychological and role adjustments, outcomes should probably centre on the minimization of role conflict and the smooth integration of the caregiving role. For example, intergenerational caregivers who are in mid-life, possibly sandwiched between two generations and occupied by multiple role demands, would probably endorse the relevance of an outcome measure that taps role captivity (Pearlin, Mullan, Semple, & Skaff, 1990). But for those who enter the role on time and at a time when they are prepared to invest in it heavily (e.g., retired, elderly spouses) measures ought to centre on knowledge of the illness and effective care practices, feelings of role competence, relationship issues (e.g., continued affection and cooperation despite the partner's diminished ability to reciprocate), as well as anticipatory coping with the eventual loss of a significant attachment figure and the attendant relinquishment of the caregiving role.

The notion of life stage also raises the issue of cohort differences in the acceptability of different types of interventions. Another insight I gained from the respite study is that caregivers deferred their use of these centre-based day programs because they felt their relative had no experience of functioning in such a group setting and therefore would not adjust easily. Many caregivers observed that such congregate care services were a relatively recent invention that would be totally alien to their relative's generation. By extension, it is likely that many older adults would find the notion of entering a support group equally alien. In fact, in a recent intervention study Pillemer (1997) attempted to randomly assign family caregivers of persons with dementia to support groups composed of other caregivers or to home visitors who themselves were veteran caregivers. Refusal rates for the support groups were so high, however, that he had to reduce the number of such groups and concentrate on the effects of the home visitors. Aside from the typical scheduling and transportation problems, Pillemer maintains that support groups were too exotic an intervention for these caregivers. They simply could not accept the idea of entering a group composed of strangers who would disclose their intimate feelings and experiences and expect the same from others. In contrast, their life experience had prepared them for a series of friendly discussions with a home visitor. They had met such people before, whether they were neighbourhood canvassers or service providers, and they knew what to expect and greeted the invitation with a greater sense of control. This premise informed the design and enhanced the impact of the peer visitor intervention with family caregivers of stroke survivors.

Selecting Appropriate and Meaningful Outcomes

Another issue that I believe we will need to work on more intensively in the coming years as we experiment with different ways of mobilizing support concerns the selection of appropriate outcome measures. My remarks are based partly on a review of the outcomes examined in the present volume and partly on my reading of the current literature. On the latter score, five critical reviews of published studies on the effects of support groups have recently been published: three examining groups for the family caregivers of elderly relatives (Bourgeois, Schulz, & Burgio, 1996; Lavoie, 1995; Toseland and Rossiter, 1989) and two summarizing the effects of support groups on cancer patients (Fawzy, Fawzy, Arndt, & Pasnau, 1995; Helgeson & Cohen, 1996). Since support groups figure prominently among the intervention programs created in the Social Support Research Program, I concentrate on some issues surrounding their impacts.

Although the evidence is mixed, the general consensus is that groups for the caregivers of elderly family members have a negligible impact on mental health outcomes, as measured by widely accepted psychiatric symptom, general distress, and burden scales, and by indices of socio-emotional functioning. Toseland and Rossiter's (1989) careful review of this literature led them to conclude that the groups should be composed of more homogeneous subgroups of caregivers, such as separate groups for spouses and adult children, and that they should continue over a longer period, experiment with alternative formats and curricula, and gauge more specific behavioural changes. The second and third reviews of these studies, one by Lavoie (1995) and one by Bourgeois, Schulz, and Burgio (1996), suggest that support groups may not address the unique circumstances and needs of individual caregivers, and therefore in many cases the outcomes that are measured are not relevant. This may reflect the fact that program planners tend to reserve to themselves decisions about outcome measures, a concern reflected in chapter 3 in the discussion of disclosure to parents of the intended aims and use of outcome measures. Although planners are willing to consult representatives of the beneficiary population about matters such as the group format, content, sequencing of activities, and leadership, they view the selection of outcomes as a highly technical decision that is reserved for those with expert rather than experiential knowledge. Whereas people who plan support groups do need to ensure that the measures they adopt are psychometrically strong and sensitive, a prior concern should be to ensure that they do not make inappropriate assumptions about the end states that matter to the participants and thereby impose a set of outcome criteria that are irrelevant or unimportant.

The selection of sensitive and relevant outcome measures is complicated by the fact that every evaluation has multiple stakeholders who differ in the outcomes that impress them. Returning to my example of respite programs, I predict that the respite program staff would be impressed by evidence that the consumers are highly satisfied with the quality of care their relative receives and with the sensitivity of staff to both the caregivers' and their elderly relative's personalized needs. Policy makers would be impressed by harder evidence. They would smile on evidence that the program was financially self-sustaining, that it prolonged the elderly person's stay in the community, and that it seamlessly integrated the delivery of other needed services to the family. Researchers would no doubt be impressed by yet another set of outcomes. Judging by their frequent appearance in the published literature and in grant proposals, I would say that researchers first and foremost embrace mental health indicators, such as symptom checklists, and rely also on quality of life measures. In short, if the program maintains or boosts the caregivers' morale by dispelling or ameliorating depressive mood or anxiety, then researchers are prepared to conclude that it made an important difference.

Finally, although their views are not usually canvassed, when they are given an opportunity to speak out, the caregivers themselves tend to identify an entirely different set of valued outcomes. It includes feeling glad that their relative is happy at the program; having an opportunity to gain some undisturbed time to themselves when they are psychologically off duty; having consistent contact with a staff member who, they believe, is looking out for them and their relative; and not having to take on extra work because of some poorly planned logistical aspect of the program (e.g., non-existent or unreliable transportation arrangements). Employed caregivers value a reduction in the number of times they must be tardy or absent from work or from the important informal networking activities that accompany work. I have never heard a caregiver say that a respite program mitigated feelings of sadness and loss, or reduced anxiety about their relative's plight, or improved the overall quality of their life. But I have heard them say that the day program gave them a chance to catch their breath, to do something concrete that they felt would improve their relative's quality of life, and to be more patient and loving towards their relative because the program allowed them time to regain their emotional composure. The more I think about what the caregivers value, the more I realize that they tend to focus on outcomes that affect their relationship with their relatives and on their sense that they are doing right by him or her, which is tantamount to saying that their sense of self-worth in the caregiving role is bolstered. At the same time, they are vigilant about anything that might add to their burdens and feel thankful for anything that temporarily eases the strains of caregiving.

The point is that most intervention researchers do not measure the end points that matter to caregivers or persons with chronic conditions, or if they do, it is more accidental than deliberate. Typically, they include a few consumer satisfaction measures and an open-ended question or two about the group's value to the participant as a 'sop' to the program staff, who want some feedback, or to break up the boredom of symptom-rating scales. They believe in their hearts, however, that this information is too soft to be taken seriously, because what really matters is a significant drop in depression or anxiety scores. Moreover, these statistically significant declines are usually clinically and behaviourally insignificant. Researchers rarely report the number of people who have moved below the threshhold for case status, mainly because the scales they use do not have clinical cut-off points. For example, they tend to measure subclinical depressed mood, but not depression. The second implication is that it is not reasonable to expect caregivers to come away from respite programs feeling less sadness about their relative or feeling less anxious about the future, because these feelings are normal reactions to their chronically stressful circumstances. Why would one want to sanitize their emotions? In fact, perhaps a more realistic and healthier outcome for the caregivers would be to have these feelings validated, normalized, and accepted. Similarly, Lavoie (1995) observes that it is unrealistic to expect a limited number of group meetings with peers to change deep-seated anxiety or depression over the illness of a loved one. In addition, he suggests that caregivers are more concerned about outcomes related to their own sense of competence and their relative's well-being than to their own emotional functioning.

In sum, in measuring the outcomes of social interventions, we have tended not only to reserve to the 'experts' decisions about the outcomes that are most meaningful, but also to overrely on indicators of emotional ill health. Moreover, the latter measures of psychiatric symptomatology have been used as absolute standards of program effectiveness, rather than considered in relation to what might be normal and even healthy emotional functioning in exceptionally harsh circumstances. It is not that these measures are altogether irrelevant, but that they are applied without sufficient recognition of their contextual relativity. More generally, as a social psychologist, I believe that it is equally important, and in some circumstances more important, to judge the value of social programs in terms of their capacity to shore up valued social roles, instil hope and confidence that progress is being made towards a more desirable future, and validate one's feelings and experiences than to judge their value in terms of impact on distress and ill health.

There is a final issue related to the search for meaningful and appropriate social and psychological measures of the outcomes of support interventions. It concerns the distinction between viewing social support as a means to an end and viewing it as an end in itself. Some strategies of marshalling support focus on supplementing people's social networks with one or more extra ties, concentrating on ways of making the new relationships as attractive and meaningful as possible. Organizations such as Big Brothers and Big Sisters have relationship formation and development as their principal goals, as do the friendly visitor programs that are offered to isolated or institutionalized elderly persons. The intent is that the new ties will give rise to perceived support, a known stress buffer, and directly contribute to morale. In these instances, support is an end in itself. Other interventions view support as the crucial mediating process that leads to desired outcomes. Examples include the deployment of home visitors to guide young mothers who may be at risk of child maltreatment or the establishment of a support group for men who have had heart attacks to improve their adherence to recommended lifestyle changes.

Intervention researchers are not always clear about which of these two outcomes they are trying to achieve, and sometimes they mistake evidence that the intervention has 'taken' for evidence that it has achieved its intended effects. For example, when researchers aim to generate support in order to reduce risk factors, then any changes they identify in either the structural properties of the participants' social networks (e.g., size, composition, density) or in the frequency, quality, or perceived supportiveness of their social interactions should be taken as evidence that the intervention was sufficiently powerful to effect these changes. Given the investigators' ultimate interest in reducing risk factors, however, they should view these changes as checks on the power of the intervention to produce the social conditions that favour the more distal psychological, emotional, and behavioural outcomes of interest. The opposite holds true as well. When researchers aim to generate support as a way of increasing a protective factor, they should take the participants' reports of increased support as evidence that they have achieved the desired outcome without looking for any more distal effects. For many people who have chronic conditions or disabilities that marginalize or isolate them, such as the HIV-infected hemophiliacs and the parents of children with chronic illnesses who are the subjects of several chapters in this volume, such support in itself is an invaluable outcome. As one of the men with hemophilia observed: '*[We] didn't believe in it at the beginning. Someone can understand you only if someone has the same thing as you. There was a lot of sharing. Everyone took the time to listen to everybody else. It can't get any better than that with regard to meeting one's needs. You know that there are people there who will take the time to listen to what you have to say*' (chap. 5).

Conclusion

The social support research program described in this volume not only reflects and buttresses the ethic of caring that is the ideological bedrock of the health professions, but also delineates a new role that professionals can assume in both clinical and community settings. It is the role of animator and facilitator of supportive social ties among populations that are in similar stressful circumstances. In fact, the research is yielding abundant details about the various ways that the helping professions can engage in the work of prevention, treatment, and rehabilitation by spurring or strengthening social bonds. The intervention research demonstrates that non-medical interventions that optimize interpersonal support can effect significant reductions in morbidity and even mortality. That message is in the vanguard of the most progressive contemporary thinking about the levers that affect public health. Witness the work of the National Forum on Health, which commissioned a number of papers on non-medical strategies of improving the health of Canadians. In the words of Marc Renaud, the chairman of the Forum's Working Group on the Determinants of Health: 'we learned that Canadians have a keen sense of what affects their health and well-being, and an awareness that health is more than health care' (Renaud, 1996).

This research program convincingly demonstrates that health maintenance and health promotion can be accomplished by carefully and collaboratively planned strategies of strengthening the social fabric and fostering interpersonal relatedness. In considerable measure, the success of the Social Support Research Program is a result of the energy, commitment, perseverance, and organizational talents of the numerous professionals and citizens who formed alliances in the common cause of promoting human welfare. I highly commend their efforts! More important, there is a larger audience that applauds their accomplishments. It consists of the many people in the community who have benefited from the supportive programs that have been designed on their behalf and the future generations of professionals who will gain instruction from this work.

References

Bourgeois, M.S., Schulz, R., & Burgio, L. (1996). Interventions for caregivers of patients with Alzheimer's Disease: A review and analysis of content, process, and outcomes. *International Journal of Aging and Human Development, 43*, 35–92.

Fawzy, F.I., Fawzy, N.W., Arndt, L.A., & Pasnau, R.O. (1995). Critical review of psychosocial interventions in cancer care. *Archives of General Psychiatry, 52*, 100–113.

Gottlieb, B.H. (1983). *Social support strategies: Guidelines for mental health practice*. Beverly Hills, CA: Sage.

Gottlieb, B.H., & Johnson, J. (1995). Impact of day programs on family caregivers of persons with dementia. Report available from the first author at the Department of Psychology, University of Guelph, Guelph, ON N1G 2W1.

Helgeson, V., & Cohen, S.(1996). Social support and adjustment to cancer: Reconciling descriptive, correlational, and intervention research. *Health Psychology, 15*, 135–148.

Helgeson, V., & Lepore, S. (1997). The hurdles involved in conducting a randomized clinical intervention. *Health Psychologist, 18*, 4–16.

Lavoie, J.-P. (1995). Support groups for informal caregivers don't work! Refocus the groups or the evaluations? *Canadian Journal on Aging, 14*, 580–595.

Miller, S.M. (1987). Monitoring and blunting: Validation of a questionnaire to assess styles of information seeking under stress. *Journal of Personality and Social Psychology, 52*, 345–353.

Pearlin, L.I., Mullan, J.T., Semple, S.J., & Skaff, M.M. (1990). Caregiving and the stress process: An overview of concepts and their measures. *Gerontologist, 30*, 583–591.

Pillemer, K.J., Suitor, J., Landreneau, T., Henderson, C.R., Jr, & Brangman, S. (In press). Peer support for Alzheimer's caregivers: Lessons from an intervention study. In K. Pillemer, P. Moen, E. Wethington, & N. Glasgow (Eds), *Social Integration in the second half of life*. Baltimore, MD: Johns Hopkins University Press.

Register, C. (1987). *Living with chronic illness*. New York: Bantam.

Renaud, M. (1996). *Non-medical strategies can improve health*. News release issued by the National Forum on Health. Montreal, 14 June.

Toseland, R.W., & Rossiter, C.M. (1989). Group interventions to support family caregivers: A review and analysis. *Gerontologist, 29*, 438–448.

APPENDIX A

Measures of Social Support for Children

The Social Support Scale for Children (SSSC) (Harter, 1985) is a self-report instrument for children that measures perceived support from significant others (parents, teachers, classmates, and close friends). The scale is based on an understanding of social support as positive regard from others (i.e., affirmational support). The scale taps the extent to which the child feels that others treat them like a person, like them the way they are, care about their feelings, understand them, and listen to their problems. Each type of supporter comprises a subscale of the instrument and each subscale contains six items for a total of twenty-four items for the complete scale. In administration to two elementary-school samples (n = 330) and two middle-school samples (n = 807), subscale reliabilities ranged from 0.72 to 0.88. Factor analysis using an oblique rotation yielded a three-factor solution for elementary-school children (who did not differentiate between classmates and close friends as carefully as middle-school children did), and a four-factor solution for the middle-school children.

The *Social Support Appraisals Scale* (SSAS) (Dubow and Ullman, 1989) assesses the extent to which children feel loved, cared for, accepted, and valued by family, peers, and teachers. The self-report measure consists of thirty-one items to which the child responds on a five point continuum (1 = always; 5 = never). The instrument uses a two-choice format (e.g., 'Some kids feel left out by their friends but other kids don't. Do you feel left out by your friends?') in order to avoid the tendency to provide socially desirable answers. A principal components analysis with a varimax rotation yielded a three-factor solution for peer, parent, and teacher support. The Cronbach's alpha was 0.88 for the overall scale and ranged from 0.78 to 0.83 for the subscales. Validity testing of the scale using correlations with the comparable subscales on the SSCC (Harter, 1985) resulted in moderate to high correlations.

The Nurturance Scale (Longfellow, Zelkowitz, & Saunders, 1982) conceptualizes support as confiding in others and measures social embeddedness in children specific to a particular type of supportive transaction. The child identifies persons with whom they would discuss nine different types of stressful situations (e.g., a bad dream). The number of situations in which the child confides in a particular person comprises the support score for that person. The average internal consistency score for the instrument is 0.68 and ranges from 0.50 for confiding in no one to 0.85 for confiding in fathers. The re-test scores range from 0.14 for friends to a high of 0.69 for fathers.

The Neighbourhood Walk (Bryant, 1985) also measures social embeddedness and is based on a dual view of social support as both relatedness and separateness from others. The items in the inventory are drawn from interpersonal sources of support (family and friends), intrapersonal support generated by the child through solitary activity, and support provided by the environment through formal activities, such as church or school attendance or seeking quiet places to be alone. The researcher conducts the interview during a walk through the child's neighbourhood as a way of stimulating the child's recall of supportive interactions. The ten interpersonal subscales measure social support from parents, grandparents, and peers. Test-re-test reliability is reported as greater than 0.85 for all scores (peer, parent, and grandparent generations).

The Network of Relationships Inventory (Furman & Buhrmester, 1985) is based on Weiss's (1974) theory of social provisions, which proposes that people look for six different types of support from others, including attachment, reliable alliance, enhancement of worth, companionship, guidance, and nurturance. The inventory consists of thirty questions for pre-adolescent children that assess perceived quality of support and enacted support through the child's perception of the six relationship qualities. In addition, the instrument captures the child's perception of the degree of relative power, conflict, satisfaction, and importance of nine different types of relationships. The internal consistency reliability score for the scale averages 0.80. Alphas for all but two of the ninety subscale scores are reported as greater than 0.60.

My Family and Friends (Reid, Landesman, Treder, & Jaccard, 1989) assesses social embeddedness and perceived quality of support in school age children using a series of twelve dialogues with the child. The child identifies supporters among family and friends and ranks the order in which they seek specific types of support from each person. The child responds to questions about the age and role of the supporters, how often they are in contact, and what activities they share. Then the child rates their satisfaction with each interaction using a colourful barometer with a sliding indicator. Median test-re-test reliabilities for a three-week interval are 0.68 for the rankings of network members and 0.69 for ratings of support satisfaction. The authors report internal consistencies for the subscales between 0.58 and 0.92.

Zelkowitz's Inventory (Zelkowitz, 1987, 1989) assesses mother's and child's perceptions of social support for preschoolers based on gratification of the child's needs for love, attention, acceptance, and learning social responsibility. Mother and child are interviewed about the composition of the child's network and the helpfulness of its members with respect to daily maintenance, occasional maintenance, nurturance, and recreation. The questions for the children's interview use different words from those used in the parent's interview, but they are conceptually congruent. Both versions of the instrument have acceptable levels of internal consistency: the Cronbach's alphas for both scales range from 0.70 to 0.96 and are stable across a two-month period.

The *Social Support Rating Scale-Revised* (SSRS-R) (Cauce, Ptacek, Mason, & Smith, 1990) is a ten-item instrument, for use with adolescents, that assesses perceived emotional support, help, and guidance from family and non-family friends who are potentially available as a source of support. Children rate each of ten classes of helper on a three-point Likert scale ranging from 1 = not at all helpful to 3 = a great deal helpful. Factor analysis has yielded four subscales: family support, friend support, school support, and support satisfaction. Test-re-test reliabilities for the scale items are reported by the authors as greater than 0.70.

Children's Inventory of Social Support (CISS) (Wolchik, Ruehlman, Braver, & Sandler, 1989) (see appendix B).

References

Bryant, B.K. (1985). The neighborhood walk: Sources of support in middle childhood. *Monographs of the Society for Research in Child Development, 50*(3), 122.

Cauce, A.M., Ptacek, J.T., Mason, C., & Smith, R.E. (1990). The social support rating scale-revised – SSRS: Three studies on development and validation. Unpublished manuscript, University of Washington, Department of Psychology, Seattle.

Dubow, E.F., & Ullman, D.G. (1985). Assessing social support in elementary school children: The survey of children's social support. *Journal of Clinical Child Psychology, 18*(1), 52–64.

Furman, W., & Buhrmester, D. (1985). Children's perceptions of the personal relationships in their social networks. *Developmental Psychology, 21*(6), 1016–1024.

Harter, S. (1985). Manual for the social support scale for children. Unpublished manuscript, University of Denver, Department of Psychology, Denver, CO.

Longfellow, C., Zelkowitz, P., & Saunders, E. (1982). The quality of mother-child relationships. In D. Belle (Ed.), *Lives in stress: women and depression.* Beverly Hills, CA: Sage.

Reid, M., Landesman, S., Treder, R., & Jaccard, J. (1989). 'My family and friends': Six- to twelve-year-old children's perceptions of social support. *Child Development, 60*(4), 896–910.

Weiss, R. (1974). The provisions of social relationships. In N.Z. Rubin (Ed.), *Doing unto others* (17–26). Englewood Cliffs, NJ: Prentice-Hall.

Wolchik, S.A., Ruehlman, L.S., Braver, S.L., & Sandler, I.N. (1989). Social support of children of divorce: Direct and stress buffering effects. *American Journal of Community Psychology, 17*(4), 485–501.

Zelkowitz, P. (1987). Social support and aggressive behavior in young children. *Family Relations: Journal of Applied Family & Child Studies, 36*(2), 129–134.

Zelkowitz, P. (1989). Parents and children as informants concerning children's social networks. In D. Belle et al., *Children's social networks and social supports.* Wiley series on personality processes (221–237). New York: John Wiley.

APPENDIX B

TABLE B1

Measures Used in the Social Support Research Program

Measure	Chapter	Concepts	Items	Scale	Adaptation to Sample/Study	Psychometric Testing
MEASURES OF STRESS						
Perceived Stress Scale[1]	3	Feelings and thoughts during past month	14	5-point Likert		Test/re-test reliability ($\alpha = 0.85$) Internal consistency ($\alpha = 0.80$)
Stress Appraisal Measure[2]	4	Primary appraisal (threat, challenge, controllability of stressful situations) Secondary appraisal (controllability by self, others)	28	6-point Likert	Stressful situations associated with cardiac condition	
Cantril Ladder[3]	6	Perception of current stress in relation to most and least stress ever experienced	1	9-rung self-anchoring ladder		Test/re-test ($\alpha = 0.70$)

Measure	Chapter	Concepts	Items	Scale	Adaptation to Sample/Study	Psychometric Testing
MEASURES OF SRESS						
Job-Caregiving Conflict Scale[4]	6	Secondary stressor: secondary role strain	4	4-point Likert		Reliability ($\alpha = 0.75$)
Role Captivity Scale[5]	6	Secondary stressor: situational intrapsychic strain	3	4-point Likert		Reliability ($\alpha = 0.75$)
Caregiver Burden Inventory[6]	6	Caregiving burden viewed in terms of constancy of care, unpreparedness for caregiving, physical impact, role conflict and negative emotions	24	5-point Likert		Reliability ($\alpha = 0.73$–0.86)
Global Perceived Stress Scale[7]	6	Measures individual's perceptions of stress-fulness of objectively stressful events	14	5-point Likert		Test/re-test (0.84–0.86)
AIDS Impact Scale[8]	7	Gay affiliation, stigma and discrimination, identifi-cation with patients, grief and loss, social reward and recognition	28 (5 impact scales)	5-point Likert	Stressful situations associated with impact of working with PWA	Reliability ($\alpha = 0.72$–0.89) Test/re-test (0.61–0.77)
MEASURES OF COPING						
Self-Report Coping Scale[9]	2	Dimensions of coping children use to manage	35 (5 scales)	Seeking social support	Support seeking behaviours used to	Test/re-test reliabilities (0.60–0.78)

		specific stressors including approach and avoidance strategies		Self-reliance/problem-solving Distancing Internalizing Externalizing	cope with stressful developmental and illness-related situations	Internal consistency (0.69–0.82)
Coping Health Inventory for Parents[10]	3	What parents find helpful or not helpful to manage the hardships associated with health problems in the family	54 (3 scales)	4-point Likert Maintaining family integration, cooperation and optimism Maintaining social support, self-esteem, psych-ological stability Understanding the medical situation through commu-nication and consultation		$\alpha = 0.79$ $\alpha = 0.79$ $\alpha = 0.71$
Ways of Coping Checklist[11]	5	Thoughts and acts people use to deal with internal and/or external demands of specific stressful encounters – problem-focused – emotion-focused	66 (8 scales)	Seeking social support Planful problem solving Confrontive coping Positive reappraisal Distancing Self-controlling Accepting responsibility Escape avoidance	How people have dealt with/managed heart disease since being in hospital	Cronbach's ($\alpha = 0.61$–0.79)
	7				How nurses in HIV/AIDS care deal with AIDS impact (gay affiliation,	

Measure	Chapter	Concepts	Items	Scale	Adaptation to Sample/Study	Psychometric Testing
MEASURES OF SOCIAL SUPPORT						
					stigma, discrimination, identification with grief, loss, social reward and recognition), and cumulative loss (exposure to numerous deaths of young people)	
Children's Inventory of Social Support (CISS)[12]	2	Structure of support networks, types of support, support satisfaction	30	Measures network size by type of supporter, functions of support (recreation/play, information/advice, emotional support, goods/services, positive feedback)		Test/re-test (0.52–0.85) Internal consistency (0.79–0.90)
Arizona Social Support Interview Schedule (ASSIS)[13]	3567	Structural aspects of support networks, satisfaction with support, need for support	30	Measures support functions of material aid, physical assistance, intimate interaction, guidance, positive feedback and social participation		Test/re-test (0.88) for network size (0.80 for support need) Internal consistency (0.70)

Norbeck Social Support Questionnaire (NSSQ)[14]	4	Functional components (affect, affirmation, aid) Structural properties of social network (size, composition) Network loss		Participants list up to 24 persons in their network, then rate (0–4) amount of affective, affirmational, and tangible support perceived to be available, specifying duration of the relationship, frequency of contact, and network loss		Test/re-test reliability range (0.85–0.92) Internal consistency range (0.89–0.97)
Personal Resources Questionnaire 85 (PRQ85)[15]	6	Part 1: Measures perceived available support and satisfaction with support received in terms of network composition relating to hypothetical life situations Part 2: Global measure of perceived available support in response to items that represent positive or negative social support functions, representing Weiss's dimensions of social support	1025	Satisfaction measured on a 6-point Likert 7-point Likert	Time frame for assessment reduced from 6 to 3 months	Internal consistency (0.87–0.90) Reassessment study test/re-test reliability (0.88–0.89)

Measure	Chapter	Concepts	Items	Scale	Adaptation to Sample/Study	Psychometric Testing
MEASURES OF HEALTH/FUNCTIONING OUTCOMES						
Loneliness and Social Dissatis faction Scale[16]	2	Loneliness	16	5-point scale indicating how much each statement is a true description for them		Internal consistency (Cronbach's $\alpha = 0.90$)
General Health Rating Index[17]	3	Indication of limits in physical and role function due to poor health, acute symptoms, and mental health	32	6 subscales Past, present, and future health, health-related worries, resistance or susceptibility to illness, tendency to view illness as part of life		$\alpha = 0.88–0.90$
Parenting Sense of Competency Scale[18]	3	Assesses parenting self-esteem	17	6-point Likert (2 subscales: satisfaction, efficacy)		$\alpha = 0.79$
Swedish Revised Version of the Preschool Behaviour Checklist[19]	3	Parental report of preschool children's positive and negative behaviours	43	5-point Likert		Internal consistency: adult competence (0.51) to externalizing problems (0.84)

					Validity: significant correlations between mother and father ratings
Michigan Family Heart Questoinnaiire (sectiions)[20]	4	*Coping* with an MI within the context of the survivor-spouse relationship	28	5-point Likert (2 subscales: active engagement & protective buffering	Not available
	4	*Survivor self-efficacy*, deals with specific tasks of recovery from an MI. *Spouse self-efficacy* was measured by 4 questions that assessed confidence in meeting specific challenges after MI. *Functional disability* was measured using 5 items (5-point Likert) such as (limitations on daily activities – working, social activities, going to church). *Pre-coronary marital adjustment* was assessed using 5 items (5-point Likert) about spouse-patient interaction pre-MI.	10	7-point Likert	

Measure	Chapter	Concepts	Items	Scale	Adaptation to Sample/Study	Psychometric Testing
MEASURES OF HEALTH/FUNCTIONING OUTCOMES						
Positive and Negative Affect Scale Schedule [21]	4	Assessment of positive and negative mood/ affect in spouses				Internal consistency: NA(0.87, PA(0.86) Test/ re-test reliability: NA(0.81), PA(0.79)
Health Complaints Scale[22]	4	Contains somatic and cognitive health complaints	24 (12 somatic complaints; 12 cognitive complaints)	5-point Likert		
Emotional/Social Loneliness Inventory[23]	5	Emotional and social loneliness and emotional and social isolation; contrasts people's perceptions of their social network with their feelings about it	15 paired	'What is true in my life' (factual) vs. 'what I feel in my life at this time' (emotional)		Internal reliability (0.82–0.86)
Caregiving Competence/ Confidence Scale[24]	6	Perceived threats of stressful situations may be mediated by perceptions of self competence	5	4-point Likert	Adapted from the *Caregiving Competence Scale*	
Barthel Index[25]	6	Assesses functional independence in terms of mobility factors and activities of daily living	15 (weight-ed)	3-point Likert		Test/re-test (0.89)

Sickness Impact Profile[26]	6	Measures perceived effects of illness on one's daily activities, feelings and attitudes Major foci: psychosocial activities, physical activities	136 items covering 12 areas of living	Yes/No	Test/re-test whole scale (0.75–0.92) Subcategories (0.82)
Life Satisfaction Index Z[27]	6	Measures general well being, zest, self concept, mood tone, congruence between desired and achieved goals and meaning of life	13	5-point Likert	Internal consistency (0.76) Reassessment study: Test/re-test (0.71–0.79)
Cantril Ladder[28]	6	Perception of current life satisfaction in relation to most and least 'satisfying life you could expect to have'	1	9 rung self-anchoring ladder	Test/re-test (0.70)
Nursing Job Satisfaction Scale[29]	7	Measures 5 dimensions of job satisfaction	35	5-point Likert	Internal consistency alpha (0.78) test-re-test satisfactory
Maslach Burnout Inventory[30]	7	Measures 3 aspects of burnout: emotional exhaustion, depersonalization, and reduced personal accomplishment	22		Internal consistency: emotional exhaustion (0.90), depersonalization (0.79), personal accomplishment (0.71) Test/re-test: emotional exhaustion (0.82), depersonalization (0.6), personal accomplishment (0.8)

Footnotes

1 Cohen (1986); Cohen & Williamson (1988); Cohen et al. (1983); Pbert et al. (1992).
2 Dewe (1993); Peacock & Wong (1990).
3 Applegate (1991)
4 Pearlin, Mullan, Semple, & Skaff (1990).
5 Pearlin et al. (1990).
6 Caserta et al. (1996); Novak & Guest (1989).
7 Cohen, Kamarck, & Mermelstein (1983).
8 Bennett et al. (1994); Visintini et al. (1996).
9 Kimes-Dougan & Bolger (1998).
10 Bradley & Brisby (1993); McDonald et al. (1999).
11 Edwards & Baglioni (1993); Falkum et al. (1997); Vitaliano et al. (1985).
12 Ellerton et al. (1996); Hough (1988).
13 Calsyn et al. (1998); Payne & Jones (1995).
14 Byers & Mullis (1987); Neatherlin (1994); Norbeck (1984); Norbeck, Lindsey, & Carrieri (1983).
15 Higgins & Dicharry (1991); Osipow & Spokane (1984).
16 Rotenberg & Whitney (1992); Vaughn et al. (1996).
17 Mahon et al. (1997); Yarcheski & Mahon (1995).
18 Dodge (1995); Johnston & Mash (1989).
19 Hagekull & Bohlin (1996).
20 James Coyne (personal communication).
21 Denollet (1993).
22 Denollet (1994).
23 Oshagen & Allan (1992); Vincenzi & Grabosky (1987).
24 Cummings et al. (1998).
25 Murdock (1992); Shah & Cooper (1993).
26 de Bruin et al. (1992); Jensen et al. (1992).
27 Fritz et al. (1997); Madigan et al. (1996).
28 Ibid.
29 Ng (1993).
30 Maslach et al. (1997); Schaufeli & Van Dierendonck (1995); Yadama & Drake (1995).

References

Applegate, J.S. (1991). Measurement as treatment: Are subjective self-ratings reactive? *Journal of Social Service Research, 14*(3-4), 45–62.

Bennett, L., Kelaher, M., & Ross, M.W. (1994). The impact of working with HIV/AIDS on health care professionals: Development of the AIDS Impact Scale. *Psychology & Health, 9*(3), 221–232.

Bradley, R.H., & Brisby, J.A. (1993). Assessment of the home environment. In J.L. Culbertson, D.J. Willis, et al. (Eds), *Testing young children: A reference guide for developmental psychoeducational and psychosocial assessments* (128–166). Austin TX: Pro-Ed.

Byers, P.H., & Mullis, M.R. (1987). Reliability and validity of the Norbeck Social Support Questionnaire in psychiatric inpatients. *Educational & Psychological Measurement, 47*(2), 445–448.

Calsyn, R.J., Morse, G.A., Kinkenberg, W.D., Trusty, M.L., & Allen G. (1998). The impact of assertive community treatment on the social relationships of people who are homeless and mentally ill. *Community Mental Health Journal, 34*(6), 579–593.

Caserta, M.S., Lund, D.A., & Wright, S.D. (1996). Exploring the Caregiver Burden Inventory (CB): Further evidence for a multidimensional view of burden. *International Journal of Aging & Human Development, 43*(1), 21– 34.

Cohen, S. (1986). Contrasting the Hassles Scale and the Perceived Stress Scale: Who's really measuring appraised stress? *American Psychologist, 41*(6), 716–718.

Cohen, S., & Williamson, G. (1988). Perceived stress in a probability sample of the United States. In S. Spacapam & S. Oskamp (Eds), *The social psychology of health: Claremont Symposium on applied social psychology*. Newbury Park, CA: Sage.

Cohen, S., Kamarck, T., & Mermelstein, R. (1983). A global measure of perceived stress. *Journal of Health and Social Behavior, 24*, 385–396.

Cummings, S.M., Long, J.K., Peterson-Hazan, S., & Harrison, J. (1998). *Clinical Gerontologist, 20*(1), 29–45.

de Bruin, A.F., de Witte, L.P., Stevens, F., & Diederiks, J.P. (1992). The state of the art of a generic functional status measure. *Social Science & Medicine, 35*(8), 1003–1014.

Denollet, J. (1993). Emotional distress and fatigue in coronary heart disease: The Global Mood Scale (GMS). *Psychological Medicine, 23*(1), 111–121.

Denollet, J. (1994). Health complaints and outcome assessment in coronary heart disease. *Psychosomatic Medicine, 56*(5), 463–474.

Dewe, P. (1993). Measuring primary appraisal: Scale construction and directions for future research. *Journal of Social Behavior & Personality, 8*(4), 673–685.

Dodge Reyome, N. (1995). Sense of competence and attitudes toward abusive interactions with adolescents in residential child care workers. *Journal of Child & Youth Care, 10*(1), 57–62.

Edwards, J.R., & Baglioni, A.J. (1993). The measurement of coping with stress: Construct validity of the Ways of Coping checklist and the Cybernetic Coping Scale. *Work & Stress, 7*(1), 17–31.

Ellerton, M., Stewart, M.J., Ritchie, J.A., & Hirth, A.M. (1996). Social support in children with a chronic condition. *Canadian Journal of Nursing Research, 28*(4), 15–36.

Falkum, E., Olff, M., & Aasland, O.G. (1997). Revisiting the factor structure of the Ways of Coping Checklist: A three-dimensional view of the problem focused coping scale. A study among Norwegian physicians. *Personality & Individual Differences, 22*(2), 257–267.

Fritz, C.L., Farver, T.B., Kass, P.H., & Hart, L.A. (1997). Correlation among three psychological scales used in research of caregivers for patients with Alzheimer's disease. *Psychological Reports, 80*(1), 67–80.

Hagekull, B., & Bohlin, G. (1996). *The Swedish revised version of the Preschool Behaviour Questionnaire*. Uppsala, Sweden: Uppsala University.

Higgins, P.G., & Dicharry, E.K. (1991). Measurement issues addressing social support with Navajo women. *Western Journal of Nursing Research, 13*(2), 242–255.

Hough, S. (1988). Social network analysis for mildly mentally retarded adults. *Psychological Reports, 63*(2), 543–546.

Jensen, M.P., Strom, S.E., Turner, J.A., & Romano, J.M. (1992). Validity of the Sickness Impact Profile Roland Scale as a measure of dysfunction in chronic pain patients. *Pain, 50*(2), 157–162.

Johnston, C., & Mash, E.J. (1989). A measure of parenting satisfaction and efficacy. *Journal of Clinical Child Psychology, 18*(2), 167–175.

Kilmes-Dougan, B., & Bolger, A.K. (1998). Coping with maternal depressed affect and depression: Adolescent children of depressed and well mothers. *Journal of Youth & Adolescence, 27*(1), 1–15.

Madigan, M.J., Mise, D.H., & Maynard, M. (1996). Life satisfaction and level of activity of male elderly in institutional and community settings. *Activities, Adaptation & Aging, 21*(2), 21–36.

Mahon, N.E., Yarcheski, T.J., & Yarcheski, A. (1997). Loneliness and health related variables in young adults. *Perceptual and Motor Skills, 85*(3, Pt 1), 800–802.

Maslach, C., Jackson, S.E., & Leiter, M.P. (1997). Maslach Burnout Inventory. In C.P. Zalaquett, R.J. Wood, et al. (Eds), *Evaluating stress: A book of resources* (191–218). 3rd ed. Lanham, MD: Scarecrow Press.

McDonald, T.P., Poertner, J., & Pierpont, J. (1999). Predicting caregiver stress: An ecological perspective. *American Journal of Orthopsychiatry, 69*(1), 100–109

Murdock, C. (1992). A critical evaluation of the Barthel Index: II. *British Journal of Occupational Therapy, 55*(4), 153–156.

Neatherlin, J.S. (1994). The effects of social support: A meta-analysis of studies that used the Norbeck Social Support Questionnaire. *Dissertation Abstracts International, Section B: The Sciences & Engineering, 54*(10–B), 50–94.

Ng, S.H. (1993). A job satisfaction scale for nurses. *New Zealand Journal of Psychology, 22*(1), 46–53.

Norbeck, J.S. (1984). The Norbeck Social Support Questionnaire. *Birth Defects: Original Article Series, 20*(5), 45–55.

Norbeck, J.S. Lindsey, A., & Carrieri, V. (1983). Further development of the Norbeck Social Support Questionnaire: Normative data and validity testing. *Nursing Research, 32*(1), 4–9.

Novak, M., & Guest, C. (1989). Application of a multidimensional Caregiver Burden Inventory. *Gerontologist, 29*(6), 798–803.

Oshagan, H., & Allan R.L. (1992). Three loneliness scales: An assessment of their measurement properties. *Journal of Personality Assessment, 59*(2), 380–409.

Osipow, S.H., & Spokane, A.R. (1984). *Applied Social Psychology Annual, 5,* 67–86.

Payne, R.L., & Jones, G. (1995). Measurement and methodological issues in social support. In S.V. Kasl, C.L. Cooper, & L. Cary (Eds), *Stress and health: Issues in research methodology* (167–205). Wiley series on studies in occupational stress. New York: John Wiley.

Pbert, L., Doerfler, L.A., & DeCosimo, D. (1992). An evaluation of the Perceived Stress Scale in two clinical populations. *Journal of Psychopathology & Behavioral Assessment, 14*(4), 363–375.

Peacock, E.J., & Wong, P.T. (1990). The Stress Appraisal Measure (SAM): A multidimensional approach to cognitive appraisal. *Stress Medicine, 6*(3), 227–236.

Pearlin, L., Mullan, J., Semple, S., & Skaff, M. (1990). Caregiving and the stress process: An overview of concepts and their measures. *The Gerontologist, 30,* 583–594.

Perkinson, M.A., Albert, S.M., Luborsky, M.R., Moss, M., et al. (1994). *Journal of Gerontology, 49*(5), S264–S275.

Rotenberg, K.J., & Whitney, P. (1992). Loneliness and disclosure processes in preadolescence. *Merrill-Palmer Quarterly, 38*(3), 401–416.

Schaufeli, W.B., & Van Dierendonck, D. (1995). A cautionary note about the cross-national and clinical validity of cut-off points for the Maslach Burnout Inventory. *Psychological Reports, 7*(3, Pt 2), 1083–1090.

Shah, S., & Cooper, B. (1993). A critical evaluation of the Barthel Index: Commentary. *British Journal of Occupational Therapy, 56*(2), 70–72.

Than, T.V., & Williams, L.F. (1994). Effect of language of interview on the validity and reliability of psychological well-being scales. *Social Work Research, 18*(1), 17–25.

Vaughn, S., Elbaum, B.E., & Schumm, J.S. (1996). The effects of inclusion on the social functioning of students with learning disabilities. *Journal of Learning Disabilities, 29*(6), 598–608.

Vincenzi, H., & Grabosky, F. (1987). Measuring the emotional/social aspects of loneliness and isolation. *Journal of Social Behavior & Personality, 2*(2, Pt 2), 257–270.

Visintini, R., Campanini, E., Fossati, A., Bagnato, M., et al. (1996). Psychological stress in nurses' relationship with HIV-infected patients: the risk of burnout syndrome. *AIDS Care, 8*(2), 183–194.

Vitaliano, P.P., et al. (1985) (The Ways of Coping Checklist: Revision and psychometric properties. *Multivariate Behavioral Research, 20*(1), 3–26.

Yadama, G.N., & Drake, B. (1995). Confirmatory factor analysis of the Maslach Burnout Inventory. *Social Work Research, 19*(3), 184–192.

Yarcheski, A., & Mahon, N.E. (1995). Rogers's pattern manifestations and health in adolescents. *Western Journal of Nursing Research, 17*(4), 383– 397.

Contributors

Sheila Banks, School of Occupational Therapy, Dalhousie University, Halifax, Nova Scotia

Karina Davidson, Department of Psychology, University of Alabama, Tuscaloosa, Alabama

Susan Doble, School of Occupational Therapy, Dalhousie University, Halifax, Nova Scotia

Steve Duck, Departments of Communication Studies and Psychology, Iowa State University, Ames, Iowa

Mary-Lou Ellerton, School of Nursing, Dalhousie University, Halifax, Nova Scotia

Benjamin H. Gottlieb, Psychology Department, University of Guelph, Guelph, Ontario

Margaret J. Harrison, Faculty of Nursing, University of Alberta, Edmonton, Alberta

Geraldine Hart, School of Nursing, Dalhousie University, Halifax, Nova Scotia

Andrew Johnson, AIDS Vancouver, Vancouver, British Columbia

Gerald Klassen, Cardiology Department, Faculty of Medicine, Dalhousie University, Halifax, Nova Scotia

Lynn Langille, Atlantic Health Promotion Research Centre, Dalhousie University, Halifax, Nova Scotia

Renee Lyons, Atlantic Health Promotion Research Centre, Dalhousie University, Halifax, Nova Scotia

Kathleen MacPherson, Departments of Community Health and Epidemiology and Medicine; QEII Health Sciences Centre, Dalhousie University, Halifax, Nova Scotia

Lydia Makrides, School of Physiotherapy, Dalhousie University, Halifax, Nova Scotia

Karen Mann, Faculty of Medicine, Dalhousie University, Halifax, Nova Scotia

Donna Meagher-Stewart, School of Nursing, Dalhousie University, Halifax, Nova Scotia

Gail G. Tomblin Murphy, School of Nursing, Dalhousie University, Halifax, Nova Scotia

Anne Neufeld, Faculty of Nursing, University of Alberta, Edmonton, Alberta

Judith Ritchie, School of Nursing, Dalhousie University; IWK Grace Health Centre for Children, Women, and Families, Halifax, Nova Scotia

Sonia Salisbury, IWK Grace Health Centre for Children, Women, and Families, Halifax, Nova Scotia

Miriam J. Stewart, Director, Centre for Health Promotion Studies, Faculty of Nursing, University of Alberta, Edmonton, Alberta

Michael J.L. Sullivan, Department of Psychology, Dalhousie University, Halifax, Nova Scotia

Dale Poel, School of Public Administration, Dalhousie University, Halifax, Nova Scotia

Donna Thompson, Mother of children with cystic fibrosis, Halifax, Nova Scotia

Patty J. Weld Viscount, Social Support Research Program, Dalhousie University, Halifax, Nova Scotia

Hermann Wolf, Physiology Department, Faculty of Medicine, Dalhousie University, Halifax, Nova Scotia